A–Z of Cat Health and First Aid

A–Z of Cat Health and First Aid

A practical guide for owners

Revised and updated

Andrew Gardiner,
BVM&S, Cert SAS, MSc, PhD, MRCVS

Line illustrations by
Jay Pressnell

Souvenir Press

First published under the title *A–Z of Cat Health and First Aid*
in Great Britain in 2002 by Souvenir Press Ltd
43 Great Russell Street, London WC1B 3PD

This revised and updated edition published 2015

Line illustrations by Jay Pressnell

ISBN 9780285642935

Typeset by M Rules
Printed and bound by Bell & Bain Ltd, Glasgow

In memory of my mother, Maisie Gardiner

No book can replace the services of a trained veterinarian. This book is not intended to encourage treatment of illness, disease, or other medical problems by the layman. Any application of the recommendations set forth in the following pages is solely at the reader's discretion and risk. You should consult a veterinarian concerning any veterinary medical or surgical problem. If a veterinarian is caring for your pet, for any condition, he or she can advise you about information described in this book.

Contents

Preface

There is a saying, 'You *own* a dog, but you *feed* a cat'.

I think this sums up quite well the intriguing nature of the relationship we have with cats. Somehow, we can never possibly 'own' them in the same way as we may think we own pet dogs – cats are far too independent, far too aloof for all that. Instead, cats may choose to share their lives with us or, just possibly, move on elsewhere if circumstances are not to their liking! Quite a large percentage of the life of a pet cat often takes place outside the home, a whole complex web of usually nocturnal activities and routines of which owners are blissfully unaware.

Most cat owners say that it is this quality of independence, mystery and resourcefulness that they find most appealing about their pets. This as well as all their individual quirks and habits of course. They are, in many ways, the ideal pet for people who do not have the time, space or energy to devote to a dog, or for those who seek out the spiritual side of life, because cats have always signified that.

My own experience of cats comes from those I have lived with, and of course from the very many cats I have treated as a veterinary surgeon. I find cats almost as varied and complex as people – there is the full spectrum of 'personalities' present, from the enormous placid lumps of feline contentment to the sleek, nervy spitfires that seem to say, 'Look at me in the wrong way and I'll fly!'

Any vet will tell you that cats can be awkward patients. For one thing, their dignity is lost, and their instincts, too, can be harmful. A sick dog may seek out reassurance and response from its 'pack-leader' owner; a sick cat may be bad tempered and irritable or may crawl under a shed to sit the illness out (or, always the worry, get progressively worse). The independence and even remoteness that we value in healthy cats can become a problem when they are not well, making feline medicine and treatment quite different from its canine counterpart.

This book, I hope, will allow owners to understand their cat's well-being better. A thorough reading of its contents will give the interested owner a good insight into cat health and behaviour, and allow the most effective nursing and first aid to be supplied to the patient under veterinary care. It should also be of value to those involved in cat rescue and welfare work, whether in this country or abroad, and the first aid sections will be especially useful when professional veterinary care is not readily available in these situations.

Andrew Gardiner, Edinburgh, UK

Author's note

I would like to thank Ernest Hecht and his colleagues at Souvenir Press for their help on this book. Illustrator Jay Pressnell's cat acted as a model for most of the cat drawings and my own cat was persuaded, with some difficulty, to pose for a few photographs. Other pictures come from cats I have treated, mainly at the Blue Cross and PDSA, and on various Greek islands when doing welfare work for the Greek Cat Welfare Society.

A. G.
January 2015

How to use this book

Please do not use this book as an alternative to seeking professional veterinary advice! It is intended to complement and expand on that, but not replace it. Although I have tried to write the book in such a way that the complex nature of cat diseases is understandable, medicine (and cats) are too unpredictable to be able to cover every conceivable situation. Vets study for years to understand animal diseases, and even then the task is often far from easy, so never rely entirely on any book, magazine article, web page or story from another owner who managed to cure their own cat of exactly the same thing using such-and-such a treatment. It's not worth the risk.

Do, however, use the book as a way of understanding your cat and its illness or injury better. Use it to ask questions of your veterinary surgeon or nurse about anything you don't understand concerning the treatment they are proposing – they will be happy to explain. If they are not, then find professionals who will! Try to bear in mind that an animal is much more complex than a machine. Diagnosis is not always easy; misleading or confusing results can be given even after extensive tests – that is in the nature of medicine and treatment, whether human or animal. Vets are denied the opportunity to have their patients explain their problems directly – much of what is relied upon comes from the owner, and this may not always be totally accurate. However, by reading and using this book, your own accuracy in describing symptoms and making observations is likely to be improved, and your cat's recovery helped as a result.

For ease of use, the book is arranged alphabetically according to diseases, symptoms or injuries. Many cat problems can be known by more than one name or might be found in the book in different ways. For example, when considering a cat that seems to be having problems passing urine, some owners might think to flick to the section on 'straining', whereas others might decide to turn turn to 'cystitis' initially. Cross-references within the book have been made to try to ensure you are always directed towards every appropriate section. Inevitably, this means that there is occasionally slight repetition between closely related sections – but this is necessary to ensure that important information is not inadvertently skipped.

For every condition mentioned, an indication of the relative urgency has also been given – this is so that professional treatment for potentially serious problems is not unnecessarily delayed.

Practical first aid

There are lots of hints throughout this book regarding how you can help your cat with home first aid and nursing, both before and after diagnosis. These techniques have been found helpful in day-to-day use, and largely use equipment and materials that are easily to hand. The Introduction also contains very useful general information on nursing sick cats and suggested items for a practical first aid kit are also given. With these things to hand, helpful first aid will be able to be started for most problems likely to be encountered with your cat.

The comments on complementary medicine in the Introduction are not intended to replace the services of a qualified veterinarian but, as the term suggests, to *complement* professional advice. There are many approaches to diagnosis and treatment; good communication between you and your vet should ensure one that you – and your cat – are happy with.

Introduction

When confronted with illness or injury in a pet cat, feelings of uncertainty, helplessness or even panic are often experienced. Suddenly, your familiar pet, usually so confident, outgoing and independent, is behaving abnormally – not the cat you are used to at all. She may be withdrawn, unresponsive to the usual things, refusing to have anything to do with food or human attention, maybe her facial expression even looks unusual. She seems to have become a different animal altogether.

In a way, the sick cat does become a different animal. When injured or ill, basic feline behavioural instincts take over and the cat withdraws more into herself – an ancient protective response designed to limit further injury and enforce rest. Approaches may be resented, even aggressively, and this despite the fact that they come from someone the cat knows well. This can be distressing for owners who want to find out what's wrong, and how to help.

The purpose of this Introduction is to give some general guidelines on dealing with sick and injured cats. These are applicable to most of the situations that are described in detail later in this book and are designed to allow you to help your cat in a safe and effective way.

Safety first

In any situation, give the first priority to safety to yourself, to anyone else who may be helping you, and then to the sick or injured cat. Be extremely careful when out of doors in situations where there is traffic, moving water or heights involved. Never attempt a rescue you are not qualified to perform – instead, seek help and monitor the situation until that help arrives.

When dealing with a sick cat at home, remember that their behavioural response can be unpredictable. Normally placid cats may strike out indiscriminately if in fear or pain, even if at first they appear to be very subdued and still. Always handle them with care, sympathy and caution. Be prepared for the unexpected.

Always seek prompt medical advice if you are bitten by a cat. Antibiotics are usually needed as cats carry various bacteria in their mouths. Your veterinary surgeon can provide a note to be handed to your doctor regarding the implications of cat bites in people.

Restraint and dealing with nervous and fearful cats

Restraint is important, both to secure a sick cat, allow safe and effective transportation or treatment, and prevent further injury. In cats, the minimum restraint for safe handling should always be used. Over-restraint can cause as many problems as under-restraint, and cats are so fast and flexible that all-out struggles to suppress them are rarely successful and may be medically dangerous for them and personally dangerous for you. Experience helps greatly in judging how best to cope with each situation, but for very distressed cats professional help should be sought. A few general pointers are as follows:

1. Clear the area of unnecessary people and noise.
2. Give the cat 10–20 minutes to settle.
3. Move slowly and take plenty of time.
4. Speak to the cat constantly.
5. Do not make sudden lunges.
6. Use food to distract the cat and win their confidence.
7. Protect your hands, arms and face.
8. Don't force the issue: if it looks impossible, back off and try later or seek help.
9. Making direct eye contact with the cat, and then deliberately blinking slowly can act as a reassurance to the cat.

Restraint in a controlled space

The simplest form of restraint is enclosure in a room or, if outside, in a place from where further escape is difficult, such as a shed or garage. This might be the technique used for extremely aggressive or unpredictable cats, whilst awaiting help from experienced handlers or whilst giving the cat time to recover from extreme stress.

Who can help in these situations, which may involve rescuing sick or injured cats in awkward or dangerous locations? The usual agencies are:

1. Local animal welfare organisations or anti-cruelty groups. Phone numbers are usually in phone books or available via veterinary practices. They often have catching or trapping equipment and experienced handlers available.
2. Fire departments for difficult rescue situations, although this very much depends on available teams and is largely done on a goodwill basis.
3. Veterinary practices – expertise may be needed to sedate cats prior to catching or trapping them.

Cats trapped for any length of time should have water and food supplied to them by, e.g. dropping or pushing food towards them.

Restraint in a box or cage

The next level of restraint is restraint in a box or cage, and this is often applicable to common first aid situations in pet cats. Most owners have a cat carrier cage or box, and this is quite suitable to contain a sick or injured cat whilst awaiting treatment or for transportation. It is much safer to have a cat in a secure carrier than to transport it by lifting, since if the cat panics while being held, she may escape, injure herself, injure people or even, if in a car at the time, result in the driver causing an accident. Cat carrier cages can have newspaper or blankets/towels put in them. If necessary, the cage itself can be covered with a blanket – very frightened cats often feel more secure when this is done. Lift the cage slowly and gently and always make sure the door or lid is securely fastened. Remember that frightened cats may scratch through wire baskets so protect your hands when lifting.

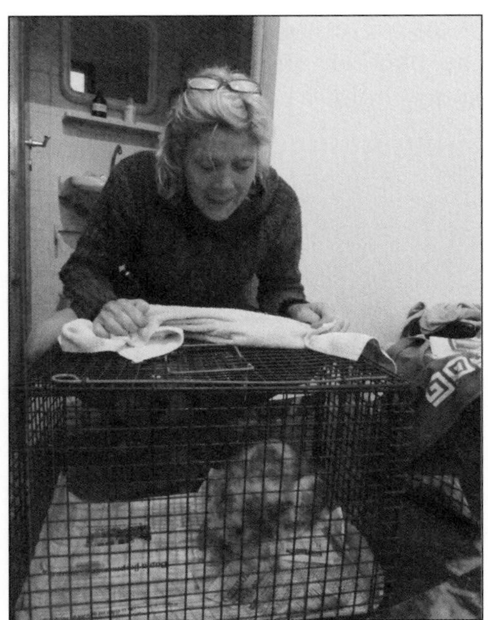

Reassuring a semi-stray cat restrained in a wire cage. (Photo courtesy of Andrea Roe.)

Getting the cat into the box or cage

- Cats may enter boxes voluntarily if the interior of the box is dark and the surroundings of the cat are bright and noisy – they see it as an escape route. Food can be put into the box to encourage the cat to enter.
- Pheromone (hormone) sprays, available from veterinary practices, are useful as cats associate these with feelings of security and may move towards the scent into the box.
- Alternatively, the cat can be forced into the box if the cat is against a wall or partition and the box is advanced slowly, open door towards the cat. The cat can be encouraged to move forwards by making some noise or disturbance behind it, by spraying water, or by touching the cat's hind quarters with a long stick or broom handle. When the cat is in, the box can then be turned or lifted to allow you to close the door on the cat. The last part of the manoeuvre can sometimes be tricky and temporarily covering the door opening with something may be necessary until the box or cage can be brought into a position where the door itself can be swung closed.
- Cat rescue organisations often have special trap cages into which cats are tempted with food. These are used with stray or feral cats, or cats which are proving impossible to capture by other means.

Lifting a sick or injured cat

If you are in any doubt about the cat's temperament or response, wear a long-sleeved coat and thick gloves. Cats are generally best lifted by 'scooping' them up around the front and back legs, since pressure under the abdomen may sometimes be painful. Carry them by holding them close in against your body with a firm but gentle pressure, using your arm to control and support the cat's body. Control both the front legs by holding near the top of the legs, above the elbow joints (see photo). 'Scruffing' cats can cause some individuals to 'freeze', and a scruff hold can be useful in, e.g., removing a cat from a small, awkward space. However, the routine scruffing of cats is discouraged in many 'cat-friendly' veterinary practices and hospitals.

Cat restraining and carrying bags are available for those involved in dealing with injured or unpredictable cats on a regular basis. A simlar effect can be obtained by wrapping the cat in a blanket or towel. The covering must be secure enough around the neck area to prevent the cat releasing the front legs. Cats wrapped in this way should still be held firmly and the front legs restrained through the blanket, since if these legs are released the cat will be able to break free from almost any hold. Most cats respond well to this kind of restraint and probably feel quite secure.

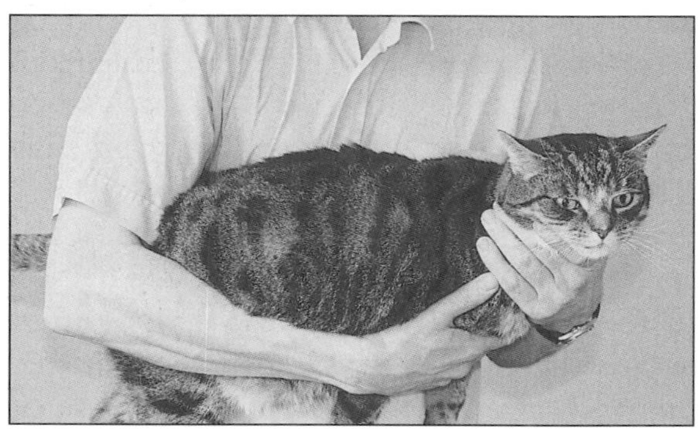

Lifting a cat correctly. The cat is being 'scooped in' against the carrier's body gently but securely, with the forelegs controlled and the head supported.

Occasionally, due to aggressive or dangerous behaviour, it is necessary to capture cats using cat catching devices. Most of these incorporate a snare loop around the neck and a long-handled pole. Catching a cat in this way commonly causes some distress to the cat, but may be the only option if the patient is to be rescued and helped from an inaccessible situation. Usually the cat can be quickly lifted and immediately transferred into a waiting cage, so that the inevitable discomfort and anxiety is momentary.

Restraint for first aid

Good restraint makes first aid and tablet administration simpler to carry out. The basic principles of calm, unhurried but firm action apply. In many cases, restraint in the sitting or crouching position is required; this is also a natural position for the cat, and one that is unlikely to be resented and fought against.

Choose a flat surface at a comfortable waist-level working height or kneel down on the floor. If using a table ensure that the surface is not slippery as this can alarm some cats and cause them to struggle if they feel their footing is insecure. Use a towel or a rubber mat. Have an assistant restrain the cat in the sitting position, using both their hands to control the front legs by holding at the elbow area. The assistant's own forearms and elbows help to support the cat and keep it stationary and level. This restraint allows the second person to examine the cat freely with both hands in order to give tablets, look at the mouth, ears, eyes, front paws etc.

If the underside of the abdomen needs to be examined, the assistant can raise the cat by lifting her underneath the elbows so that the cat stands up on her hindlegs on the surface. This exposes most of the abdomen. To examine the top of the back or tail area, the cat is held lengthwise along the assistant's body, again controlling the front legs.

Throughout this restraint, the cat should be soothed and talked to, and the underside of the chin can often be rubbed or tickled by the person holding.

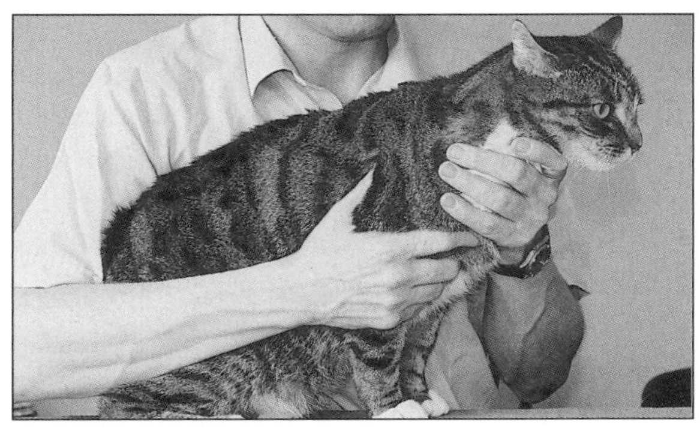

Restraint in the sitting position on a non-slip surface. Note the use of the right forearm to support and control the cat's body and the right hand to gently control and restrain the front legs; the other hand can help here if needed, by sliding down from the neck area. The cat, though nervous (seen from ear position and facial expression), does not resent the restraint.

Nervous cats may respond well to having their head or body covered with a blanket or towel while being restrained. (A word of caution – some cats panic when their heads are covered, so be aware of this.) The towel also serves as a useful screen for the occasional swipe or attempted bite! In the sitting position, a towel can be wrapped around the cat from the neck down, and the assistant can hold this firmly, with only the head exposed for examination or tablet administration. Always concentrate on controlling and limiting movement of the forelegs.

If you are having continued problems with a frightened, nervous and aggressive cat, it is best not to persist as this could endanger yourself and the cat. Instead, make the cat secure in a carrier or cage and seek professional advice. Sedation is likely to be necessary and will allow the necessary examination and tests to be carried out in a safe, effective way.

General nursing of cats

Sick, injured or recovering cats require peace and quiet, well away from bright lights, noises and excited children or animals. The best temperature is a pleasantly warm room temperature for people – additional warmth is obtained from blankets, well padded warm water bottles or warm packs, if needed. Food should be tempting and within easy reach. There should also be water and a litter tray nearby.

Sick cats often have very poor appetites. They may reject their usual cat food and attempting to force them to eat is pointless. Try any of the following, which often seem palatable to poorly cats.

- Tinned fish, especially sardines in tomato sauce.
- Smoked ham.
- Prawns.
- Cooked chicken or fish.
- Special convalescence foods obtainable from veterinary practices.

Warming the food helps release aromas which will tempt the appetite.

Cats need to be checked on, unobtrusively, every hour or so, and it can be helpful if you note down some basic medical observations about them, such as:

- Number of times vomited or diarrhoea passed.
- When normal faeces and urine are passed.
- Amount eaten and drunk.
- Breathing rate at rest, and whether this appears normal (see **Breathing problems**).
- Overall demeanour and responsiveness.
- Any other symptoms you see.

Sick cats often appreciate attention, stroking, gentle grooming and bathing of the mouth, eyes and nose with water and cotton wool. This frequently seems to improve their demeanour significantly, and many cats will eat during or after this treatment. It is an important psychological stimulation and is all part of good nursing.

Administration of medication

It is important that your cat receives any medication supplied by your vet according to the treatment instructions given. This will usually be written clearly on the packaging of the product or the tablet bottle label, but if in doubt ask for clarification as some dosing patterns can seem quite complicated at first. Make sure you know exactly what you are to do, and when.

If there are anticipated problems, e.g. an elderly or infirm owner, difficulties with the dosing schedule owing to work patterns, or any other such problems, discuss these with the veterinary staff in advance. Other treatment options such as long-acting injections, a different type of tablet or even a period of hospitalisation, may be better. Usually, a satisfactory compromise can be reached which will suit both owner and cat.

Ensure all medication is stored correctly, well out of the reach of children or other animals. Some products, once opened, must be kept in the fridge and the use of disposable gloves when handling animal medicines is a good habit.

Missed doses

With certain drugs, a missed dose is ignored and the next dose is given at the time it would normally be due. With other products, a missed dose is corrected by giving another dose as soon as possible after you realise you have missed one; and with yet other drugs, a missed dose may be corrected by giving a double dose at the next dosing time. Always check with your vet as to what action to take, and never give double doses unless specifically instructed to as this could be potentially dangerous with certain drugs. When no advice is easily available, the safest course of action is generally the first: simply give the next dose when it is due.

Administration of tablets

There is no doubt that cats are less amenable than dogs when it comes to giving tablets. Many dogs will eat palatable tablets straight from the hand like sweets, or else can easily be persuaded by a piece of cheese or butter wrapped around the tablet. These methods do work in some cats, but certainly not all – many cats seem inherently suspicious of attempts to trick them in this way! Giving the drugs can rapidly become a nightmare for owner and cat alike, and is obviously much worse with drugs that need to be given two or even three times a day. In some cases, it may be frankly impossible to follow treatment regimes initially suggested and, in these cases, further discussion with the vet is required. Don't feel bad about not being able to cope. Some cats cannot be tabletted even by vets.

What are the best methods available for giving tablets?

Over the mouth

This is undoubtedly the most dependable method. The tablet is placed in the mouth, behind the base of the tongue, and is immediately swallowed by the cat. It sounds easy; it *is* easy in some cats, who genuinely do not seem to mind this process at all. The author once had a hyperthyroid cat who required three tablets daily for the last years of her life. She was so easy to treat that it could be done almost one-handed – she seemed to look on it as receiving affectionate attention.

Probably about 25 per cent of cats fall into this 'very easy-to-dose' category. A further 50 per cent can be tabletted in this way, but doing so requires a little skill and practice. The remaining 25 per cent cannot be dosed like this without extreme distress on the part of the owner and/or cat. It is not worth persisting with these patients. Try another method (see below) – there is no point in turning treatment into trauma.

Give a tablet by mouth as follows:

1. Adopt a relaxed and positive attitude beforehand. You are going to succeed easily!
2. Have the cat sitting quietly. If you can find someone to assist you here, this helps greatly by restraining the cat's shoulders and elbows in the relaxed sitting position (see p. xxi). They must control the front feet and steady the cat, but ever so gently. Over-restraint winds many cats up. Reassure the cat.
3. The person giving the tablet holds the tablet in fingers or (often easier) a pair of plastic forceps or tablet administrator – these are obtained from vets or pet shops.
4. Using their left hand (if right handed), the person giving the tablet gently takes the cat's head and tilts it back a little so that the nose points to the ceiling at about a 45-degree angle.
5. At this point the lower jaw tends to fall open slightly. The tip of the forceps or finger touches the lower jaw near the incisor teeth and presses down gently. The mouth almost invariably opens without much force.
6. The head is tilted back just a little further for a second and the tablet is gently dropped onto the tongue. Try to place the tablet on the centre of the tongue, but near the top.
7. The cat's mouth is closed for a few seconds.
8. Licking of the nose by the cat indicates success. Give the cat lots of attention.
9. A spat-out tablet indicates failure!
10. After one failed try, there tends to be a reduced success rate with each subsequent attempt to give the tablet, i.e. unfortunately you become less and less likely to succeed. The tablet gets wet and sticky, feline tempers start to fray and stress levels rise. At this point, back off and allow things to settle down before trying again.

Note: don't be tempted to 'throw' the tablet into the back of a cat's mouth. Cats have an extremely sensitive larynx which can easily enter into a spasm, which is both unpleasant and dangerous for the cat.

In food

This is quite a useful method, especially for those living alone. Whilst some cats can be tabletted single-handed, especially if you are able to kneel behind them on the floor and cradle them between your knees, it does take practice. Giving tablets in the food is often possible (but always check with your vet first) – it usually does not affect the action of the tablet, and some drugs must be given around the time of feeding anyway.

It is important, however, to go about this in the right way – otherwise the discerning cat will eat the food, but not the tablet you have tried to hide in it. Bear in mind the following points.

1. You are most likely to succeed when the cat is hungry. In cats normally given free access to food, it may be better to lift food bowls when on medication so that you are always guaranteed a hungry cat when it comes to tablet time.
2. Tablets are far easier to disguise in wet food. If your cat is not normally fed tinned food, get some tins or a very palatable human food like sardines in tomato sauce (many cats love this), tuna, or pâté.
3. Powder the tablet doses very finely between two spoons (keep these for cat use only).
4. Mix the powder into a SMALL mount of the chosen food, e.g. one tablespoonful.
5. Offer this to the cat.
6. When all of it is eaten, feed more food without any tablets in it.
7. For the constantly suspicious and intelligent cat, you can give a tiny amount of unadulterated food to get the taste buds going before presenting the medicated food immediately after it.

Multiple medications

A few unfortunate cats may require several different sorts of tablets daily on an ongoing basis. Obviously, one wants to make this as easy as possible for both cat and owner as there is no point in prescribing a regime which simply cannot be carried out for practical reasons. Treatment of certain heart conditions may require two or three different drugs daily. Aware of this problem, some vets are combining the various drugs into a single gelatin capsule, so that instead of different individual tablets needing to be given, only one composite capsule is required. These capsules have to be made up on an individual basis for each cat, and may constitute an additional expense, but the effort can be worth it for the problem cat.

Liquid medication

A number of drugs are available in liquid form, and these may be easier to use. The liquid can be given via a dropper or mixed into food. Antibiotics, some wormers and anti-inflammatory painkillers may be given this way.

Long-acting injections

These are an alternative to tablet medication in some cases. Long-acting antibiotic injections may be used and are very convenient.

Other drugs such as steroids are available in long-acting injection form, and these can last many weeks and may be used in inflammatory conditions of the mouth or skin. They have obvious advantages in that no-one needs to worry about tablets, but their disadvantages are a higher propensity for side-effects, especially with long-term usage, and the fact that once the injection has been given, the steroids cannot be 'taken out' of the cat again should another condition arise in which steroids are unhelpful. Tablets, on the other hand, can be stopped promptly and are much sooner out of the cat's body. Despite these problems, long-acting steroid injections may have a role in certain cats and certain medical problems.

Injections given by the owner

Owners of diabetic cats soon become proficient at giving the painless subcutaneous injections that are needed to keep their pets alive. The procedure is exactly the same for other drugs, except that larger needles and larger injection volumes may be required. While this may seem an alternative for the cat that is difficult to treat with drugs by mouth, most vets are reluctant to use this method except in diabetes – preferring to find another solution if possible as this avoids health and safety issues with drugs and injection equipment in the home.

Surgery

In a few instances, cats can be spared the need for on-going medication by surgical operations. Two common examples of this are in the treatment of over-active thyroid gland and megacolon, but various other conditions also come into this category, e.g. some chronic ear conditions. The aim would be to cure the underlying condition by means of a surgical operation and eliminate the need for on-going drug treatment. Surgery of this type often involves removing abnormal tissue. It constitutes a larger one-off expense but if successful should mean that the cat can then be discharged from treatment.

Complementary medicine

Much of the information in this book is designed to help complement treatment or advice provided by the veterinary surgeon or veterinary nurse. In this sense, complementary medicine includes many aspects of good nursing and care, such as creating a comfortable environment for the sick cat in terms of temperature, noise level, bedding, providing tempting food, or feeding special, 'prescription' diets specific to a cat's needs because of a disease they are suffering from, and so on. Other aspects focus on providing psychological support for the cat which is geared towards the cat's individual personality and temperament. For some cats, that may mean lots of human attention when ill; for others, very minimal levels of interaction may be best. Many cats cope best with fairly minimal levels of interaction and a quiet, comfortable environment. These aspects can make a significant difference to a cat's recovery from illness or injury. Veterinary nurses are highly experienced in this area, but owners, who know their cats best of all, can also make a large contribution if they are sensitive to their cat's needs.

Other forms of complementary medicine are more like forms of treatment and may be prescribed if they are thought appropriate. There is some overlap here between complementary and alternative medicine. Therapies such as massage/physical therapy and physiotherapy and even hydrotherapy (tolerated very well by most dogs and some cats) may be used under veterinary advice. A search on the Royal College of Veterinary Surgeons 'Find a Vet' search engine (http://findavet.rcvs.org.uk/find-a-vet/advanced-search/) produces a list of over 700 veterinary practices who provide some form of complementary medicine. If you are interested in seeking complementary medicine advice you should do so through one of these practices, or by speaking to your own vet who may be able to arrange a referral.

All forms of complementary medicine should be used under professional veterinary advice. Certain forms of treatment, e.g. homoeopathy, are controversial within the veterinary profession since their modes of action may not be known, or else the evidence base may be questioned. Although some veterinary surgeons use these treatments, many others may not. It can be dangerous, even life-threatening for your cat, to seek or use complementary medicines on your own, or on the advice of someone who is not also a qualified veterinary surgeon, even if they claim high success rates and cures. Only veterinary surgeons have the medical training and breadth needed to see the whole picture and to choose from a wide variety of treatment approaches and to know when specific interventions are needed to avoid complications or treat dangerous symptoms.

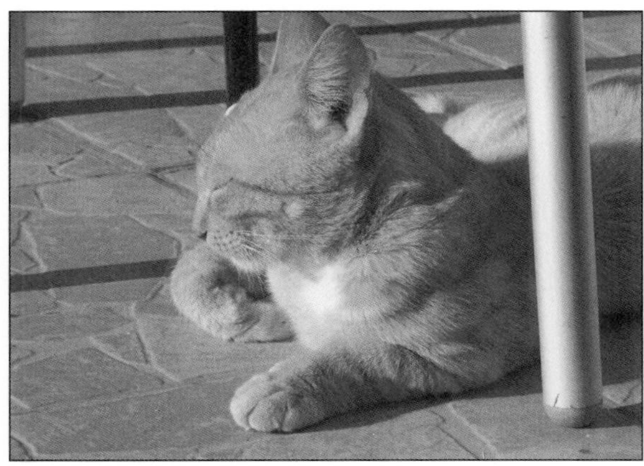

Don't put your cat at risk by using treatments without veterinary advice.

A

Abortion

Abortion is the loss of developing kittens from the womb before pregnancy has finished. It can occur at any stage of the pregnancy and has a variety of causes, including trauma, infections, and abnormalities in the reproductive system of the female cat.

The abortion may go unnoticed, or else the female cat may be noticeably ill beforehand.

☎ Urgency

Any illness occurring in a pregnant female should be attended to promptly as abortion is always a potential risk. Once abortion has occurred, the cat should definitely receive a veterinary examination to ensure that further complications are not present.

✚ First aid & nursing

Only general supportive care is relevant. Keep the cat warm, quiet and offer tempting food until the veterinary appointment.

Veterinary treatment

- Cats ill after abortion may require some on-going treatment for problems such as infection, high temperature and dehydration. A hospital stay may be needed.
- If future breeding is intended, the cause of abortion may need to be investigated. This could entail blood tests (for internal problems, virus infections, etc.), X-rays and ultrasound examinations. Quite extensive investigation may be required, and sometimes a cause cannot always be determined.
- Note that most pet cats are neutered (spayed) at a young age and so do not become pregnant and therefore cannot suffer from abortion in the first place.

Related or similar conditions

- ▶ **Birth**
- ▶ **Neutering**
- ▶ **Oestrus and mating**
- ▶ **Pregnancy**
- ▶ **Pyometra**

Abscess

An abscess is a painful swelling caused by infection, usually occurring underneath the skin. They are common in cats, and are often found around the head area, legs or the hindquarters. Penetrating wounds (e.g. bites, sharp injuries from wire, etc.) often cause abscesses as they act like an injection of harmful bacteria. Bites are by far the commonest cause in cats and fighting male cats are especially prone to them. The incidence is much higher in male cats that have not been castrated (neutered).

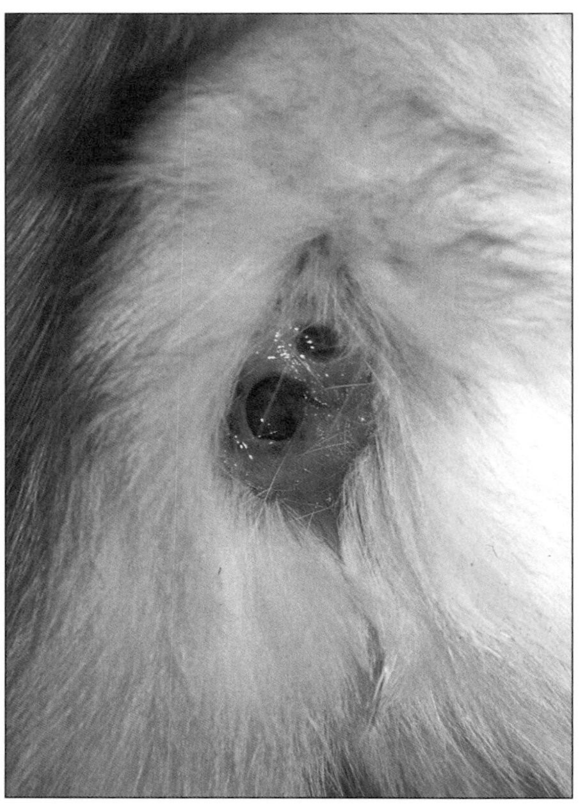

Abcess resulting from a bite.

Another cause of a persistent abscess could be a 'foreign body' embedded underneath the skin. Air rifle pellets, tooth fragments (from bites), splinters or thorns may all act as a persistent source of irritation and infection, leading to constant inflammation and discharge from a wound.

Abscesses usually take several days to develop, during which time the cat may be subdued, irritable or in pain. Cats may have a high temperature and no appetite. The affected area may be tender and inflamed, gradually swelling in size with discoloured and abnormally textured skin on the surface. Usually the hair is thinned or lost but sometimes the only sign is extreme sensitivity over the area where the abscess is developing.

Most abscesses near the surface eventually rupture, discharging foul-smelling yellowish fluid (pus). Rupture, though thoroughly unpleasant and messy, usually improves the symptoms considerably and the cat will be in much less discomfort.

Other sites for abscesses are in the mouth, throat, between the toes and (less commonly) in internal organs, where they are very serious.

☎ Urgency

Subcutaneous (under the skin) abscesses are not life-threatening but should be treated promptly to ensure a good response. A routine daytime appointment will normally be advised by the veterinary surgeon.

✚ First aid & nursing

You can really help the situation with some simple first aid. Abscesses should be encouraged to rupture and, once ruptured, should not be allowed to close over before infection is controlled, otherwise the whole unpleasant process could be repeated.

Before rupture, warm compresses (e.g. cloths, cotton wool) held against the abscess will relieve discomfort and aid 'pointing'. Take a large wad of cotton wool, soak in warm water, squeeze out and then hold against the inflamed area for 5–10 minutes 3 or 4 times daily.

After rupture, regular bathing (3–4 times daily) with large amounts of warm saline solution will remove discharges and encourage continued drainage. Use the cotton wool pad technique described above but leave the cotton wool wetter before applying. Alternatively, you could spray the area

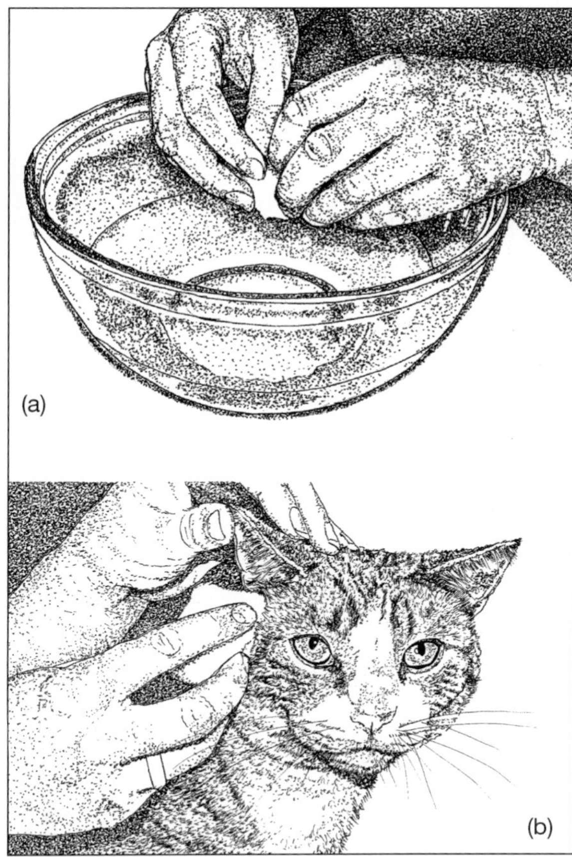

(a) Soaking the cotton wool; (b) Applying it to the cat's face. Hold gently in place for a few minutes before wiping away any discharge.

using a plant sprayer or (if the cat will allow) shower with plain water using a shower head. Wear disposable gloves.

Bathing usually needs to be kept up for several days. One teaspoon of salt can be added per pint of warm water for a gentle effective bathing solution.

> **Note:** Some cats are so uncomfortable and angry with painful abscesses that first aid should not be attempted. Take them to the vet as soon as you can.

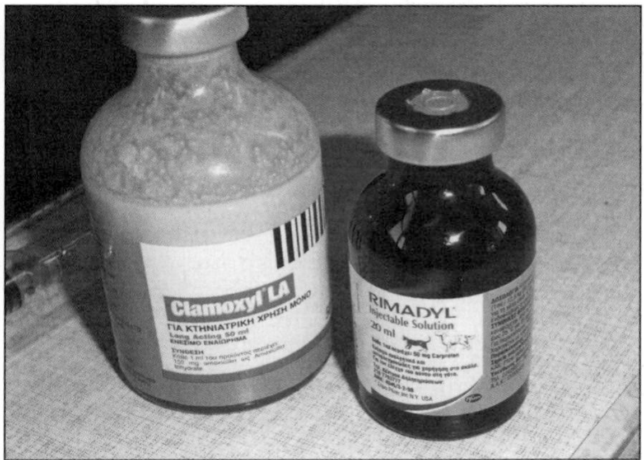

Antibiotics and painkillers are commonly used to treat abcesses.

Veterinary treatment

- Antibiotics are often supplied by injection given at the veterinary clinic, and usually followed up with a course of tablets for a week or so, or a long-acting injection may be used.
- Antiseptic flushing solutions may be given (or instructions to use saline).
- Large abscesses are often lanced and soft drains may then be inserted for a few days to promote drainage. This operation usually requires a short general anaesthetic and possibly a day or two of hospitalisation.
- If a foreign body is suspected, X-rays and an operation to try and locate and remove it may be recommended.
- Painkillers may also be prescribed.

Tip

First make sure the water or saline you use is not too hot. Wrapping the cat in a large towel to control the front and back legs, and the help of someone else to hold and steady the patient (who may not be all that patient!), will often make the job a lot easier. Remember than an abscess is likely to be less painful *after* it has ruptured, even although it may look worse at this time.

When using compresses and bathing, proceed very slowly and gently, gradually building up the time you spend treating the cat and gradually applying a little more pressure through the wet cotton wool. This allows the cat to get used to what you are trying to do. If it all turns into a struggle, abandon the exercise and try again later but proceed even more slowly this time! Some cats enjoy water and will allow wounds to be sprayed or even showered.

Related or similar conditions

- **Bites**
- **Fever/high temperature**
- **Infections**
- **Pain**

Accident

The commonest accident involving pet cats is a road traffic accident, but other relatively common ones are falls, burns, electrocution and coat contamination with dangerous substances such as oil. Sadly, cats are also occasionally the victims of malicious airgun injuries.

The possibility of internal injury must always be considered in any accident, especially those involving motor vehicles. These serious injuries do not always show up at the time of the accident, but they can be life-threatening. The priority is to try to prevent the cat's condition from deteriorating further while professional help is sought.

Note that it is almost always better to take the cat to the veterinary clinic rather than have the veterinary surgeon come out to the scene of the accident. By learning basic first aid principles (see below), you can do much of what the veterinary surgeon would be doing at the scene anyway. Valuable time will then be saved and the cat can be safely transported to a clinic where all the necessary personnel, equipment and drugs will be to hand.

☎ Urgency

Any accident where the cat is experiencing difficulty breathing, appears unconscious, is bleeding heavily or is unable to move is a serious emergency and immediate veterinary telephone advice should be sought, preferably at the same time as basic first aid is being applied.

Apparently minor accidents, where the cat is able to stand and walk and appears generally normal (if a little shocked), can still sometimes be serious. If a heavy blow was received, especially on the abdomen or chest areas, advice should be sought as soon as practicable even if the cat seems normal.

Close attention should be given to all accident victims for 24–48 hours as their condition can change rapidly and delayed onset shock can be serious.

✚ First aid & nursing

First ensure that you are not in danger yourself, especially if the accident has occurred near traffic.

The 'A-B-C' resuscitation routine should be followed. Place the cat in the 'recovery' position on a blanket, coat or jersey to provide padding and conserve heat.

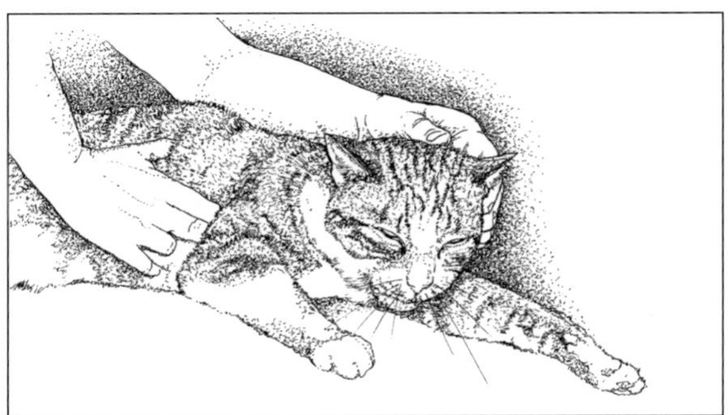

Recovery position, unconscious cat. The right fingers feel for a heart beat.

A Check that the cat has a clear airway.

Carefully open the mouth in unconscious cats; draw the tongue well forward and remove any obvious obstructions seen in the mouth/ throat. Swab away excess saliva or blood. (Take great care not to get accidentally bitten. If possible, wedge the mouth open or have someone hold the jaws apart while you inspect for obstructions. Many semi-conscious cats are capable of biting).

B Check for breathing by carefully observing the chest for movement or detecting air flow at the nostrils (put a mirror in front of the nostrils and look for condensation, or hold a wisp of tissue or cotton wool in front of the nostril opening). If there is no breathing, begin artificial 'mouth to nose' respiration immediately

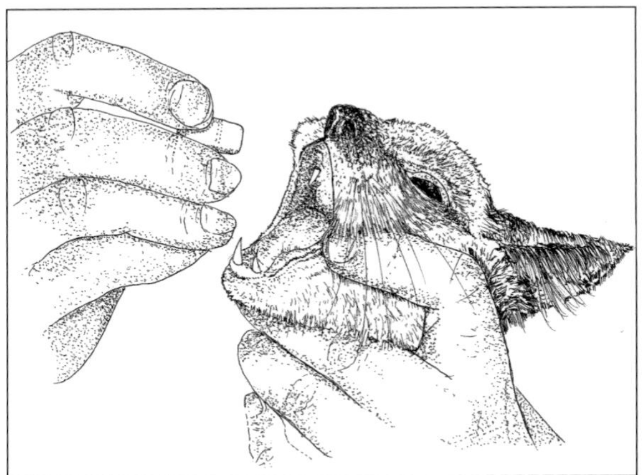

Checking mouth, removing obstructions. Swab away any blood or fluid, taking great care not to be bitten.

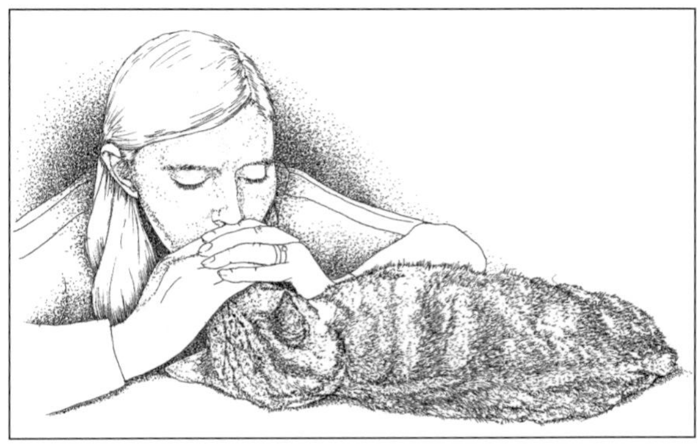

Artificial respiration: mouth to nose through cupped hands. Use approx. 10 breaths/minute.

C Check the circulation. Apply pressure or bandages to serious bleeding wounds. Minor bleeding wounds or grazes, where the blood seeps gradually, are not important at this point, but stronger arterial bleeding of bright blood or rapid flow of darker (venous) blood

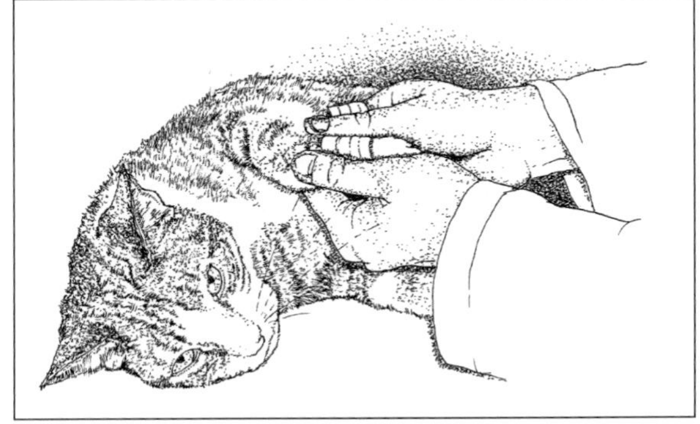

Applying dressing to bleeding wound. Bandage on or hold firmly in place.

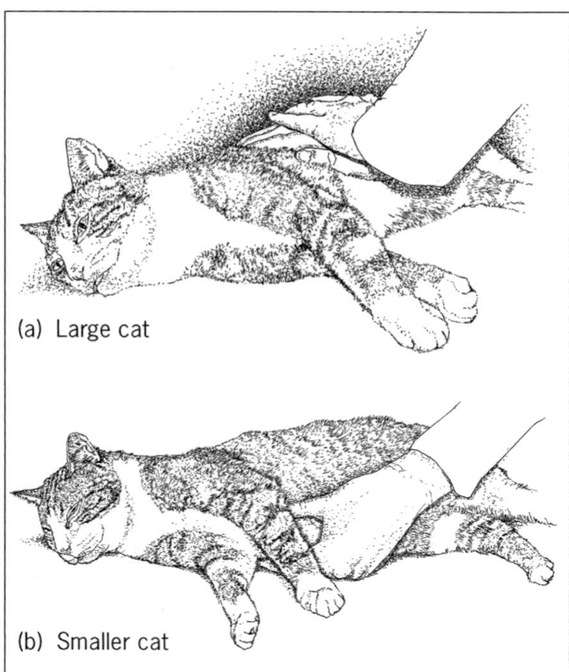

Two ways of performing external heart massage (compress once every 1–2 seconds).

must be attended to. Feel the chest behind the elbow for a heart beat; if there is no heart beat, compress the chest between the fingers and thumb of one hand to provide external heart massage. Keep checking for breathing and a heart beat as artificial respiration and heart massage is performed.

When spontaneous breathing returns, observe the cat carefully. Attend to any minor bleeding wounds and cover the cat with blankets, coats or jerseys to conserve heat. Carry the cat wrapped in a blanket for safety and comfort.

Veterinary treatment

- Resuscitation often involves intravenous fluids (a drip) and a supply of air enriched with oxygen once the animal is hospitalised.
- Drugs such as antibiotics, painkillers and steroids may form part of the initial treatment and stabilisation.
- X-rays are often used to diagnose fractures and serious internal injuries.
- Emergency surgery is occasionally needed for severe haemorrhage, though most surgery is delayed until after the animal is stabilised if possible. This may take several days.

Tip

Take care as cats in pain may be unpredictable and aggressive. See the guidelines for dealing with fearful or aggressive cats (see p. xviii), to ensure you can help the cat in a safe and effective way.

Related or similar conditions

- **Burns**
- **Electrocution**
- **Falls**
- **Fractures/dislocations**
- **Shock**

Aggression

See also **Behaviour problems**.

Uncharacteristic aggression in cats is often caused by pain, and you should always consider that this might be the case. Often, a veterinary examination will be needed. Common sources of pain leading to aggression in cats are: tooth pain, gum inflammation (gingivitis), abscesses, wounds, arthritis, fractures, ear problems and sprains/strains.

Cats with a fever/high temperature are

frequently irritable and aggressive and episodes of colic or gastric irritation due to fur ball may cause similar signs especially if the abdomen is handled, such as when the cat is picked up. In older cats (over 7 years) an overactive thyroid gland may need to be considered (hyperthyroidism). This condition frequently causes hyperactivity and aggression, in addition to other symptoms.

Aggression can also be caused by behaviour problems. This can be due to a change in home environment, the addition of new animals to the household or neighbourhood or to sudden changes in routine. Sometimes behaviour seems to change after a cat has been away for a while, e.g. in a cattery or a veterinary hospital, and then returns home.

Rarer causes of aggression include liver disease and brain damage and, in countries where the disease is present, rabies.

☎ Urgency

A cat that seems in severe pain should always be treated urgently. It will help your veterinary surgeon if you are able to indicate where the pain seems to be coming from. Observe the cat carefully to try to find out which area of the body is causing the problem but do not do anything which may provoke an attack.

When behavioural problems are the cause, the condition is of a less urgent nature as investigation and correction is likely to take some time. It is important here to highlight any changes in the cat's lifestyle or routine in the days or weeks leading up to the aggressive behaviour. Keeping a detailed diary of when and where the aggression occurs, and anything that seems to provoke it, may help in diagnosis and recognition of important trigger factors.

Overactive thyroid gland, liver disease and brain tumours all require special diagnostic tests to identify them. Frequently, other symptoms are present as well.

✚ First aid & nursing

Do not try to give any 'human' drugs such as aspirin, paracetamol or ibuprofen to the aggressive cat in pain. Cats are very sensitive to these drugs as they are unable to detoxify them in the same way as people. Inadvertent paracetamol poisoning frequently leads to death in cats.

The best first aid measures for the aggressive cat are to keep the patient quiet and relaxed, perhaps in a darkened room or in a well-padded cat cage or carrier, whilst arrangements are made for veterinary attention or advice.

Reduce stimulation from children, noises and bright lights. Cover the cage or box with a blanket or towel if necessary and lift or move it gently and slowly.

Veterinary treatment

- It is frequently necessary to sedate very aggressive cats in order to examine them fully and perform appropriate tests and treatments. As sedatives work better and are safer when the patient is as relaxed as possible, the measures outlined above can greatly help the process and make the veterinary surgeon's job easier.
- Correction of the source of pain (e.g. removal of diseased teeth, repair of fractured bones, suturing of wounds) and administration of painkillers usually restores the cat's temperament to normal.
- Behaviour problems may need detailed investigation and an individual programme of treatment. This can be a

lengthy process and specialist advice may need to be sought.

- Other medical conditions such as overactive thyroid gland, liver disease or brain problems may be able to be treated or controlled, thus improving the cat's behaviour.

Related or similar conditions

- **Arthritis**
- **Behaviour problems**
- **Ear problems**
- **Fever/high temperature**
- **Pain**
- **Thyroid gland (overactive)**

Airgun injury

Because of their independent lifestyles and tendencies to sit still in certain places, cats are, sadly, quite frequently the targets of airgun rifle attacks. The injuries caused depend on the closeness of the range at which the weapon was discharged, and the area of the body aimed for. Airgun pellets are also occasionally picked up incidentally on X-rays when other problems are being investigated, so it is very likely that many more cats are shot than are detected.

The entry wound can be very small and hard to find on the cat's hairy body; also they tend to seal over quickly. This is why cases may go undetected if no serious internal damage has resulted. As far as the unsuspecting owner is concerned, the cat may simply be a little off colour, nervous or irritable for a day or two, possibly showing signs of aggression or pain. The pellet remains within the cat, usually causing no serious problem, although occasionally persistent, draining abscesses can result from the effect of the 'foreign body' within the cat's tissues.

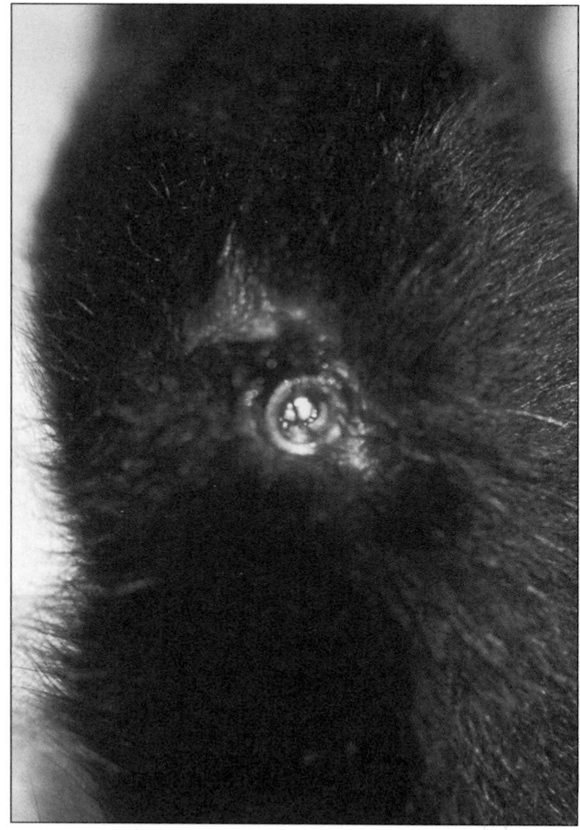

Airgun pellet lodged in the skin.

Pellets penetrating the abdomen, chest or head can however be immediately serious or life-threatening.

☎ Urgency

If you have seen the attack taking place, or suspect it, then you should contact your veterinary surgeon immediately for advice. The most urgent cases are those cats which are bleeding heavily, having difficulties breathing or lapsing into and out of consciousness (shock). Any injury to the eye is also a serious emergency and the potential always exists for vital chest damage if the chest wall is punctured or for internal organ damage if the abdomen is hit.

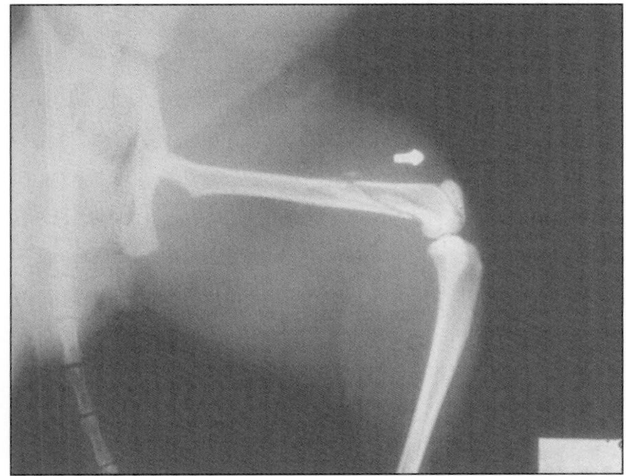

X-ray of a cat's hind leg. The cat returned home very lame and an X-ray revealed an airgun pellet above the stifle (knee) joint. The pellet is embedded in the muscle but has also caused a fracture of the thigh bone (femur). The pellet resembles a white arrow on the X-ray.

Many pellets, especially if fired from a distance, do not penetrate far into the body and can sometimes be felt lodged in muscle just underneath the skin. Owners sometimes detect these small hard nodules some time after the event, when the entry wound has closed over and healed. The cat appears quite normal in other respects. A routine veterinary appointment in these cases can confirm the presence of a pellet and allow notification of the appropriate authorities. It may not need removed if causing no problem.

If you know your cat has been shot, the police should be contacted with, if possible, details of where and when the attack took place and descriptions of the people carrying it out. The local branch of animal welfare charities should also be informed, as well as neighbouring veterinary practices.

+ First aid & nursing

If necessary, apply the ABC routine of resuscitation (see under **Accident**) and transport your cat urgently to the veterinary centre. Do not attempt to remove any visible pellets. Leave them where they are and let the veterinary surgeon investigate the severity of the damage caused.

Severely bleeding wounds should have a pressure dressing applied or held in place. If the eye is affected, a moistened pad should be held over the injured area if the cat will tolerate this.

Veterinary treatment

- In severely injured cats, resuscitation followed by diagnosis and treatment for serious internal chest or abdominal injuries may be needed.
- Removal of the eye is often required in cases where this sensitive organ is damaged.
- Antibiotics and painkillers may be used.
- Intravenous fluids (a 'drip') are often used where there has been blood loss or shock.
- Chronic abscesses associated with an embedded pellet may not resolve until the pellet is removed surgically.

Related or similar conditions

- ▶ **Abscess**
- ▶ **Anxiety/fear**
- ▶ **Shock**
- ▶ **Wounds**

Allergy

An allergy is a disorder which occurs when the body reacts in an unusual way to a substance. Most allergies cause inflammation of one type or another. Depending on where this inflammation occurs, different symptoms can be produced. Inflammation in the respiratory tract may cause coughing, sneezing or asthma. Inflammation in the skin may cause scratching or hairloss/**Baldness** (alopecia). Inflammation in the bowel can cause **Diarrhoea**. Inflammation around the eyes can cause eyelid swelling or watering of the eyes.

By far the commonest allergy in cats in that associated with **Fleas**. Cats can become extremely sensitive to flea saliva, so that when even a single flea bites, a hugely exaggerated skin reaction can occur, with intense itching, inflammation and hairloss occurring all over the body surface.

Raised skin blotches of 'nettlerash' can occur when a cat has brushed against or lain among plants to which it is allergic. The eyelids and paws are often inflamed.

Many other allergies are possible, to household products, foodstuffs, chemicals (including drugs), plants, pollens in the air, and even to house dust. Identifying the source of an allergy can sometimes be a problem, requiring patience and detective work since, as in people, individuals can vary widely in what they are allergic to.

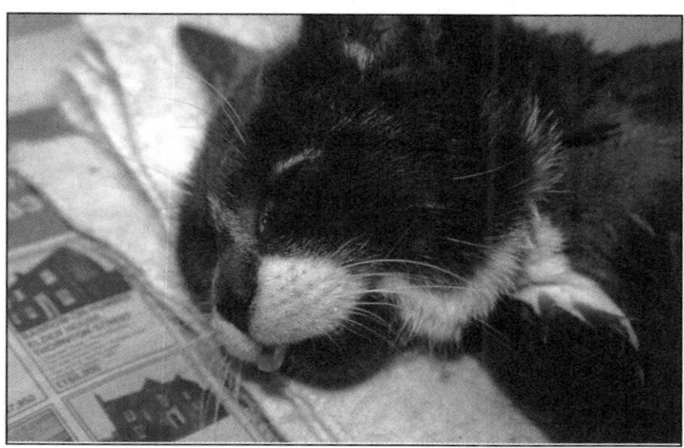

Cat suffering from an acute allergic reaction causing swelling of the face.

☎ Urgency

Most allergies do not give rise to life-threatening problems, the exception being a very acute form of allergy known as anaphylaxis. When this occurs, it causes collapse, respiratory problems and shock. It must be treated as an emergency.

Other allergies tend to lead to sneezing/coughing, skin problems and occasionally vomiting/diarrhoea, and a routine veterinary appointment should be made as long as there is no interference with normal breathing, swallowing and eye function.

✚ First aid & nursing

For the rare occasion when anaphylaxis occurs, the ABC routine of emergency resuscitation should be followed (see under **Accident**), and immediate veterinary advice sought.

For other allergies, if you suspect you know what caused the reaction, remove your cat from the vicinity. Mild symptoms will often disappear over a few hours. Cool water can be used to bathe inflamed skin and eyes and the cat should be kept in a cool, well ventilated place and observed carefully.

If fleas are suspected, the house should be vacuumed, all the cat's bedding washed, and advice sought regarding flea treatment products for all cats and dogs in the household. The soft furnishings in the house will also need to be treated to destroy flea eggs and larvae.

Veterinary treatment

- Severe allergic symptoms causing shock or collapse may be treated using potent drugs such as adrenalin or steroids, especially when the respiratory system is involved or threatened.
- Flea allergy (by far the commonest allergy in cats) requires veterinary flea control and possibly skin treatment to settle the irritated skin.
- Suspected dietary allergies require the feeding of carefully controlled test diets to exclude certain proteins from the diet in order to see if these are causing symptoms. If so, the symptoms will improve but this can take many weeks to show and food allergy can be a difficult and frustrating condition to prove.
- Other skin allergies may require the use of diagnostic tests to try to identify the substance being reacted to. Sometimes, anti-allergy injections may be able to be given to limit sensitivity to the substance.
- Allergic reactions caused by adverse effects of medical drugs are fortunately rare, but if you suspect this has happened, stop the medication and contact the veterinary surgeon for advice.

> **Note:** Always use flea control products with caution. It is possible to poison cats by over-dosing, or by using products too frequently or mixing different products. Do not use products or formulations designed for dogs. In general, it is safest to only use prescription products obtained from your veterinary surgeon in the correct formulation and dose frequency. Some suggestions for non-chemical means of controlling fleas are given under **Fleas**.

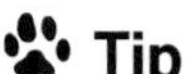

Tip

No matter what your cat is allergic to, decreasing the 'allergic load' within the house can be helpful. Cats with asthma, for example, are always worse when smokers are present in the house. Carpet cleaners, aerosol sprays and plug-in room fresheners should be avoided or used in one room at a time only, and consideration given to using a low dust cat litter, e.g. wood chips, rather than Fuller's earth or other grit products.

Related or similar conditions

- **Asthma**
- **Baldness**
- **Fleas**
- **Skin problems**

Anal glands

The anal glands are two small scent glands located on either side of the anal opening at the 4 and 8 o'clock positions. During defaecation, they normally empty by releasing their contents on to the faeces. Cats suffer from anal gland problems much less frequently than dogs, where it is common. However the glands can occasionally cause problems in cats, becoming impacted or infected.

Symptoms are irritation/discomfort at the anal area, tail clamping or signs of irritability, restlessness and pain. Cats may sit down and drag their bottoms along the ground in the same way that affected dogs do. Anal gland abscesses can also occur. These are very uncomfortable and may result in symptoms of aggression in affected cats. The abscess may rupture to the surface, producing an unpleasant discharge. Rupture is usually associated with an improvement in symptoms as pain is relieved.

☎ Urgency

Anal gland problems, though uncomfortable, are not life-threatening and a routine veterinary appointment is usually advised.

✚ First aid & nursing

Warm compresses can help – take a large pad of cotton wool, soak in warm (not hot) water, and apply this gently to the area for 5–10 minutes at a time. Some cats may not tolerate this if in discomfort and distress. In these cases, it is best to leave the cat alone in a quiet place.

Ruptured abscesses would benefit from salt water bathing (1 teaspoon salt to 1 pint [560 ml] warm water). This can be achieved using the cotton wool pad technique mentioned above, or else by gently running the salt water over the area from a spray bottle (or use plain water from a shower head). Again, not every cat will allow this but it is helpful if they do! A ruptured abscess is always messy and unpleasant to deal with, though usually less painful than before rupture. Wear disposable gloves.

Veterinary treatment

- Impacted glands can be expressed by the veterinary surgeon, usually bringing about rapid relief of symptoms.
- Abscesses or deep infections may require an anaesthetic to allow surgical drainage, followed by a course of antibiotics and, usually, painkillers.

Related or similar conditions

- ► **Abscess**
- ► **Constipation**
- ► **Pain**
- ► **Worms**

Anemia

Anemia means a shortage of red blood cells. Red blood cells are the specialised cells which transport oxygen from the lungs to all the tissues and organs of the body. Without this vital supply of oxygen, all normal body functions eventually cease.

Anemia can arise after serious bleeding, either internally or externally, if enough red blood cells are lost. Any form of severe trauma or accident could result in anemia in this way. Poisoning is another potential cause of anemia since certain poisons destroy red blood cells. Additional common causes include viral and other infections – feline leukaemia virus for example – which may cause destruction of red blood cells within the body, and heavy parasite infestation, especially in kittens, who may lose significant volumes of blood to blood-sucking parasites: **Fleas**, **Lice** or **Ticks**.

Liver disease and **Kidney disease** can both cause anemia due to poor rates of production of red blood cells and cats with **Cancer** may become anemic due to some of the complications of chronic disease.

Anemic animals are weak, tire easily, have pale gums and may experience difficulty in breathing due to shortage of oxygen carrying by the blood. Overall, anemia is a serious condition which must be recognised and treated promptly. In particular, the veterinary surgeon will try to find out exactly why the cat has become anemic in the first place.

☎ Urgency

Anemia can develop rapidly (e.g. after severe blood loss) or slowly (e.g. in response to chronic disease of the liver or kidney, or cancer) but once symptoms appear, they should be treated promptly. Most cats become anemic due to chronic diseases developing over a period of weeks or months. They tend to cope with this quite well at first, by adjusting their behaviour and activity levels.

Animals that are anemic and in shock after road traffic accidents or similar injuries require emergency treatment and resuscitation. If other problems are controlled this type of anemia is fully reversible.

Animals that are anemic due to chronic diseases must be diagnosed and treated promptly to avoid further and possibly irreversible deterioration. If poisoning has occurred, time is of the essence and emergency treatment should be started as soon as possible after the intake of poison.

✚ First aid & nursing

For cats involved in accidents, apply the ABC resuscitation routine (see under **Accident**) and seek veterinary help immediately. If you know a poison has been taken in, seek veterinary help without delay. See also under **Poisoning**.

In other cases, a veterinary diagnosis of the anemia is essential. Prior to the appointment, the cat should be kept warm, stress-free and encouraged to eat and drink. In kittens with severe parasites, manual removal of the parasites using a comb or tweezers is safer than applying chemical products to an already weakened animal. The veterinary surgeon will make a decision as to which insecticide, if any, to use at this stage.

Veterinary treatment

- Initial efforts will be made to diagnose the cause and type of anemia, and are likely to involve blood tests and possibly other tests.
- Severely affected cats may require a drip or blood transfusion to save their lives whilst other forms of treatment can begin to take effect.
- In all cases, good nursing, rest, stress reduction and promotion of the appetite are vital to recovery and convalescence.

Related or similar conditions

- ▶ **Bleeding**
- ▶ **Feline infectious anemia**
- ▶ **Feline leukaemia**
- ▶ **Kidney disease**
- ▶ **Poisoning**

Anxiety/fear

See also **Behaviour problems**.

Anxiety can occur to some degree in most cats during strange or unfamiliar experiences, e.g. travel, visiting the veterinary surgery, during thunderstorms. The extent to which anxiety is shown depends on the character and personality of the cat, and also their prior experiences in life.

Some cats remain completely unfazed by new experiences or situations; for others, life is generally more anxious. These cats seem frightened by many different things, or perhaps by one thing in particular but it is severe enough to cause serious distress. Signs of severe anxiety in cats include

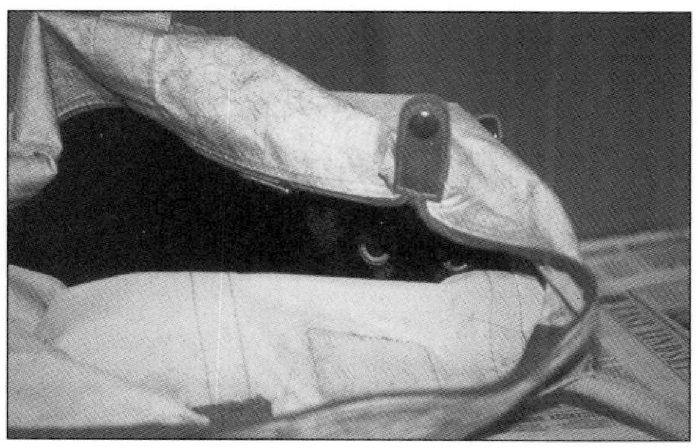

Admitted for a routine operation, this black cat gained some extra security by remaining in his owner's slightly unusual cat carrier while in the hospital cage. He observed the goings-on without feeling unduly threatened.

hiding away, making strange miaowing sounds, uncharacteristic aggression, poor appetite and panting. In severe cases, urine and faeces may be passed.

Another general sign of anxiety can be urine marking, where a cat passes urine (or occasionally faeces) in inappropriate places in the house. This problem is discussed further under **Spraying (urine)**.

Anxiety and stress can worsen or trigger other diseases. Two conditions thought to be worsened by stress in cats are **Cystitis** and inflammatory conditions of the bowel (**Enteritis**). In addition, some anxious cats exhibit their problem by **Overgrooming**, leading to hair loss.

☎ Urgency

Anxiety only becomes an urgent medical problem when it occurs in a cat which cannot tolerate stress. In these cases, severe anxiety can on rare occasions be fatal. Cats suffering from heart disease, severe anemia, overactive thyroid gland, asthma and respiratory problems do not cope with stress well. They do not have the extra capacity within their bodies to handle the effects of this and can collapse. Therefore all efforts must be made to avoid stressful circumstances which could result in deterioration if a cat suffers from one of these problems.

For otherwise healthy cats, anxiety is not an emergency although it is undoubtedly unpleasant. The measures described below can help considerably.

+ First aid & nursing

Important first aid involves reassurance, removal from the source of stress and placing the cat in a cool, quiet, dark place. A very useful measure in the hot, stressed and panting cat is to direct a cool air fan over the cat cage/carrier to increase air circulation. Dampening the head, ears and body with cold water will also help to promote heat loss through evaporation. Noise, bright lights and hot temperatures should be avoided. The presence of a person or other animal which the cat knows well can provide extra reassurance.

Should collapse occur, the ABC resuscitation technique (see under **Accident**) must be followed and urgent veterinary help sought.

Veterinary treatment

- Although sedative drugs are available, these should not be considered a permanent answer for the anxious cat. Longterm, they have side-effects which may be undesirable. Instead, efforts should be made to identify the source of anxiety and to remove or alter this, possibly by changing the cat's routine or environment, or arranging necessary movements/ appointments, etc. such that anxiety is minimised.

- Synthetic pheromone sprays or plug-ins are available for certain anxiety-related problems in cats. These chemicals resemble the natural pheromones which cats deposit on surfaces when they run their faces along them. Their use has been shown to help some anxiety-related problems in cats. They are available from the veterinary surgeon if the cat's anxiety problem seems of a type which will respond.

Related or similar conditions

- ▶ **Aggression**
- ▶ **Behaviour problems**
- ▶ **Overgrooming**

Appetite (abnormal)

Cats do not eat unusual objects ('foreign bodies') as frequently as dogs, nevertheless a wide variety of things are still occasionally consumed. Needles are often swallowed when cats play with them attached to threads; similarly, other long strands such as cassette tapes and pieces of string/elastic bands may be swallowed. Very unusual foreign bodies may also be encountered.

Unusual tastes may appeal to certain cats and this can occasionally cause problems if the substance they lick is toxic. Antifreeze comes into this category and some house plants, such as the leopard lily, are poisonous if eaten. Some cats simply enjoy foods not normally associated with cats' appetites, e.g. melon, celery, but this is just an individual preference and in the absence of other symptoms is usually nothing to worry about.

Appetite is abnormal if it is excessive (as in overactive thyroid gland and diabetes, especially if connected with weight loss) or very poor (as in kidney disease and many other infections and chronic diseases). Occasionally, liver disease can give rise to unusual appetites/cravings for normally unappetising things. Usually, other symptoms of illness will also be present.

☎ Urgency

The urgency depends on the symptoms being shown. Frequent vomiting, incoordination, weakness or fits demand immediate

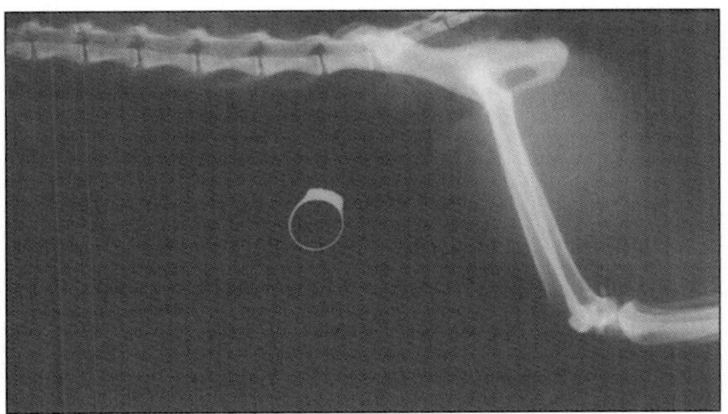

X-ray of a cat's abdomen. She had been vomiting persistently for several days. Her X-ray revealed the cause of the problem and also solved the mystery of a missing wedding ring.

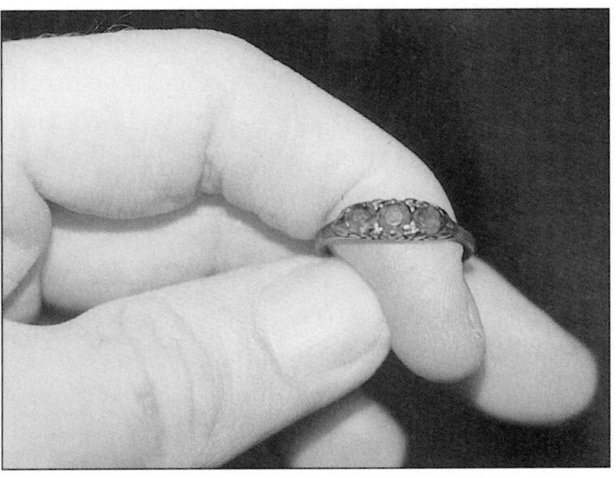

The ring after removal from the cat's small intestine.

attention since these symptoms are associated with severe diseases or toxicities which must be diagnosed and treated rapidly. Some 'foreign bodies' can result in life-threatening intestinal obstruction.

Abnormal cravings should normally be investigated but they are not urgent in the absence of other major symptoms.

Increasing appetite in the face of weight loss is a frequent finding in cats with overactive thyroid glands, and also in diabetes. Blood tests are needed. These symptoms generally appear over the course of several weeks or months.

A poor appetite should also be checked out since this may represent an underlying problem that needs treated. Various things can cause this from tooth pain to kidney disease, as mentioned above.

✚ First aid & nursing

If a cat is vomiting frequently, food should be withheld and only tiny amounts of water or glucose solution offered until the veterinary appointment. Do not delay excessively as cats can quickly become dehydrated with severe vomiting.

Sometimes, if a cat has eaten string or tape, an end maybe found protruding from the mouth or anus. On no account should this be pulled. Seek veterinary attention straight away. Often, linear strands become lodged around the base of the tongue and the veterinary surgeon will check for this.

Cats with very poor appetites can be tempted using strongly scented foods which can be warmed up to release more aroma. Sardines and similar tinned fish are often appealing, and many sick cats seem to like fish in tomato sauce. Chicken, smoked ham or other meat can also be tried. Offer small amounts at a time and try hand feeding/coaxing.

If you suspect a toxic product or plant has been eaten, try to find out the name and seek advice immediately. With chemicals, if possible, take the label to the veterinary surgeon. You should not attempt to make a cat vomit by giving, e.g. strong salt solution. The cat will likely resist, there is a risk of inhalation, and caustic substances can cause more damage as they are vomited up. Seek professional help instead.

Veterinary treatment

- Blood tests are often used to help diagnose abnormal appetite caused by overactive thyroid gland, diabetes, kidney or liver disease.
- In the case of swallowed 'foreign bodies', surgery may be needed to remove the offending object. Surprisingly, needles usually pass through the bowels uneventfully without causing any damage but may need removing from the anal area at the end of their journey.
- Threads, strings, tapes etc. can be serious as they can cause bunching up and resulting severe damage of the intestines. These usually require surgery for removal. Always suspect a problem if your cat becomes ill after playing with a thread, string or tape.
- Toxicities are treated with general supportive treatment (drips, etc.) and specific antidotes if available.

Tip

Eating grass is considered normal in cats and is not a sign of other illness. Occasionally, vomiting may occur afterwards if the grass stems were particularly rough. Many pet stores sell small tubs of grass which can be made available to indoor cats.

Related or similar conditions

- **Diabetes**
- **Foreign body**
- **Thyroid gland (overactive)**
- **'Wool' eating**

Arthritis

Arthritis means inflammation of the joints and surrounding tissues. It is a common cause of lameness in older cats, and can also occur in younger animals following bone or joint injury. In severe cases, the affected joints will be thickened and painful with a restricted range of motion.

Arthritis can affect any joint and also the spine. In cats, common joints affected are the elbows, carpus (wrist), stifle (knee) and tarsus (ankle) joints.

Common symptoms are stiffness and limping, especially after rest, and general irritability and pain. Many cats with arthritis of the spine do not groom themselves adequately, leading to poor coat and matting of hair, especially along the back. They may resent touching or stroking of the back.

Cats tend to cope with mild arthritis relatively well. When symptoms are shown, the problem is usually fairly severe.

☎ Urgency

The problem is not urgent in nature as arthritis develops slowly over months to years. Often, however, an exacerbation of the problem may occur after a fall, accident or incoordinated movement. Symptoms can then become very severe, with total lameness or pain on movement. The painful cat may show aggression when touched or picked up.

✚ First aid & nursing

Rest and warmth are important. Ensure that feed and water bowls and also litter tray are within easy reach. Do not allow companion animals to aggravate the arthritic patient by trying to play, etc. Ensure that plenty of thick bedding is available and that the cat does not need to jump up or down to reach this.

Veterinary treatment

- X-rays may be used to confirm arthritis and differentiate it from other bone or joint conditions, e.g. bone cancer, joint dislocation, etc.
- Anti-inflammatory drugs can be very effective in relieiving pain and discomfort. Due to potential side-effects, especially with long term usage, the lowest effective doses should always be aimed for.

Remember that the aim is to improve quality of life. Although high drug doses may eliminate symptoms entirely, they may occasionally cause harmful side-effects. A balance should be sought between relieving pain and discomfort and using minimum amounts of potent drugs.

Tip

Do not be tempted to give human painkillers such as aspirin, paracetamol or ibuprofen to arthritic cats! Cats are extremely sensitive to these drugs and they can readily prove fatal.

In overweight cats (obesity), weight loss is vital because otherwise the pain from arthritis will be difficult or impossible to control. Often, achieving a normal body weight is all that is required to relieve the symptoms in mild or moderate cases. Most adult cats weigh from 3.0 to 5.0 kilogrammes, depending on their stature.

Related or similar conditions

- **Bone/joint problems**
- **Grooming (poor)**
- **Obesity**
- **Pain**

Asthma

Feline asthma (sometimes called feline bronchitis) is an allergic-type respiratory condition which causes difficulty breathing, wheezing and coughing/gagging. Usually, symptoms first appear in young to middle aged cats and can be made worse by cigarette smoke, carpet cleaners, furniture polish, air fresheners and perfumed cat litter.

Many cats show exaggerated breathing effort at rest and wheezes can be heard. Severe respiratory distress, similar to an acute asthmatic attack in people, can also occur. Cats with asthma are free of additional symptoms which suggest other forms of respiratory diseases such as pneumonia or lung tumour.

Cat flu is another possibility which can lead to similar signs, although cats with this problem tend to sneeze more, and often have a nose discharge and runny eyes. They sound extremely congested when they are breathing.

☎ Urgency

Mild to moderate cases are not urgent and a routine appointment should be sought. However, severe attacks can occasionally occur during which extreme respiratory difficulty is seen. These count as emergencies since death is possible during the attack.

✚ First aid & nursing

In mild cases, improve ventilation and move the cat away from places where aerosols, cleaners, perfumes or smoke are present. A cool environment helps; also avoid stresses and noise. Placing the cat in a cat cage or carrier. If possible, direct a cool air fan across the cage.

Future use of perfumed cleaning products and aerosols should be avoided if possible since they can aggravate the condition, as can cigarette smoke. Also examine the type of cat litter used. Some products create a lot of dust particles and these can be very irritating for asthmatic cats. Experiment with different cat litters including wood pulp, sand, paper or earth. Do not use any litters which release perfumes or scents as they become damp.

Severe cases require urgent veterinary attention. Avoid stressing the cat if at all possible. If collapse occurs, use the ABC resuscitation technique described under **Accident**.

Veterinary treatment

- X-rays are likely to be used in any cat with severe breathing problems in order to help with diagnosis. The very seriously affected cat may be placed in an oxygen tent initially until stable enough for further tests or examination.

- Other diagnostic techniques such as bronchoscopy (looking at the airways using a small camera) may be suggested.
- Blood tests will probably be recommended.
- Several drugs are used for asthma but most cats with severe symptoms require the use of steroids to reduce inflammation in the airways. Usually, the response is good, however the cat may need to stay on these drugs permanently to keep symptoms at bay. Due to potential side-effects, the veterinary surgeon will try to find the lowest dose which works.
- Bronchodilators are sometimes used in addition to the above. These drugs help open up small airways and reduce the spasm which causes the unpleasant asthma-type symptoms.
- Drugs can be given by tablet, injection or by the use of adapted inhalers, which are often well-tolerated in cats and are easy for owners to use at home.
- If infection is suspected, a course of antibiotics may be given.

Tip

Anything you can do to reduce 'allergens' (smoke, dust, perfumes, etc.) in the house is likely to help your cat a lot if it suffers from asthma.

Related or similar conditions

- **Breathing problems**
- **Cat flu**
- **Heart disease**
- **Pneumonia**

B

Bad breath

The two main causes of bad breath (halitosis) in cats are tooth/gum problems and kidney disease. However a cat that is ill for a long time with almost any problem could develop bad breath as a result of poor overall condition. As such, bad breath may only be a general indication of poor health in some cats.

Mouth ulcers, caustic burns to the mouth and severe virus infections, such as feline leukaemia virus (FeLV) and feline immunodeficiency virus (FIV), may also cause bad breath and gum inflammation, as may tumours in the mouth or throat areas.

General symptoms often associated with bad breath include mouth pain, poor appetite, dribbling, pawing at the mouth and irritability. Affected cats may not be grooming properly because of a sore mouth, resulting in matted coats and poor overall coat condition.

☎ Urgency

Bad breath is not usually an emergency but if the mouth is so sore that the cat stops eating and drinking, an appointment within the next 24 hours is required to prevent dehydration and other problems.

+ First aid & nursing

Providing soft or liquidised food and warming this up may help. Keeping the mouth and lips clean by bathing with tepid salty water (1 teaspoon to 1 pint [560 ml]) can help prevent matting of fur from saliva and food residues.

Mouth washes/rinses, while not tolerated by all, or many, cats, can be useful to help keep certain problems under control. Only solutions designed for cats, and obtained from the veterinary surgeon, should be used. Special toothbrushes and toothpaste are also available. Given time and patience, many cats will tolerate tooth brushing (which helps reduce tooth and gum disease and tooth loss), but some individuals find the process too stressful, as do their owners!

Veterinary treatment

- In order to examine the mouth and throat thoroughly, and without pain or distress to the cat, a general anaesthetic may be needed.
- Dental surgery, including extraction of diseased teeth, may often be necessary. Some cats are prone to feline gingivitis/stomatitis (severe chronic inflammation of the gums and mouth) – a problematical condition which can be extremely difficult to control.
- Blood tests are often taken for severe/recurrent gingivitis due to the association with serious viral illnesses in cats

(especially feline immunodeficiency virus, FIV). Blood tests also check out kidney and liver function, both of which can indirectly lead to bad breath. Occasionally, undiagnosed diabetes may be detected, which has been causing debility and mouth problems.

- Caustic burns to the mouth may be treated by resting the mouth completely by means of placement of a feeding tube into the nose or oesophagus. Most cats tolerate these tubes very well and they ensure that a good plane of nutrition can be kept up while the injured tissues are healing. They are usually left in place for several days to a week, but tubes in the oesophagus can be left for many weeks without any problems (see p. 151 which shows a cat with a nasal feeding tube in position).

Related or similar conditions

- ▶ **Feline immunodeficiency virus (FIV)**
- ▶ **Kidney disease**
- ▶ **Mouth and tooth problems**

Balance (loss of)

Loss of balance can be caused by a large number of problems in cats. Most of these require a veterinary diagnosis at an early stage. This may entail a variety of different tests.

Ear problems which cause severe pain, infection or inflammation of the middle or inner ear can affect the sensitive organs of balance located there. Cats may hold their heads to one side, shake their heads frequently and appear uncoordinated or walk in circles. Ear pain is thoroughly unpleasant and affected cats can become quite frantic in their efforts to gain relief.

Brain injury or brain tumour may also affect balance. Brain injury is usually sudden in onset (e.g. after a fall or accident), whereas brain tumours may lead to a more gradual onset of symptoms. Although people may also use the term 'stroke', the condition does not exist in cats in the exactly the same form as in people, nevertheless it is a useful shorthand description for problems which can affect older cats and cause loss of balance and inability to stand in severe cases.

Idiopathic vestibular syndrome is a similar condition to 'stroke' but can affect cats of any age. This can be a sudden onset and severe condition showing loss of balance, falling over, rolling and head tilt as well as rapid flickering movements of the eyes. Although the symptoms are alarming, improvement usually occurs over several days. However it may take a few weeks for the cat to return to normal and some cats are left with a slight head tilt. The exact cause of this problem is unknown and, although several treatments may be tried, it is thought that symptoms disappear of their own accord, given time. Other similar conditions need to be ruled out however.

Other severe illnesses and poisoning may also initially appear as a loss of balance, and cats having fits will be unbalanced. Finally, bone or joint problems and spinal injury can cause similar symptoms due to the effects of pain or paralysis.

As can be seen, a diverse range of problems has to be considered here. Relevant information from the owner regarding previous health, the onset of symptoms, any trauma or accident and any other symptoms present, can help narrow down this long list of possible diseases.

☎ Urgency

Owing to the unusual and dramatic symptoms, most owners usually seek urgent attention if their cat starts showing symptoms of loss of balance.

✚ First aid & nursing

First aid consists of keeping the cat (and yourself) calm, removing obstacles which the cat could stumble into and, if necessary, confining the cat in a cage or a carrier whilst attention is sought. A quiet, darkened room will reduce stimulation to the cat and help with symptoms.

Veterinary treatment

- Close examination of the ears, possibly under anaesthetic and incorporating X-rays, may be required. Additional X-rays may be required for trauma cases where bones/joints or the spine is suspected to be damaged. For suspected brain tumours, a CT or MRI scan (if available) may be recommended.
- Blood tests are likely to be used in cases of poisoning and in cats having fits, to try to detect underlying organ damage (especially that affecting the liver and kidneys).
- Other tests may be recommended depending on the symptoms in individual cats and the vet's suspicion as to what might be going on.
- Treatment may be surgical (certain ear problems, fractures and some causes of spinal damage) or with drugs (poisoning, fits).
- Good nursing is required for the unbalanced cat to prevent injury and allow normal feeding and use of the litter tray.

Related or similar conditions

- ▶ **Bone/joint problems**
- ▶ **Brain damage**
- ▶ **Ear problems**
- ▶ **Fits**
- ▶ **Poisoning**

Baldness (alopecia)

Baldness (the medical term for loss of hair is alopecia) is quite a common symptom in cats, although usually only a portion of the cat's coat is affected. The hair is lost due to scratching or grooming (licking) by the cat. Occasionally, hair falls out of its own accord due to hormonal causes. Note that hair shedding from a cat is only a medical problem if it results in true patches of baldness; otherwise it is usually assumed to be normal casting of dead hair strands, which occurs continuously in housed cats, and is something which is lived with by all cat owners.

Common sites for baldness are along the top of the back towards the tail base, on the underside of the abdomen, especially between the hind legs, along the flanks and down the forelegs. By far the commonest cause of baldness in cats arises due to fleas and the very common allergic skin disease associated with them (usually called flea allergy dermatitis, FAD; or flea bite hypersensitivity, FBS). Until proved otherwise, most cats with hair loss are assumed to be suffering from fleas! The symptoms and treatments are discussed fully under **Fleas**. Fleas must always be ruled out first, otherwise attempted treatment of the skin may prove time-consuming, frustrating and expensive.

Other skin parasites, including mange mites and ringworm, may cause skin problems and hair loss in cats. Food allergy is another potential cause. This tends to be considered once parasites (fleas, mites, ringworm) have been ruled out. Overall, it is not common.

Overgrooming due to behaviour problems (sometimes called psychogenic alopecia) occurs in cats, often in cats of a nervous disposition. In these patients, no obvious cause for the licking of fur can be found but the cat persists in doing it, sometimes until large areas of hairless coat result. The skin underneath usually looks normal and non-irritated. This diagnosis tends to be reached once other possibilities have been ruled out.

☎ Urgency

Baldness is a non-urgent condition and a routine veterinary appointment should be sought.

✚ First aid & nursing

Little in the way of first aid is appropriate. It is best not to apply anything to the cat's coat prior to your appointment (creams, shampoos etc.) even if the skin does look dry or cracked. This could make diagnosis harder as the veterinary surgeon will be looking for fairly subtle signs of the cause of the problem and applied products could mask this vital evidence or wash it out.

Flea products purchased from pet stores should be used with care. In general, a veterinary diagnosis should be sought before applying any product to your cat's skin or coat since toxicity can occur, either by direct absorption through the skin surface or as a result of the cat licking their coat after a product has been applied. Note that mixing different products can prove fatal. Owners may be tempted to do this, or to give repeated doses, if the first product or application seems ineffective. Young kittens should always receive a veterinary examination and professional advice on parasite treatment followed.

It is very useful to let the veterinary surgeon know the answers to several important questions (see box). These can help narrow down the large list of possible diagnoses which may be causing the baldness in your cat.

10 important questions

1. How long have symptoms been present?
2. Are there other pets in the house (cats, dogs)? Do they have skin problems?
3. Does the cat gain access to outdoors?
4. Does the cat appear itchy?
5. Have carpet or furnishing cleaning products been used recently?
6. Are there any skin problems in humans in the household?
7. Have any flea products been used on the cat recently?
8. Has the cat's diet been changed recently?
9. Has the cat's bedding been changed recently?
10. Have you noticed any other symptoms in your cat?

Veterinary treatment

- A careful search for fleas will always be made as these are so common. Other skin parasites are checked for in hair pluckings, skin scrapes or skin biopsies. Unless parasites are eliminated from the patient, contact animals and the environment, the skin problems will not clear up, so do not be surprised if your veterinary surgeon seems very focused on parasitic causes initially.
- Blood tests may be indicated for hormonal problems and special diets may be tried for suspected food allergy. Diets need to be adhered to strictly for around 2 months before any effect can be judged.
- Common drugs used to treat skin problems in cats are antibiotics (when there is skin infection), steroids (for itch and self-inflicted damage) and hormones. Steroids are often very successful in reducing the damaging 'itch-scratch-itch' cycle, but the aim is always to wean the cat off these or get down to very low dosages for the long term, due to potential side-effects.
- Some skin problems cannot be cured, only controlled by careful use of drugs, environmental or food alterations.
- Note that skin problems caused by overgrooming may be improved by taking measures to reduce the stress levels in the susceptible cat.

Related or similar conditions

- ▶ **Allergy**
- ▶ **Fleas**
- ▶ **Overgrooming**
- ▶ **Skin problems**

Behaviour problems – general

Behaviour problems comprise a variety of disorders which cause alteration in what is considered to be 'normal' behaviour patterns for pet cats. There is however a very wide spectrum of 'normal' behaviour in cats, associated with different individual character traits, learning experiences and interactions between other pets and human beings in the household. This is what makes each cat an individual, with its own cat personality, habits and idiosyncracies. Thus the term 'behaviour problem' only tends to be used when the behaviour causes inconvenience, distress or concern to the owner, or actual physical symptoms in the cat.

The commonest behavioural problems encountered in pet cats in veterinary practice are listed below. These are discussed in more detail in the relevant sections. The complex nature of some behaviour problems means that specialist help is often needed. The commonest conditions referred to veterinary surgeons are:

- Toileting problems, especially **Spraying (urine)**, which can be a major problem

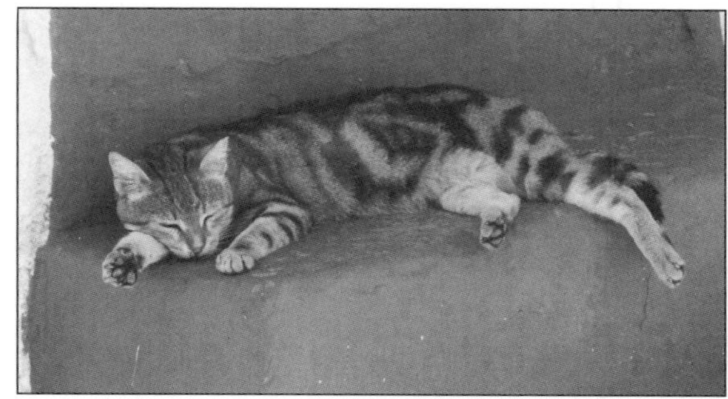

Cats are individuals and behaviour patterns consequently vary quite a lot.

for cat owners, requiring in-depth understanding of several aspects of cat behaviour.
- **Anxiety** states, possibly leading to Overgrooming by the cat, causing large hairless areas on the coat.
- **Aggression** to cats, other animals, or people.
- Poor **Socialisation** – this may result in aggression or simply in cats that avoid interaction with owners or other pets and do not enjoy being handled, lifted, groomed or spoken to.
- Fear – in cats, fear tends to show as aggression or as withdrawal behaviour (hiding away/poor socialisation). The fear may also relate to a very specific thing, e.g. children, loud noises, the cat carrier basket, etc.

Many owners have their own ideas about behaviour problems, e.g. 'He passed urine on my bed to get back at me for leaving him alone yesterday.' Note that this is nearly always incorrect, and can lead to confusion, even worsening of the problem.

Quite often, unusual behaviour has a medical cause. Good examples are the aggressive cat which is actually in pain, the restless, irritable cat suffering from overactive thyroid gland, or the cat with defective vision. Cats with damage to the nervous system may also show unusual behaviours such as incoordination, fits or head tilt as well as uncharacteristic responses such as 'seeing things', unusual fears and aggression. For this reason, a comprehensive medical examination, possibly including blood tests, may be advised for a cat with an apparent behaviour problem.

☎ Urgency

Most true behaviour problems (problems arising 'psychologically' within the cat) are not urgent. They have developed over a period of weeks to months, sometimes vary in severity and cause differing levels of concern to different owners. A routine appointment should be sought and the nature of the problem explained in advance to the veterinary staff as, often, behavioural consultations are designed to be longer than the standard time for examination. This is to allow for full discussion of the cat's history, symptoms and provisional treatment plan.

✚ First aid & nursing

For most behaviour problems, first aid is not appropriate. The only action an owner can take is to remove the cat from any obvious source of aggravating stimulus, e.g. other animals, loud noises, and avoid these situations until medical advice is sought. Try to identify trigger factors, patterns and any measures you have discovered which seem to improve the problem. All this will help the vet get to the source of the trouble. It is always difficult to be truly objective, and to avoid misinterpreting the cat's behaviour by trying to understand it from a human point of view, but this is essential if an accurate understanding is to be reached.

Veterinary treatment

- Treatment for behaviour problems can involve behavioural therapy (modifying behaviour by changing the cat's environment or its social interactions with other animals and people), drug therapy and, in certain cases, surgery.

- Surgery is used when there is an underlying problem which an operation can help with, e.g. an overactive thyroid gland, a source of pain that can be removed (e.g. a tumour), or perhaps neutering of previously unneutered animals if the behaviour is thought to be associated with sexual hormones or patterns.
- Drug therapy can be helpful in certain specific conditions such as urine marking (usually it needs to be combined with behaviour therapy), some anxiety disorders, and in medical problems which result in altered behaviour states, e.g. diabetes, fits. Drugs will of course help when strange behaviour is caused by the cat's response to any general disease, such as the intense itch/pain of ear mites, or severe discomfort and bad temper from diseased teeth.
- Behaviour therapy is a large and complex area, but is important in many cases because in order to try to alter/improve behaviour, one must first understand why it is happening. Difficult cases may be referred to vets specialising in this field. Investigation can be quite a lengthy process, and requires very close cooperation and understanding between vet and cat owner. The owner has to acquire an in-depth knowledge of cat behaviour, and how this can be factored in to try to improve matters. It can be extremely rewarding to see the results, but they may take several weeks or months to appear. It is vital that all people in the house understand the aims and objectives of any behaviour therapy programme, otherwise one individual could undo all the good work that others are striving to achieve.

Note: Punishment is notoriously ineffective for behaviour problems and should be avoided at all times, irrespective of how frustrating the problem may be or how appropriate punishment may seem in the circumstances. It is not helping the situation.

Tip

It is a good idea to prepare a written summary of the problem, noting down all the things that are of concern, the timing and so on. Provide as much detail as possible. In some cases, owners have taken video footage of their cat at home, which can be extremely helpful in understanding intermittent behaviours only exhibited in the cat's home environment.

Some useful initial questions to note

1. When did the problem start? Did anything seem to trigger it?
2. How often does it occur? Are there any patterns you have noticed?
3. Have there been any major changes in the household, e.g. flitting, additions or losses of animals or people, changes in the cat's routine, a new cat in the neighbourhood?
4. Is the behaviour associated with a particular individual or animal in the household?
5. What things have you tried to control the problem, and what has been the result?

Continued

6. Is the cat showing any other physical symptoms, e.g. weight loss, drinking to excess.
7. Start keeping a daily diary, note down the time and occurrence as far as you are aware of every time the unusual behaviour happens. Note down anything you think might be contributing.

Related or similar conditions

- **Aggression**
- **Anxiety/fear**
- **Bereavement**
- **Brain damage**
- **Overgrooming**
- **Spraying (urine)**

Bereavement

Although cats are notoriously independent and often quite solitary animals, most vets recognise that bereavement occurs in some cats. A fairly common situation is an elderly cat owner who dies, leaving behind their pet cat, who is also old. The cat then goes to live with someone else, perhaps a relative or family member, but seems withdrawn and uninterested in life. Minor medical problems may become more severe and in extreme cases the 'will to live' may be lost. The change of environment (e.g. a new house/ area, perhaps with children) adds further stress and worsens the situation.

Similarly, when a close animal companion of the cat dies, be it a cat, dog, rabbit, or in fact any species, effects of grief/ pining can be seen and may last several weeks or even months. Some cat owners often say that their pet has 'never been right' since the bereavement occurred, especially if the two pets had been together all their life. Subtle, or sometimes dramatic, changes in the cat's behaviour, demeanour and interest in life have taken place.

☎ Urgency

Bereavement is not an urgent condition. In fact, as in people, time may be all that is needed to give the cat an opportunity to accommodate to the loss and change.

+ First aid & nursing

Try to treat the bereaved cat largely as normal. Stick to usual routines, which will give security to the cat, and if the cat seems to respond to this, provide a little more interaction than normal. Leaving the basket, bedding, bowls and toys of the deceased pet around for a time, though probably distressing to the human beings involved, may help the bereaved cat by providing familiar scents. Similarly, something with a previous owner's scent on it may help.

Veterinary treatment

- No specific medical treatment is normally recommended for bereavement grief in cats, though general recommendations along the lines of those mentioned under First Aid above will probably be supplied.
- Sometimes, the stress of the bereavement results in worsening of current medical problems or in the appearance of disorders that have been existing at a 'subclinical' level. In this case, normal veterinary diagnosis and treatment will be followed.

Related or similar conditions

- **Anxiety/fear**
- **Euthanasia**
- **Old age problems**

Birth (parturition, kittening)

The duration of pregnancy in the cat is, on average, 63 days. Later stages of pregnancy are marked by significant abdominal swelling, mammary (breast) development and reduced exercising ability.

Most cats have no problems during the birth process itself. Unlike dogs, body size and conformation (shape) is relatively constant in cats, and physical problems in the delivery of the kittens are consequently fairly rare. However, Caesarian sections are occasionally needed if problems do develop and the pregnant and kittening cat should always be kept under close, if unobtrusive, observation.

The majority of pet cats have been neutered (spayed) at a young age, usually around 5–6 months or younger (neutering can be carried out from 12 weeks, so-called 'early neutering'), and so will never have kittens, but occasionally people are surprised when a cat they assumed was neutered (e.g. if obtained from a friend or rescue organisation) turns out to be pregnant!

☎ Urgency

Cats having kittens only require medical care if problems develop. Recognition of when to seek help is important, and many owners, if inexperienced in this area, can become confused. Most often, owners suspect problems are present when in fact none is. See below for the normal progress and timing of birth in the cat, and what to look out for if things are not going as expected.

If concerned, it does no harm to seek telephone advice from the vet, but do not be surpised if, after receiving details, he or she advises further observation and waiting. As mentioned above, the majority of cats have few problems if left largely undisturbed.

The normal birth process

In cats, normal birth can last from 1–36 hours without any particular problems being present. It is not always possible to tell when the birth process has stopped since there may be 'rests' of quite long periods (e.g. several hours) in between delivering individual kittens. However, by recognising the important phases below, you will be able to decide when an interruption to the sequence may indicate a problem.

Stage 1 of birth

The queen cat usually becomes restless, even agitated, and may make miaowing sounds and knead the bedding of her nest place. She usually licks around the perineum (area beneath the tail) and there may be some clear discharge from the vagina. Heavier breathing or panting may be noticed.

These preliminary signs can last for a long time (occasionally 24–36 hours) and still be quite normal. In most cats, progress to Stage 2 of birth occurs after a few hours. Veterinary advice requested at Stage 1 will often be along the lines of: 'Reassure the cat if she needs it but avoid undue disturbance. Offer food and water but don't be surprised if she doesn't take any. Make sure there is a secure, safe area for her to have the kittens in.'

Stage 2 of birth

This is when the kittens are produced. At this point, contractions of the uterus and abdominal muscles occur and the start of these contractions signals the end of Stage 1 above.

The queen may be very restless at this time; she may miaow loudly and vary her position frequently. Straining continues until the kitten is born, usually within 30 minutes of strong straining. Most kittens are delivered in a 'diving' position with head and forelegs first, but back leg delivery is also possible.

Initially, the membranes surrounding the kitten are seen at the vagina. These rupture and release birth fluids. The queen may nibble at the kitten as it is being delivered and rupture the birth sacs in this way – she is not attempting to eat the kitten at this point.

If the kitten is delivered still covered in its membranes, and the queen does not show any tendency to remove these, they can be gently broken and pulled away from the kitten's head to allow breathing. Do this promptly if the queen does not within 1–2 minutes. Puncture the sac with your nail or tear between fingers to reach the kitten inside. Resuscitate if necessary (see diagrams on p. 30).

Stage 3 of birth

After the birth of a kitten, its placenta (connection to the uterus) is passed. The kitten is connected to the placenta by the umbilical cord, which the queen may rupture by chewing. If the queen does not successfully sever the cord, this should be tightly tied with thread several centimetres from the kitten's abdomen, and then torn or cut with scissors below the knot, i.e. the knot remains between the broken or cut cord and the kitten (to stop any blood loss on the kitten's side).

The queen may eat the placenta – this is quite natural. Sometimes there is a delay before the placenta is passed, or the placenta from the previous kitten's birth may be passed along with the next kitten to be born.

Kittens usually come at intervals of around 10–15 minutes to one hour and the complete Stage 2 process above is repeated each time. Note however that there can also be lengthy delays in the process, extending to 2, 4 or 8 hours, without there being any problems. In these delays, the queen may attend to and feed the kittens already born and rest or eat. Litter size varies but is often around 3–6 kittens.

Signs of problems – when to seek help

- No kittens after 30–40 minutes of strong straining, i.e. the cat seems permanently stuck in Stage 2 of labour.
- Kittens that remain in their birth sacs – remove them, if the mother does not do so quickly, to enable them to start breathing.
- Kittens that are inactive after birth – most move vigorously. Attempt resuscitation as described in the diagram.
- Kittens that get stuck when partially delivered. Gentle traction in a downwards direction can be made using a warm, damp towel to grip the kitten's body. This should aid delivery. If it does not, a more severe birth obstruction is possible and professional advice should be sought.

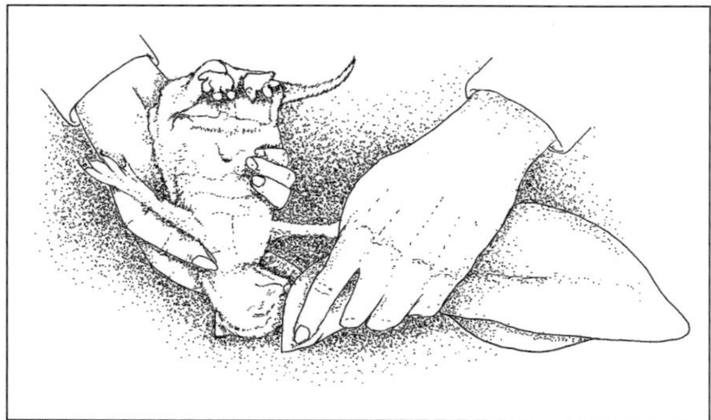

Resuscitating a kitten: wipe fluids away from the mouth/nose area while in a head-down position.

+ First aid & nursing

Birth is a natural process and first aid is not normally required. Good preparation is however helpful. Most importantly, the cat must have access to a quiet, secluded area in which to form a nest and have kittens. Often, she will choose a suitable place herself, e.g. in an airing cupboard, under a bed, in a drawer or in a quiet corner. You may be able to influence this choice of location by leaving a strategic cupboard door open and making a comfortable area within it – but don't be surprised if the cat spurns this and chooses somewhere of her own! Ensure that excited children do not disturb or touch the pregnant or kittening female cat; this can interfere with the normal flow of events and lead to problems. The best approach when birth has started is quiet observation every 20 minutes or so, no more frequently than that.

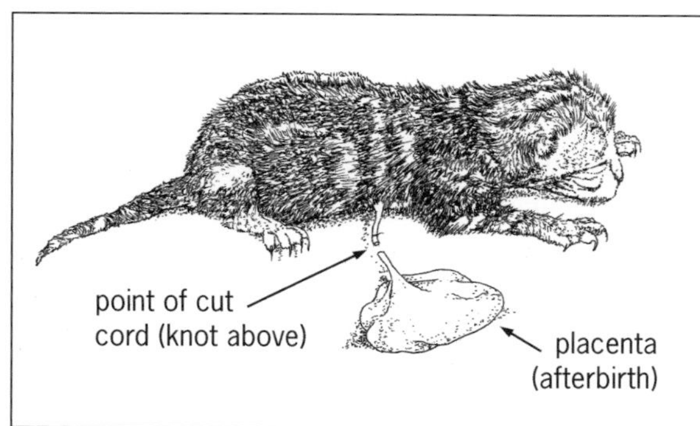

Cutting the umbilical cord below a thread knot.

It does no harm to leave a saucer of water, some food and a litter tray within easy reach of the cat. She may use these between delivering kittens or at the end. The temperature in the nest area should not be excessive. Normal room temperature is fine. Cotton sheets are the best type of bedding and make sure there are no obstacles under or in which newborn kittens could become jammed.

Having a towel ready may be useful to rub and stimulate any kittens that are not breathing well, but in most cases the normal actions of the cat will provide the necessary stimulus to gasp and breathe.

Veterinary treatment

- In cases of problems with the birth process, e.g. a kitten unable to be delivered, exhaustion of the dam, bleeding, etc. veterinary attention will be needed. Drugs are sometimes tried to promote uterine contractions if the problem is simply muscular weakness due to prolonged straining with a large litter. Otherwise, and if a kitten is incorrectly presented or stuck in the birth canal, Caesarian section is usually required.
- Certain drugs can be given to promote the 'let down' of milk. These are often used after Caesarian section, when they also assist with contraction of the now empty uterus.

Related or similar conditions

- **Abortion**
- **Oestrus and mating**
- **Pregnancy**
- **Pyometra (womb infection)**

Bites

Bites are a frequent injury in cats, especially in fighting males. Unneutered males will usually get into fights more frequently due to territorial disputes, but all cats may on occasion suffer from a bite from another cat. Some of this depends on the temperament of the individual cat and the presence of other cats in the area. Fights may be more frequent when a new cat joins the neighbourhood and upsets the current 'pecking order'.

The usual places that are bitten are the tail or tail base, the forelegs or around the head area. Bites can be received from other species too, especially dogs, foxes and possibly other animals, e.g. rats.

Small bites may go unnoticed due to the cat's dense fur. The cat may be irritable for a day or two, then recover. Often, quite severe signs of pain may be seen, and the formation of an abscess after a cat bite is a common event. Very severe bites inflicted by a large animal such as a dog can be extremely serious. Deep puncture wounds, extensive bruising and chest or abdominal trauma can result, with potentially fatal consequences arising from shock and bleeding.

Bites of any type characteristically cause a puncture wound. These are a problem because, although the skin break is small, the damage underneath can be large, especially if an abscess occurs. In muscle areas, a condition called cellulitis may develop – this is a very painful problem and affected cats will be miserable, often with a fever/high temperature.

> **Note:** Cats' mouths carry many bacteria. If you are ever bitten by a cat you should seek medical advice promptly. Your vet will be able to write a note advising the doctor of likely bacteria involved, which will affect the choice of antibiotic used.

The potential for disease transmission occurs with bites. Usually, infection develops due to bacteria (leading to abscess or cellulitis), but important viruses can be transmitted by bites, especially rabies (not in the UK), feline leukaemia (FeLV) and feline immunodeficiency virus (FIV).

☎ Urgency

If you notice a bite wound and the cat is otherwise well, a routine veterinary appointment should be arranged and the cat kept indoors and watched carefully until that time. If you suspect more serious injury (e.g. crushing type bites across the chest inflicted by a dog), do not delay to seek advice and emergency attention. Any interference with breathing (e.g. rapid shallow breaths or very deep slow ones), reluctance to move or difficulty in rousing the cat are very important signs that something serious may be going on.

+ First aid & nursing

Wounds can be gently bathed in tepid saline (1 teaspoon salt to 1 pint [560 ml] water) to clear discharges. Soak a large wad of cotton wool and hold this against the wound for 5 minutes every hour or so, as described under **Abscess**. Other forms of antiseptic are best avoided until a diagnosis has been made.

Veterinary treatment

- This is largely the same as for abscesses. Antibiotics and painkillers are often prescribed. If fractures or internal damage are suspected, hospital observation, X-rays or other tests or treatment may be needed depending on what is found. An over-riding concern in severe attacks by larger animals is the risk of internal chest or abdominal damage, e.g. lung or bladder rupture.
- Drains may be inserted to promote release of pus from developing abscesses near the surface.

Tip

Take care when handling as cats in pain may resent attention. Follow the advice given for handling and treating cats on page xviii. Very distressed cats are best left alone until seen by the vet.

Related or similar conditions

- ▶ **Abscess**
- ▶ **Bleeding**
- ▶ **Infections**
- ▶ **Shock**
- ▶ **Wounds**

Bleeding (haemorrhage)

Severe loss of blood (haemorrhage) is life-threatening and produces a state of medical shock (loss of blood pressure and oxygen starvation to the brain and other organs). If not rapidly reversed, shock leads on to death. This physical form of shock, involving loss of blood pressure and oxygen, is worsened by the mental shock that severe injury or trauma can also cause.

Major, life-threatening bleeding usually occurs externally, after a serious wound which damages a large artery or vein. Internal haemorrhage is also possible after any severe blow to the body or occasionally as a result of other diseases. This 'hidden' haemorrhage can be difficult to pick up unless the animal is being observed carefully. It may occur after severe falls, road traffic accidents, as a complication of surgery and in certain medical problems where blood clotting ability is poor or has been affected by toxins (poisons).

Warning signs of possible internal bleeding after an accident

- Irregular breathing
- Pale gums
- Cold extremities (ear tips, paws, tail)
- Unresponsive, progressing to comatose condition

Less severe bleeding is a common and necessary part of any minor injury. This type of bleeding usually stops within 10 minutes in response to blood's natural tendency to clot and seal small disruptions in blood vessel walls.

It can be difficult to assess the amount of blood loss since a little blood seems to go a long way, and to those unused to accident situations, understandable panic may set in. Expert advice is usually needed to be on the safe side. Minor, non-life threatening bleeding is much more common than major haemorrhage however.

☎ Urgency

Major bleeding, where bright red blood appears in spurts or when darker blood rapidly wells up from a wound, is always an emergency. Veterinary advice should be rapidly sought, but first aid can save the animal's life (see below) and should be applied first.

Similarly, because of the risk of medical shock, any cat which shows the signs mentioned above for internal bleeding should be seen immediately.

Minor bleeding should also be treated by first aid means. It is less urgent, but nevertheless should be checked out since sometimes the damage is more extensive than it first appears.

✚ First aid & nursing

With any severe bleeding, the important thing is to apply firm even pressure to stem the flow of blood, thereby conserving blood pressure and keeping the cat alive. The exact method of applying the pressure is not important, as long as it is effective. Common techniques are:

1. Bandages can be applied. These are ideally taken from a first aid kit but can also be improvised. A pad (cotton wool, tissue, handkerchief, etc.) is placed over the wound and layers of bandage wound round firmly over it. On areas where it is impossible to bandage, the dressing can be firmly held in place while help is sought. If blood seeps through the bandage, do not remove it. Instead apply further firmer layers. Bandages are the best method of dealing with bleeding in a first aid situation.
2. On limbs (or the tail) a firm tourniquet can be applied above the bleeding point. Tourniquets can be improvised from bandages, pieces of string, etc. They should be tied just firmly enough to stop the flow of blood. Tourniquets should only be used when a bandage fails to control the bleeding.
3. Bleeding from the ear is best dealt with by applying a pad to the bleeding point and holding this is place. Cotton wool helps stem the flow as wisps of material allow the blood to clot within it. Any movement of the head is likely to set the bleeding off again.

In all cases the cat should be kept calm and placed in a secure cat carrier or held, perhaps wrapped in a blanket. Keep the patient warm – use a padded hot water bottle. 'Bubble wrap' conserves heat very well and can be wrapped around the cat underneath a blanket. Additional layers help retain heat.

Veterinary treatment

- Major blood loss is treated using intravenous fluids (a drip), oxygen therapy and intensive care. Sometimes, if blood is available, a transfusion will be carried out.
- Severe bleeding wounds may require surgery to inspect and repair them, but this will normally be after the cat has been stabilised.
- Bleeding due to poisoning may be able to be treated using specific antidotes or drugs to help counteract the effect of the toxin if it is known what poison was to blame. A common one is Warfarin (rat poison) which a cat may take in by

eating a dead rodent. If you know poison has been taken in, try to find and take the label to the veterinary clinic with you.

Related or similar conditions

- **Accident**
- **Collapse**
- **Shock**
- **Wounds**

Blindness

Blindness is the end result of serious eye disease. It can, however, also be caused by disease or injury to the brain or nervous system (so-called 'central blindness' – because it relates to the central nervous system). In central blindness, the eye functions normally but the brain cannot decode the messages received from it, so the cat is still effectively blind.

Any severe condition or injury affecting the eye may lead on to blindness. The eye tolerates sharp injuries far better than blunt blows, which are liable to disrupt the structure of the eye much more dangerously. Other causes of blindness include tumours (arising in the eye or spreading there from elsewhere), glaucoma, severe inflammation (iritis/uveitis), high blood pressure and cataract.

Blindness may apparently be sudden in onset or else can develop over a period of time. Since cats often adapt well to failing vision, the blindness may appear to be sudden in onset, whereas it has in fact been developing more slowly but has gone unrecognised.

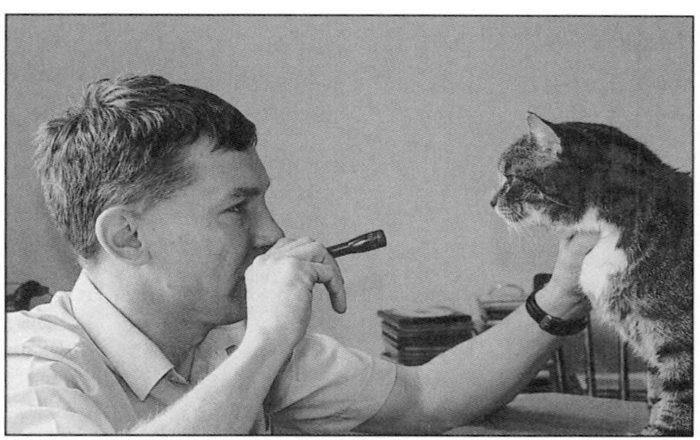

Initial examination of the eye to test for basic light reflexes.

How do I know if my cat really is blind?

Because of their excellent hearing, it can be difficult in certain cases to know if a cat is blind. The following methods should help:

1. Watch the cat very carefully. Does he or she bang into objects occasionally, or else rely entirely on sensations from the whiskers instead of the eyes?
2. Drop cotton wool balls or similar objects in front of the cat. Does he or she see them? Try to make sure no noise is made as the objects fall. Pass objects across the cat's line of vision, taking care not to create air currents.
3. Construct a small obstacle course using up-turned boxes, waste paper bins, etc. and see if your cat can negotiate this (see diagram, page 35). Try the test in both bright and dim lights.

Blind or partially sighted cats often cope well in familiar surroundings but if the environment is changed (e.g. furniture moved about) they may become confused.

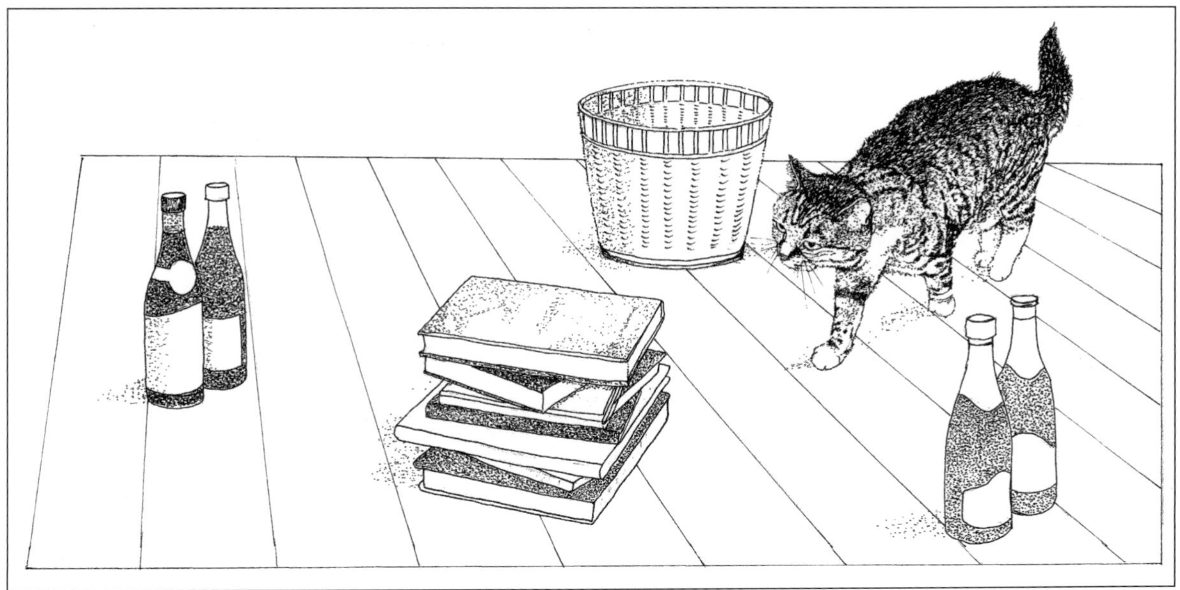

Construct a simple obstacle course to test vision and note how the cat copes.

☎ Urgency

Sudden blindness should be assessed urgently as it may sometimes be possible to limit the severity with appropriate treatment. In many cases this is unfortunately not possible however.

Any physical injury of any type to the eye must also receive immediate attention if the best chance of preserving vision is to be taken. This is discussed more fully under **Eye problems**.

More gradually failing vision should be checked out through a routine appointment as soon as it is noticed – again, with the aim of limiting the damage to the failing eye.

✚ First aid & nursing

No first aid is really appropriate unless there is an eye injury present. The blind cat may be distressed and should be put in a small well padded space (e.g. cat carrier) and reassured whilst awaiting treatment.

Veterinary treatment

- The main aims are to assess the severity of the vision loss, see whether this is likely to be permanent, and try to treat any identified underlying causes.
- Examination of the eyes will obviously be needed, but a variety of blood and other tests may be called upon to establish what underlying problem has led to disease in the eye.
- For the chronically sore and nonfunctional eye, surgical eye removal is by far the best option. Cats cope well, are free of pain, and lead a good quality of life.
- For cats which end up blind in both eyes, a careful assessment and discussion of quality of life will be needed. Individuals vary and some cats can lead a good life if care is taken regarding their surroundings and safety. In old cats with many other problems, this may be the time to consider euthanasia.

Related or similar conditions

- ▶ **Brain damage**
- ▶ **Eye problems**
- ▶ **Old age problems**

Blood blister (haematoma)

This condition is commonest in the ear flap, where it results in a large soft swelling on the flap, known as an aural (ear) haematoma. However, haematomas can occur in any location – they are simply collections of blood-based fluid which accumulate underneath the skin. Usually, trauma is the cause.

In the ear, the trauma is caused most often through frequent head shaking or scratching resulting from ear problems, especially ear mites. The constant shaking eventually ruptures a small blood vessel in the space between the skin layers on either side of the ear. Blood leaks out and forms a swelling, which can distort the shape of the ear considerably and cause some discomfort. Occasionally, haematomas are found on both ear flaps if ear problems have been particularly severe.

Haematomas do not usually rupture, but if one did, considerable mess would be produced due to leakage of bloody fluid from the ear. This would be worsened by shaking of the cat's head. Blood loss is minor; however repeated shaking tends to ensure that it gets spread around a great deal and may be alarming to see.

Sometimes, after a haematoma has healed, the ear remains distorted in shape due to fibrosis – a condition some vets call 'cauliflower ear'. Although this looks odd, the function of the ear is usually unaffected, though regular gentle ear cleaning may be required.

☎ Urgency

Although it can look frightening, haematoma is not an emergency condition. However, because of the discomfort involved, an early routine appointment should be sought to alleviate the cat's irritation.

✚ First aid & nursing

If there is constant scratching, fitting an Elizabethan collar will help protect the ear until veterinary attention can be sought (see the cat on p. 151).

If the ear is full of impacted wax and debris, applying a gentle ear cleaner (e.g. Leo Cat ear cleaner) or a few drops of olive or almond oil to the ear will help loosen the material. Many cats enjoy having the base of their ear gently massaged after application of drops in this way.

Veterinary treatment

- The underlying cause of the haemtoma must be found and this will require ear cleaning and examination, possibly under anaesthetic. Often, ear mites prove to be the culprits, but inflammation in the ear (otitis), foreign bodies (e.g. grass awns), polyps and tumours all may cause ear pain and shaking, leading to a haematoma.
- The haematoma itself may need to be drained of its fluid, which could require minor surgery.
- Ear drops, antibiotic tablets or other treatments may also be supplied. Make sure these are applied exactly as directed.

- For polyps and tumours, surgery may be needed.

Tip: Avoid cotton buds

Do not insert instruments, cotton buds or objects into the ear canal in an attempt to clean it. In doing this, you are much more likely to impact any material that is there, and the lining of the ear could also be damaged. Simply apply any drops, massage the ear base, and allow the cat to shake his head if he wants to. Quite often, material comes out when the head is shaken! See the photograph on page 73 for how to apply drops properly.

Related or similar conditions

- ▶ **Bleeding**
- ▶ **Ear problems**

Blood pressure (low or high)

Every organ and tissue in the body depends, for its healthy function, on an adequate blood supply. Oxygen and nutrient-rich blood is delivered to the tissues, and waste products removed from them, via the circulatory system (the heart and blood vessels).

Rather like a central heating system, the pressure within the circulatory system must be just right. If pressure is too low or 'leaky', it cannot 'drive' the system (radiators, or tissues and organs) and normal processes may slow down or completely stop. If pressure is too high and stays at this level for a long time, there is the danger that something may 'explode' and damage or threaten life.

Low blood pressure

The commonest cause of low blood pressure in cats is severe blood loss, for example caused by bleeding after a road traffic accident. This blood loss could be external bleeding (into the environment) or, just as dangerous, internal bleeding, for example into the chest or abdomen. Huge amounts of blood can be lost internally and 'silently'. A severe and sudden loss of blood pressure is more dangerous than a more gradual one, partly because there is less chance of noticing this and intervening, and less chance of the cat's body compensating. Sudden loss of blood pressure commonly causes fainting (loss of consciousness as the blood flow to the brain diminishes). Other causes of low blood pressure include toxic or allergic reactions, problems with the pump in the circulatory system (the heart), and any other cause of the general medical condition which vets refer to as 'shock'.

Signs typical of low blood pressure are a depressed or unreactive cat who seems cold to the touch (especially on peripheral areas such as the feet and eat tips). Gums may be very pale (a condition called pallor) as well as cold and dry. A weak pulse may be present. These symptoms are a consequence of the body trying to maintain central or core blood pressure to the vital organs by temporarily diverting blood away from less important structures on the periphery. However this can only work for so long before all structures start to get damaged.

☎ Urgency

Suspected low blood pressure is an emergency and veterinary advice should be sought immediately.

✚ First aid & nursing

Whilst transporting the cat to the vet, it is important that body temperature is maintained or increased. Use dry blankets, towels or bubble wrap. Warm (not hot) water bottles can be very useful to start to get the cat's temperature up. If driving, turn up the heating in the car on the way to the veterinary practice. Ensure that the cat's neck is not kinked and that there is a clear airway at all times. If the cat vomits, place the cat is a head down position to prevent inhalation of the vomit. Talk to the cat to try to maintain consciousness.

Veterinary treatment

The initial focus will be on returning blood pressure to normal or near normal by giving intravenous fluids (a drip) or blood transfusion, oxygen and drugs to try to establish normal pressure. The cat will be warmed up.

Whilst this is going on, attempts to diagnose the underlying cause of the low blood pressure will be made so that specific treatment can be started when the cat is stabilised. This may entail blood tests, X-rays or other imaging (e.g. CT scan).

Related or similar conditions

- ▶ **Hypothermia**
- ▶ **Shock**
- ▶ **Heart disease**
- ▶ **Accident**
- ▶ **Poisoning**
- ▶ **Bleeding**

High blood pressure

High blood pressure is common in both cats and people. On its own, high blood pressure tends to exist without any external signs until an organ or tissue gets damaged. That may take years of living with high blood pressure. Think of an over-pressurised central heating system that can contain the increased pressure for a long time until 'something gives'. Most cats with high blood pressure are older individuals, very often suffering from kidney disease or over-active thyroid gland. The raised blood pressure has occurred because of these underlying conditions. A few cats may have high blood pressure on its own, without any underlying condition, but this is rarer in cats compared to people.

High blood pressure can damage several vulnerable organs, notably the eyes, kidneys, heart and brain. This damage from raised pressure can then complicate any underlying condition, creating a vicious circle effect. Signs of this sort of damage occurring may include partial or complete blindness, bleeding into the eye, kidney failure, brain damage (showing, for example, as fits), and heart disease.

☎ Urgency

The problem is not an emergency unless rapid deterioration is seen, e.g. sudden blindness or collapse from heart problems. Many cases of high blood pressure in cats are picked up during the routine screening of older cats (over 8 years) and the screening of cats who have medical conditions associated with high blood pressure, e.g. kidney disease and over active thyroid.

✚ First aid & nursing

Any cat with vision loss or deterioration need to be kept in a safe place until he or she can be seen by the vet. For cats with kidney disease, heart disease or over active thyroid gland, refer to the appropriate sections of this book.

Veterinary treatment

The cat's blood pressure will be monitored regularly to determine if the high blood pressue is consistent and requiring treatment. Most cats tolerate this painless procedure well once they have become used to it. Just as in people, repeated measurment and acclimatisation tends to reduce the 'white coat effect' of blood pressure being raised during the measurement process. Obviously, in many cats visiting the vets, blood pressure will be raised because of travel and stress. However this is taken into account when interpreting readings.

Particular attention is paid to the eye in diagnosing and monitoring high blood pressure.

Various drugs, alone or in combination, are used to treat high blood pressure. Individual cats vary a lot, both in terms of underlying diseases that are present, and also their response to treatments, so it is often a case of fine tuning over weeks or months to attain the best balance of treatment for the individual. Your cat with high blood pressure may not receive the same treatment as your neighbour's. On-going monitoring is vital.

In some cats, high blood pressure reveals an untreated underlying disease (e.g. over active thyroid gland) and, once that condition is dealt with, the blood pressure returns to normal and does not itself require treatment.

Related or similar conditions

- **Thyroid (overactive)**
- **Heart disease**
- **Kidney disease**
- **Eye problems**

Bone/joint problems – general

Bone and joint problems usually show as lameness or stiffness or as sensitivity when the limbs are touched. Sometimes general signs of irritability and pain will be all that is noticed. The cat may spend more time resting and be reluctant to play or interact with other animals or people. Symptoms may appear worse in cold damp weather.

The spine consists of a series of small bones (vertebrae) linked by joints, and neck/spinal pain can result in a reluctance to move or turn around. Spinal pain is often due to arthritis in older cats. In younger animals, trauma may be a more likely explanation.

☎ Urgency

Arthritis is not an urgent condition. It comes on slowly and may wax and wane in severity. It is discussed fully under **Arthritis**.

Any fracture or dislocation caused by trauma (e.g. a road accident) should be treated urgently, as this is likely to be extremely painful and there is always the risk of more serious internal injury such as bleeding or chest damage.

Bone tumours develop slowly but may suddenly start to show severe signs, hence can give the impression of a sudden condition if the weakened bone fractures.

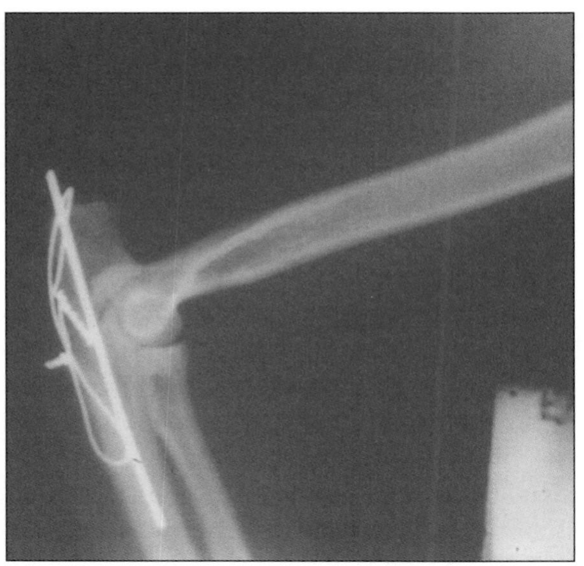

X-ray showing surgical repair of a broken elbow joint using a stainless steel pin and wire. The point of the elbow had been fractured after a fall from a high wall.

+ First aid & nursing

Do not administer human painkillers to cats. Fatal overdosing can easily result and the administration of human drugs will limit what treatment the vet can then provide.

The best first aid measure is to restrict the cat's activity (e.g. in a cat carrier) whilst attention is sought. Take care, since bone problems can be extremely painful and a frightened cat in pain may bite or attack in panic. Guidelines for handling frightened cats in pain are given on page xviii.

In most cases, confinement in a well bedded cage or carrier is safest and most practical however. The cat will find the most comfortable position in which to lie, sometimes choosing to lie on the injured leg in order to splint it and prevent painful movements.

Veterinary treatment

- Often, X-rays are used to find out what the problem is. This will then allow appropriate medical or surgical treatment to be planned.
- Fractures will usually be repaired using special metal implants (or, in the case of the pelvis, cage rest will often be advised). Dislocations may also require surgery.
- Painkillers may be prescribed as for arthritis.
- Bone tumours are always serious as they have frequently spread to other organs in the body by the time a diagnosis is made. However, quality of life may be able to be maintained for a considerable period of time. This depends on the type of tumour, its location and suitability for treatment, and the response to drugs or surgery used. Each case is different.

Tip

Whenever matted hair is found along the back, spinal pain or arthritis should be considered. This is likely to be what is preventing normal grooming in this region.

Pain in the jaw joints may show as reluctance to eat or as head shyness. The jaw could be broken or dislocated – common injuries after a fall. The jaw may appear asymmetrical or there may be drooling.

Related or similar conditions

- **Accident**
- **Arthritis**
- **Falls**
- **Fractures/dislocations**
- **Sprain/strain**
- **Tumour**

Brain damage

Brain damage can result from trauma (e.g. a fall, a road accident), from infection, from the effects of deprivation of oxygen and certain toxins (poisons) and from the result of increased pressure within the brain. Tumours involving the brain can also result in damage and altered brain function. The symptoms here depend on which part of the brain is being affected by the growth.

Certain common medical problems result in the accumulation of waste products within the bloodstream. These act like toxins and may affect brain function. This can be a feature of severe kidney and liver disease, for example, and cats with uncontrolled diabetes may show incoordination and fits, mimicking brain damage or disease.

Kittens may be born with congenitally damaged brains. In some cases, these problems are not compatible with life and the kitten dies when very young; in other instances, the kitten survives but may show abnormal behaviours or perhaps have a tendency to have fits.

Signs of brain damage can vary a lot, from very subtle alterations in behaviour to uncharacteristic aggression or fear. Incoordination, weakness, circling or fits are all possibilties. In attempting to diagnose these, the vet will try to eliminate those diseases which can produce signs that may be confused with primary brain disease.

☎ Urgency

This depends on the nature of the symptoms. A cat that is having fits or that is severely agitated because of incoordination or apparent blindness should be assessed as soon as possible. While most fits pass over quickly (within 10 minutes) they occasionally extend for a much longer time – a severe state which must be treated urgently as life is in danger. Similarly, any cat that has encountered severe trauma (e.g. a fall or road accident) should be treated as an emergency because treatment given at this time may prevent irreversible damage. More subtle signs such as personality change and short periods of weakness or incoordination should be checked out at a routine appointment.

✚ First aid & nursing

The main concern is to protect the uncoordinated cat from damaging himself and to try to limit anxiety, fear and panic. The cat should be placed in a well padded cage or box, put in a quiet, dark and cool place and observed carefully. If a cat is found having a fit in a room, switch off television and lights and move dangerous objects away from the cat. Obtain veterinary advice as soon as possible.

If trauma has occurred, and it is safe to do so, basic first aid for wounds and bleeding should be carried out, but bear in mind that minor injuries are not of vital importance at this stage and these are best not interfered with if to do so would agitate the cat further or risk damage to yourself.

Severely agitated cats may be safely lifted wrapped in a thick blanket, with the person lifting wearing thick gloves and a long sleeved coat. Cover the cat's head with the blanket, wrap the cat up and hold firmly. Transfer as quickly as possible to a secure carrier.

Veterinary treatment

- The priority will be to try to establish what is going wrong, and where. Clinical examinations, blood tests and X-rays may all be called upon and, increasingly, brain scans are being used in animals with suspected brain damage. Once the nature of the disease is understood, treatment can be decided upon.
- Most brain tumours carry a poor outlook, but many of the other problems which result in symptoms of brain malfunction can be treated, provided the damage to the brain is temporary and reversible.
- Fits (see under appropriate section) may be able to be controlled with appropriate medication.

Related or similar conditions

- ▶ **Accident**
- ▶ **Balance (loss of)**
- ▶ **Behaviour problems – general**
- ▶ **Blindness**
- ▶ **Fits**
- ▶ **Liver disease**
- ▶ **Poisoning**

Breathing problems

Breathing difficulty arises due to problems in the respiratory system or, less commonly in cats, the heart. A large variety of problems can occur here. Unfortunately, the symptoms produced by all these problems are often rather similar, making this sort of disorder quite hard to diagnose initially. Clues can be obtained from such things as the age of cat, her previous health history, whether there has been any trauma or accident, etc.

Recognising the normal breathing pattern

Cats in veterinary surgeries are often stressed – they may have travelled some distance in a basket, been surrounded by unfamiliar noises and scents and will be handled by strangers. For these reasons, they may be breathing faster than they normally would; very stressed cats will open their mouths and pant in these circumstances. Sometimes this stress breathing pattern confuses or masks symptoms, so it can be very helpful for an observant owner to monitor breathing at home and report changes to the vet. This is especially useful when monitoring responses to treatment.

What is normal breathing? If you observe your cat while she is resting (and preferably not purring!) you will notice a gentle rise and fall pattern of the chest area:

- As the cat breathes in, the chest expands outwards.
- Exhalation results in the chest collapsing inwards again.
- There is usually a short pause, then the whole cycle is repeated. This comprises one complete breath pattern ('in-out-pause').

If you count the number of breaths per minute it should be somewhere between 15–30 in the resting healthy cat. Breathing should appear effortless, with no exaggerated effort, wheezes, snorts or snuffles. The mouth should remain closed and there should be no strong movements occurring in the abdomen (stomach) area to help move air in or out of the chest.

Breathing problems usually alter the above pattern in one way or another. Common problems are:

- Breathing that is rapid and shallow.
- Breathing that requires extra effort (shown by extra movements of the abdomen).
- Breathing that is noisy, interrupted by coughs, wheezes, etc.
- Mouth breathing in a resting cat.
- Breathing that seems to be worse when the cat adopts certain positions, e.g. lying on one side.

Common causes of breathing problems include:

1. Cat flu
2. Asthma/feline bronchitis
3. Feline infectious peritonitis (FIP)
4. Pneumonia
5. Rhinitis/sinusitis (inflammation in the nasal passages)
6. Polyps (growths) in the nose or throat
7. Heart disease

These are discussed in the appropriate sections.

☎ Urgency

The respiratory system is a vital one and serious problems here can be rapidly life-threatening. Some of the conditions (e.g. cat flu) are relatively common and not serious, but others (pneumonia, heart problems, foreign bodies causing obstruction of the airway) are potentially very serious. If you are in any doubt, always seek professional advice for breathing problems.

✚ First aid & nursing

The priority is to maintain a 'clear airway' to allow the cat to draw in and expel air.

If a cat is collapsed, follow the 'B' for breathing routine described under **Accident**, to ensure the airway is clear and artificial respiration can be given. This simple technique can be life-saving.

In chronic infections and cat flu, frequent bathing of discharges around the nostrils may be needed. As well as helping with breathing, this will encourage the cat to eat as most cats will not eat well unless they can smell their food adequately.

In warm weather take great care to ensure that the cat with respiratory problems does not become overheated, especially when travelling to the veterinary clinic. At home, use cool fans and bathe the paws and ears with cold water. While travelling, open windows in the car (provided of course the cat carrier is secure). Watch carefully for signs of breathing distress (open mouth panting, fast breathing).

Veterinary treatment

- Breathing problems require careful investigation with clinical examination, X-rays and possibly other tests such as blood or fluid sampling to arrive at a diagnosis.
- In extreme situations, the animal may be ventilated on oxygen using a breathing tube inserted into the windpipe (as for anaesthesia). This is simply an improved method of artificial respiration carried out when appropriate facilities are to hand.
- Suitable drug therapy (or, occasionally, surgery) can be worked out once a diagnosis has been made.

- For serious problems, periods of hospitalisation may be needed to stabilise the cat and allow them to become settled on treatment and for diagnostic tests to be worked through a step at a time.

Related or similar conditions

- ▶ **Asthma/feline bronchitis**
- ▶ **Cat flu**
- ▶ **Feline infectious peritonitis (FIP)**
- ▶ **Heart disease**
- ▶ **Pneumonia**
- ▶ **Rhinitis/sinusitis**

Bronchitis

See advice under **Asthma** and **Breathing problems** above. Bronchitis is often treated in a similar way as **Asthma**.

Bruising

Bruising occurs whenever damage disrupts blood vessels and surrounding tissue. The damage causes the leakage of blood into tissues, as well as inflammation. Most traumatic injuries cause bruising to some degree and very severe bruising can occur where damage occurs across thick muscle layers since many larger blood vessels will be present here and susceptible to injury.

Crushing type injuries cause more bruising than sharp penetrating ones, and this is one of the reasons why bite wounds can be so painful – as well as the direct punctures from the teeth, pressure from jaw closure results in widespread bruising of the tissues in the area surrounding the bite. The pain produced is of two different types at once and very unpleasant.

Bruising is easy to recognise in people as the blood accumulating underneath our skin readily discolours it. As the bruise gets older, the colour changes, sometimes producing a variety of shades as the pigment in the leaked blood is broken down into all its constituent chemicals. In cats, the thick hair coat masks most of the appearance of bruising. Often, however, when hair is clipped off, the full extent of bruising can be seen and this commonly extends over a much wider area than initially appreciated.

Injuries sufficient to cause bruising are painful, although the pain tends to ease somewhat before all the discolouration of the bruising disappears, which takes quite a long time.

☎ Urgency

Unless it occurs in areas where the coat is thin (e.g. underside of abdomen) you are unlikely to recognise bruising directly. Instead, the cat will appear in pain when bruised areas of the body are touched. Flinching, muscular twitches and hissing/spitting are common symptoms when these areas are handled. The cat is likely to be grumpy and possibly off food. In most cases, a routine appointment should be made unless there is anything else to suggest more serious injury, e.g. breathing difficulty.

✚ First aid & nursing

Rest is the most important thing. Avoid handling the bruised cat too much; most cats will prefer to lie quietly in a warm place. Do not administer any human painkillers.

Veterinary treatment

- Once injuries such as fractures, dislocations and wounds are ruled out, usually only 'symptomatic' treatment is indicated for bruising, i.e. painkillers. The bruising itself disappears given time. Homoeopathic arnica or arnica cream is said to be effective for bruising. One 6c or 30c tablet can be given twice daily for 2–3 days. This should not replace veterinary attention.

Related or similar conditions

- **Bites**
- **Bleeding**
- **Pain**
- **Sprain/strain**

Burns

The pain from burns, and the extent of damage to skin and underlying tissues, can be very severe and unpleasant. Additionally, burn injuries are often much worse than they at first appear. Often, the full extent of the damage is not apparent until several days after the injury occurred since there is a delay between the burn occurring and the worst of the skin damage becoming visible. Also, as with bruising, the thick hair coat of cats may mask much of the injury, leading the owner (and vet) into a false sense of security. All burns are serious – and painful. Even a tiny patch of scalded skin can be very uncomfortable on ourselves.

Burns can arise from household accidents involving hot water – the commonest cause – as well as from contact with fire, electricity or caustic chemicals. Many burns occur in kittens as they explore their surroundings. It is easy for them to slip and fall into a hot bath, spill over a mug of coffee or knock boiling pans from the cooker. Burns on all four feet are particularly painful as the cat is forced to use the injured area immediately after the accident.

Any cat receiving burns after a house fire is also likely to have inhaled significant quantities of smoke, so treatment for this problem will be needed too.

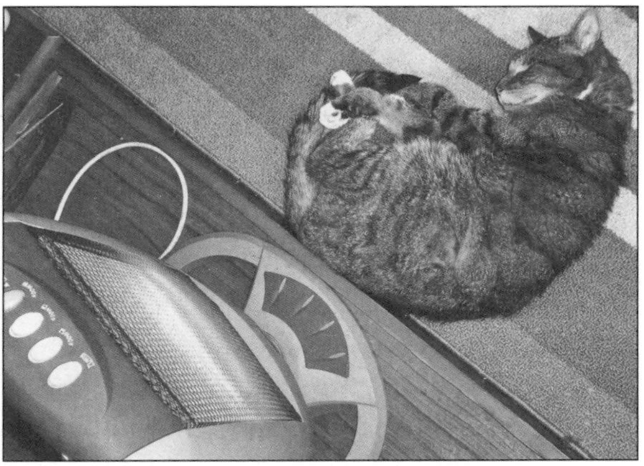

Cats love heat but burns can be serious and painful

☎ Urgency

Except for the most minor ones (e.g. singeing of the coat due to sitting too close to a fire, where there is no actual skin injury) burns should be dealt with urgently, mainly because adequate pain control will be needed and early treatment can help limit skin damage.

+ First aid & nursing

Immediate application of cold is required and this should be kept up until professional help is obtained.

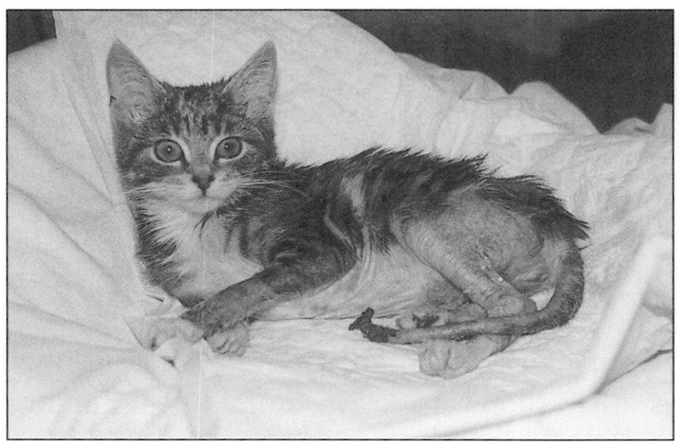

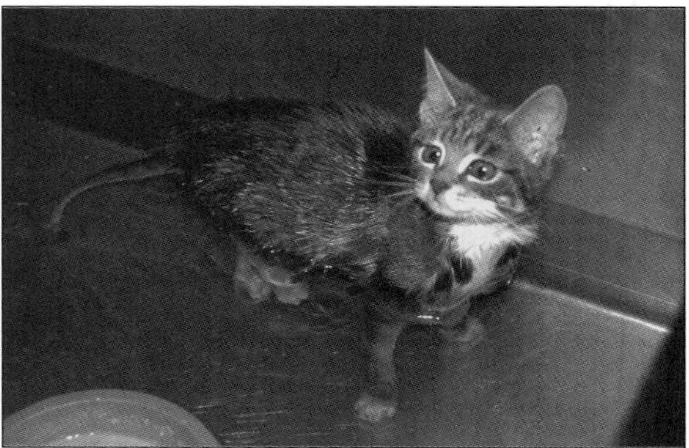

'Spider' fell into a bath of hot water, and received extensive second degree burns to her abdomen and legs. Intensive nursing treatment included hydrotherapy in order to try to prevent contractures developing in the healing skin. Amazingly, after her initial bad experience with water, she did not mind the later stages of treatment when she had to exercise in a water bath each day.

Burns on the feet can be treated by standing the cat in iced water in a basin. If possible, aim for a minimum of 20 minutes in the water after the burn. Then seek veterinary help.

Burns on the body can have ice cubes, frozen peas or cold water applied to them. It is necessary to replenish the source of cold frequently for the best effect. Iced water can be sprayed on using a plant sprayer.

Do not apply any other products to burned skin until the situation has been assessed by a veterinary surgeon.

Veterinary treatment

- Treatment for shock and smoke inhalation may be needed if there has been a house fire.
- In other cases, intravenous drips may be used to treat shock and dehydration or if there are burns to the mouth area.
- Painkillers will often be needed, however burn pain is notoriously difficult to manage and, often, anaesthesia is necessary for dressing changes, which may be required daily for many days in severe cases.
- Once the extent of the damage becomes apparent (this may take several days), efforts can be made to manage the wounds and decide how best to get them to heal. If contractures become a problem, surgery may be needed at a later stage (usually several weeks to months later).
- Badly burned cats require intensive care involving dressing changes, hydrotherapy, supported nutrition and management of pain. The process can be lengthy and expensive, but many cats do very well.

Related or similar conditions

▶ **Breathing problems**
▶ **Pain**
▶ **Salivation**
▶ **Shock**

C

Cancer

Cancer is an emotive word but, medically, it means an abnormal growth of cells which has the potential to enlarge (forming a tumour) and spread into nearby and even distant areas of the body. In doing this, normal function of the tissues invaded by the tumour cells may be affected, causing signs of illness and organ failure.

Cancer (or neoplasia, as it is often medically referred to) can affect virtually any cell type of the body – hence there are a large variety of different cancers, in different locations, and of differing degrees of seriousness and severity. Some of these, such as cancer of the ear tips in cats with white ears, are potentially curable with prompt treatment. In other instances, the tumour or cancer may be very advanced

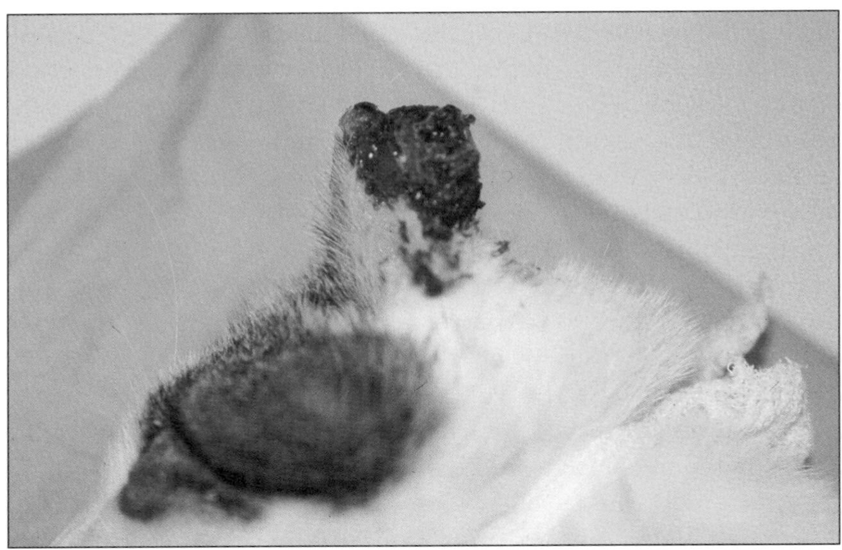

Cancer of the ear tip, caused by exposure to ultraviolet rays in sun-bathing cats, is common. It causes the ear tips to initially become red and inflamed. Later, ulcerated areas appear which may bleed. The condition extends down towards the base of the ear. Early treatment involves removing most of the ear flap, and limiting exposure to sun.

by the time of diagnosis, and a complete cure is not possible. One problem is that the body can cope well with some cancers, showing very few symptoms until a certain point is reached – but by the time these symptoms appear, the cancer is already beyond effective treatment. This is usually the case with liver cancer, for example, as the liver copes extremely well until a very large percentage of its function is destroyed, but then it suddenly fails. When the liver problem is picked up because of the symptoms produced, the disease has already progressed beyond the point where a cure could be obtained, although general supportive treatment may be able to be offered to improve quality of life.

Growths or tumours on or under the skin surface are usually easily detected as swellings which grow in size. Those on the surface may ulcerate. Skin growths can appear in any location. Not all such growths are malignant – benign tumours are relatively harmless in that they do not spread widely within the body, but they can still cause problems if they arise in an awkward area, e.g. the eyelid.

Internal tumours are harder to detect. They are sometimes picked up when the abdomen is felt (palpated) by the vet, or after X-rays and other tests. Internal tumours may be suspected in chronic diseases of older cats which cause weight loss and vague signs of illness not obviously caused by other problems. Occasionally, internal tumours are noticed quite incidentally, when the cat is being treated for an unrelated problem.

☎ Urgency

Even very malignant cancers are gradual diseases, showing their symptoms over weeks or months, hence few forms of cancer require emergency treatment. The exceptions would be cats that seem to deteriorate suddenly when it is known that they are already suffering from cancer, and problems of skin tumours starting to bleed, perhaps after they have been accidentally knocked.

✚ First aid & nursing

In most cases, a diagnosis of cancer will have been made during routine appointments and advice will then be given on general care. It is important that all cats suffering from cancer are not unduly stressed, that they are kept on a good plane of nutrition and that medication is given as directed. Symptoms such as lethargy, poor appetite, vomiting, diarrhoea and breathing irregularities need to be watched out for as these can indicate worsening of the disease or temporary complications.

Veterinary treatment

- Initial emphasis will be on diagnosing the type and severity of the cancer, which can then allow a prognosis to be given. Not all tumours are malignant, and for those that are, successful treatment may be possible if spread elsewhere in the body has not occurred.
- Skin lumps are often removed in their entirety and submitted for analysis, but sometimes, if removal could be awkward, a small biopsy may be taken first to allow further treatment to be planned better.

- If a tumour has not spread and is removed completely with 'safe surgical margins' (i.e. a boundary of healthy tissue all around it) the cancer will be cured, even if that tumour was a malignant one. Unfortunately, it is not always possible to be sure that a tumour has *not* spread – there is no definite test, but many cats are cured of cancer by successful surgery of this type.
- Cancer not amenable to surgery may be able to be treated or controlled by drugs or radiation. This very much depends on the type of cancer, its sensitivity to treatment, possible side effects, and the age and general health of the cat, as well as the wishes of the owner.
- For those cats with an untreatable cancer, once quality of life deteriorates, euthanasia is the kindest option and this should be discussed with your vet in advance of the time needed, so that everyone is clear when will be the right time to take this difficult decision.

Tip: Skin lumps

Owners are understandably often worried about skin lumps they find on their cat. Is it a tumour? If so, is it a dangerous one or can it be treated?

The only definite way of answering this question is to have the lump removed or biopsied. A pathologist will then look at the tissue and give a diagnosis.

There are however some general guidelines that vets often use when assessing lumps and trying to determine their malignancy, as follows:

Probably benign skin lump

- Mobile and loose in skin: can be 'picked up' through the skin
- Well demarcated with clear edges
- Grows slowly
- Surface smooth
- Not painful to touch

Possibly malignant skin lump

- Fixed to underlying tissues of skin: cannot be easily 'picked up' through the skin
- Poorly demarcated: difficult to tell where growth starts and stops
- Grows rapidly
- Surface angry or ulcerated
- Possibly painful to touch

Sometimes, your vet may ask to monitor a lump, to return after a few weeks or so to assess its size and appearance. It is best to measure the lump: use a ruler, make a sketch of the shape of it, or take a photograph. This way, you can be sure that changes that may be occurring are genuine, and not in your imagination. The vet may well make these measurements, etc. in the clinic and add them to the case notes. Most cases of lumps being monitored turn out to be benign. If the vet was seriously worried at the start, removal or biopsy would have been suggested then.

Related or similar conditions

- ▶ **Abscess**
- ▶ **Euthanasia**
- ▶ **Feline leukaemia virus (FeLV)**
- ▶ **Old age problems**

Canker

Canker is a term often used to describe ear problems which result in itchiness, inflammation and increased ear wax. See under **Ear problems**.

Castration (male cats)

Castration is the surgical operation to neuter male cats in order to prevent breeding and the reproductive behaviours associated with this. Most pet male cats are neutered since unneutered toms tend to stray, get into fights, and indulge in urine-marking behaviours which owners find unpleasant. In addition, there is the welfare aspect of unwanted kittens to consider. If you have an unneutered tom cat, and he goes outdoors, you do not know how many pregnancies he may be responsible for, and how many unwanted kittens may suffer as a result.

The incidence of certain diseases, especially **Feline immunodeficiency virus** (FIV) and **Feline leukaemia** (FeLV) is higher in unneutered toms. All in all, the arguments for neutering are strong and generally are considered to outweigh the 'unnatural' aspects which concern some owners. Responsible cat owners usually have their pets neutered as well as vaccinated.

☎ Urgency

Routine castration is a non-urgent operation. However once a young male cat starts to mark out territory with urine, most owners view neutering with some urgency, if the marking occurs in and around the house! Most toms are neutered any time after 5–6 months of age. Neutering earlier than this is possible, and may be carried out by rescue organisations and animal shelters.

✚ First aid & nursing

Before any elective operation, food should be withheld for 10–12 hours. This is to allow the stomach to empty and reduce the risk of vomiting while under general anaesthesia, which can be dangerous. Free access to water can be allowed up until the morning of the operation.

Cats receiving an operation should be fit and healthy. If your cat happens to be off colour on the day of the surgery, be sure to let the vet know. The operation may be postponed. After a general anaesthetic, recovering cats should be kept warm and quiet for 12–24 hours, and kept indoors. A light meal can be offered on the evening after the operation. The neutering operation in male cats is simple and quick, and most cats recover rapidly. Cats that appear subdued, lethargic or in pain may be experiencing complications, and advice should always be sought if there are any worries of this type after any surgical operation.

Veterinary treatment

- The operation is a short one but requires a general anaesthetic.
- No stitches are used unless there is a problem with an incorrectly positioned testicle.
- Painkillers should normally be given afterwards, often by a single injection at the time of the operation.
- Most cats return to normal behaviour after 12–24 hours.

Related or similar conditions

▶ **Neutering**

- **Spraying (urine)**
- **Surgery**

Cat flu

Cat flu is a viral illness of cats causing respiratory problems, nose and eye discharges and sneezing. It is a common condition, rarely fatal (except in young kittens or debilitated cats), but causes considerable problems for infected cats as the viruses tend to persist in the cat's system after recovery. Symptoms can then recur throughout the cat's life, especially during times of stress (e.g. going into a boarding cattery or veterinary hospital). 'Carrier' cats can also be infectious to other cats.

Severely congested cats may refuse to eat as they are totally unable to smell their food, and are then in danger of becoming dehydrated. Their breathing may be noisy with copious nasal discharges and sinusitis. They are frequently miserable and lethargic.

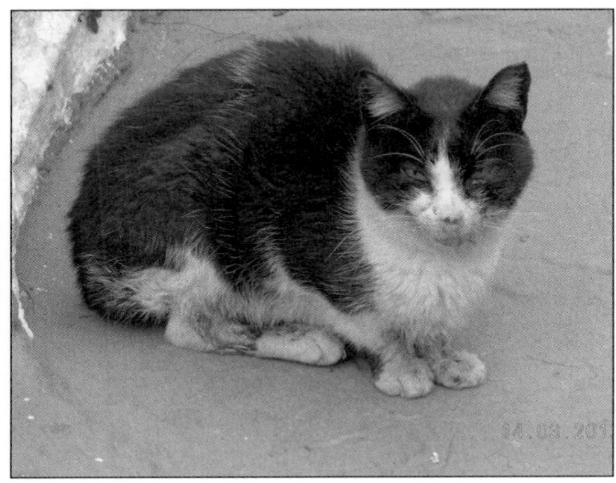

Greek cat suffering from chronic cat flu.

Two main viruses (feline calicivirus and feline herpes virus) and several bacteria can be involved in this condition, and vaccination against the main viruses is recommended in all cats, starting at around 8 weeks of age. Vaccination is less likely to be effective if a cat has already experienced the disease, but is still recommended as it may lessen the severity of future attacks.

☎ Urgency

Typical symptoms of cat flu are not an urgent problem unless the cat has refused food and water for several days and has become dehydrated. In normal circumstances, a routine appointment should be made. Also check the vaccination record card to see when the last booster vaccination was received.

Vaccine questions and answers

All cats should have an up-to-date **Vaccination** record made out in their name and detailing the diseases that are protected against (usually the viruses of cat flu, feline enteritis and possibly also feline leukaemia [FeLV] and chlamydia infection). This card should be stamped or signed and dated by the veterinary clinic giving the vaccines or boosters. If you acquire a cat and he or she does not have a vaccination record, you should not assume that vaccination has been carried out. Perhaps a vaccine was never given or only done so years ago. Although blood tests can be done to check immunity levels, they are expensive, and most people are guided by their vets and decide to have a vaccination course repeated to ensure protection is adequate.

Is a booster needed every year?

Currently, most vets recommend yearly boosters. It is possible that some cats retain immunity to certain diseases for longer than a year, possibly even a lot longer. However there is no easy means of checking this, and it is possible that immunity to cat flu viruses may weaken even before a year has elapsed in some cats. Vaccine manufacturers currently recommend yearly boosters to top up immunity, and so that is the policy most vets follow.

If you have an indoor cat that never goes out or comes into contact with other cats, you could discuss the possibility of less frequent booster vaccinations with your vet. Bear in mind, however, that if your cat has to enter a cattery at any time, or travel abroad under the Pet Passport scheme, an up-to-date vaccine history would be required.

Since entering a cattery can be stressful for many cats, there is a good argument to have a booster vaccination several weeks beforehand, unless the yearly booster was received within the last 6 months. This is because stress tends to make cats more susceptible to both shedding the virus (if they are carriers) or picking it up (if they have never been infected).

✚ First aid & nursing

Cats with cat flu require a lot of nursing. Frequent bathing to remove discharges from the eyes and nose is needed, usually every few hours or so. Water that has been boiled and allowed to cool is best, and damp cotton wool is used. Medicated wipes are best avoided as they may irritate the very inflamed and sensitive tissues.

It is important to tempt the appetite as these cats frequently will stop eating due to loss of the sense of smell arising from severe rhinitis (inflammation of the lining of the nose). Often, warming the food up helps to release a stronger smell and powerfully scented foods like sardines can be tried. Many cats enjoy tinned fish in tomato sauce. The best idea is to offer frequent small tempting meals rather than surrounding the convalescing cat with bowls full of food it may not feel like eating.

Severe congestion can sometimes be aided by steaming. Put the cat into a cage or box carrier, cover this with a large towel or blanket, and then place a bowl of hot water under the towel but *outside* the carrier itself to create a mini steam room. Leave one side of the basket (that opposite the steaming bowl) uncovered by the blanket to ensure conditions do not become unpleasantly hot and humid.

Alternatively, allow the cat into the

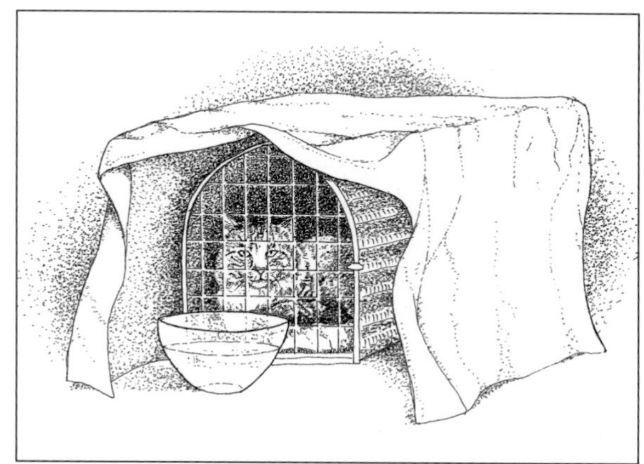

Steaming for nasal congestion caused by cat flu. Twice daily is sufficient.

bathroom when a shower or bath is being taken! (It will be safest to keep the cat in its basket at this time, especially if you are using a hot bath).

Veterinary treatment

- There is no specific treatment for the viruses implicated in cat flu. Emphasis remains on prevention of the disease by vaccination, starting in kittens at around 8 weeks of age.
- In cases of cat flu or flare ups, bacterial infections frequently become superimposed on the virus disease and these, at least, are amenable to treatment with antibiotics, which may lessen the overall symptoms somewhat. Decongestants are sometimes also tried to relieve stuffiness, and multivitamins may be prescribed.
- For dehydrated cats which are not eating, fluid therapy using intravenous drips may be required otherwise complications of reduced food intake and dehydration occur.
- Flare ups of cat flu may last 1–2 weeks. Unfortunately, they do tend to recur in the future as the virus persists at a low level in the respiratory system, often seeming to come active at times of stress or other illness.

Related or similar conditions

- ▶ **Appetite (poor)**
- ▶ **Breathing problems**
- ▶ **Cough**
- ▶ **Eye problems**
- ▶ **Fever/high temperature**
- ▶ **Pneumonia**

Chlamydia infection

Chlamydophila felis is a bacterium which causes mainly conjunctivitis in kittens, sometimes also with mild signs of sneezing and nasal discharge. Affected cats have an eye discharge and a reddened eye with swollen eyelids. The condition may start off in one eye and then affect the other one. The symptoms can be long lasting and may form part of a cat flu infection.

☎ Urgency

Chlamydia itself is not a life-threatening problem but, since the symptoms mainly affect the eye, prompt attention should always be obtained as it is possible some other disease is occurring which could permanently damage the eye if not assessed and treated early.

✚ First aid & nursing

The eyes should be kept open by bathing with water than has been boiled and allowed to cool. Artificial tears (e.g. Lacrilube; Visco-Tears) can be used to keep the eye moist and comfortable before veterinary treatment. The cat should be kept indoors and appetite tempted. The disease is very infectious so other cats should be checked for signs as well.

Veterinary treatment

- Antibiotics in the form of eye ointment and, usually, tablets are required. Lengthy treatment is required as the bacterium can be very difficult to eliminate completely – usually at least a month's treatment is used.

Tip

A vaccine is available for this disease. Vaccination is more often carried out in catteries than in individual companion cats which usually recover quickly when treated.

Related or similar conditions

- **Cat flu**
- **Eye problems**

Choking

Choking can be a confusing symptom since it is often difficult to distinguish between choking, coughing and retching. Indeed, sometimes a cat may seem to do all three of these. Generally, choking involves obstruction to the respiratory system with consequent problems *inhaling* air into the system. Coughing is a forceful *expulsion* of air from the respiratory system in response to irritation, and retching involves the digestive system – often, retching results in the production of saliva and may lead on to regurgitation of hair, grass or vomit. Retching is a frequent symptom in cats and many owners confuse this with choking. It is much more common than choking.

True choking may occur if a cat inhales or swallows a 'foreign body' which lodges in the throat or windpipe, if food or bony material gets stuck in the throat, or if the neck is compressed by being trapped or crushed, e.g. by a large dog. It is obviously a serious situation as oxygen starvation and death can quickly follow. The larynx of the cat is extremely sensitive and choking can lead on to a dangerous condition of laryngeal spasm, which can shut off the airway completely, risking life.

☎ Urgency

First aid may prove life saving as the delay involved in transporting the cat to a veterinary practice in genuine emergencies may in some situations be too lengthy.

✚ First aid & nursing

If the cat is fully conscious and breathing, the best option is to seek professional help as soon as possible unless it is very obvious what is causing the choke and you feel able to remove it safely. Transport the cat in a stress-free way and ensure a good air supply. Warn the practice you are coming.

If you do attempt removal of anything causing an obstruction, help will usually be needed to support the cat and control the front limbs. Often the best procedure is to wrap the patient firmly in a towel leaving only the head exposed. The head is angled back slightly and one finger used to depress the lower jaw. The other fingers are then free to remove the object, or else plastic tweezers could be used. Take care not to get bitten. This is not an easy procedure in most cats, but may be worth trying if you can clearly see the object causing the problem.

If the cat has collapsed (fainted) due to lack of oxygen, opening the jaws can be much easier. Open as widely as possible to get a clear view (no damage is caused by brief, wide opening of the mouth) and remove the object using fingers or tweezers. A torch or directed light may help. Fluid can be swabbed away with cloth or tissues (avoid cotton wool as this tends to disintegrate and stick to the throat area). Even in unconscious cats, it is safer to have an assistant keep the mouth widely open or else wedge it open by placing something between the back teeth, as semi-conscious cats will occasionally still bite. Once you are sure the throat area and airway is clear, begin the 'ABC' mouth-to-nose resuscitation routine as described under **Accident**. Provided the obstruction has been removed, resuscitation in this situation can be successful if applied quickly.

Veterinary treatment

- True choking often requires the use of an anaesthetic to examine the throat area, as only a very superficial examination is possible in the awake cat.
- X-rays and further tests may be needed, as appropriate.
- In severe cases, stabilisation in an oxygen tent and the use of antiinflammatory and other drugs may be needed.

Related or similar conditions

- ▶ **Asthma**
- ▶ **Breathing problems**
- ▶ **Collapse**
- ▶ **Cough**
- ▶ **Heart disease**

Coat contamination

This is a serious, common and often underrated problem in pet cats. The problem arises when the hair coat or paws become contaminated with paint, oil, wood treatment, antifreeze or other noxious chemicals. Cats' tendencies to sit or lie in enclosed spaces, e.g. under parked cars, and their habits of roaming widely around neighbourhoods, mean that they quite frequently come into contact with these substances.

The immediate instinct is for the cat to lick off the unfamiliar substance and, being fastidiously clean animals, they will often lick incessantly at contaminated areas of the coat or paws. Unfortunately, this means that they can consume considerable quantities of dangerous substances which may damage the mouth, throat, oesophagus, stomach and other organs, as well as get absorbed into the body generally. Thus the problem quickly becomes one of toxicity (poisoning), of a similar type to that affecting 'oiled' seabirds after environmental accidents.

The poisoning symptoms shown depend on exactly what was consumed, but can include vomiting, incoordination, salivation and fits.

☎ Urgency

This is an urgent situation, although it may not appear so due to delayed onset of action of the toxicity. The more substance the cat takes in, the more serious can be the consequences. The cat will not appear ill at the time of licking the coat but the problems are potentially building up. Any cat with a contaminated coat must therefore be treated urgently to decontaminate the coat and prevent further intake of the substance.

✚ First aid & nursing

The first action is to prevent any further licking of the coat and paws. The easiest way of doing this is to fit a buster collar (also known as an Elizabethan collar) around the cat's neck to prevent grooming. It is a good idea to have a buster collar in the home first aid kit for cats, since they are helpful in several circumstances. They are obtainable from pet shops and veterinary practices and most cats prefer the transparent variety. A collar or loop of bandage must be secured around the neck to hold the buster collar itself in place.

If no collar is available and the contamination is limited to the paws or lower legs, putting bandages on (or even socks) can prevent licking. Failing this, the cat will need to be held constantly before being washed or while being taken to the veterinary practice as it is vital that further licking does not occur.

Washing

It is not possible to wash all cats safely – some can only be treated under sedation. If you can wash the cat at home, repeated use of detergent-based liquids (washing up liquid) is needed, with copious lathering and rinsing. For badly contaminated cats, this may need to be repeated several times. It can be a lengthy process but it is vital that all traces are removed, including between the toes. Often, a more thorough job can be carried out under sedation or anaesthesia, but an initial wash at home may help considerably.

Veterinary treatment

- Sedation or anaesthesia is often needed to allow repeated washing, rinsing and decontamination, which is the vital part of the treatment.
- Intravenous fluids (a drip) may be given to support the cat and help eliminate absorbed toxins from the body. This can be life-saving in severe cases.
- Blood tests, to check on organ damage (especially liver and kidneys), may be advised and treatment, if necessary, arising from these results.

Related or similar conditions

- ▶ **Liver disease**
- ▶ **Poisoning**
- ▶ **Ulcers (mouth)**
- ▶ **Vomiting**

Colds

See **Cat flu** above.

Colic

Colic is the pain that result from spasms occurring in the stomach or bowels. It is a difficult problem to diagnose in cats as this type of pain is largely subjective, however it may be suspected if there is pain when the abdomen is touched or when the cat is picked up, or if the symptoms seem to come on after eating. Colic typically occurs in 'waves', with periods of less pain in between. Sometimes, gurgling noises may be heard coming from the abdomen. It is likely that cats troubled by fur balls may experience colic from time to time.

☎ Urgency

The problem is not an urgent one unless the cat seems in severe pain, or the symptoms include repeated vomiting. Indeed, many bouts of colic pass over by themselves within an hour or two.

✚ First aid & nursing

After a bout of colic it is wise to feed a bland diet for a day or two. Cooked chicken or fish is suitable. Milk should be avoided (milk can cause colic symptoms in some cats and is not anyway required in adult cats, who lose the ability to digest it properly). If you know what may have triggered the episode (e.g. a change of food) then avoid that in the future.

Veterinary treatment

- Colic may be treated using antispasmodic drugs, or by attending to underlying problems, e.g. fur balls, inflammatory bowel disease/colitis, inappropriate diet.
- Experimentation with the diet may be successful in many cases. Once you have found a suitable food, stick to that for the future as it could mean that drug therapy is not needed.

Related or similar conditions

▶ **Constipation**
▶ **Diarrhoea**
▶ **Fur ball**

Collapse

Cats may enter a state of collapse for various reasons. Diseases or injuries involving the heart and respiratory systems are the commonest causes, and are emergency situations where prompt action by the cat owner can save a life (see under **Accident**)

Cats suffering from chronic diseases such as kidney or liver failure or certain cancers may enter a state of collapse if they suddenly deteriorate. Usually a more gradual worsening of the condition would be noticed beforehand by the owner. Unfortunately, ill cats do tend to seek refuge in secluded places. If they cannot get home, they may crawl under sheds, etc. where there is a risk of hypothermia and dehydration.

Poisoning may also cause collapse, but often signs of fits or twitching would be seen. Untreated or unstable diabetes can also bring about collapse.

☎ Urgency

Any cat in a state of collapse is obviously in an urgent situation and treatment must be received quickly. Apply basic first aid and seek veterinary help.

✚ First aid & nursing

The 'ABC' resuscitation routine, as described under **Accident**, should be followed in all collapsed cats. In doing so, you may save the cat's life as the time delay involved in travelling to a veterinary clinic may prove too long. Resuscitation could take place or continue, if needed, on the way to the clinic.

Veterinary treatment

- Initial attempts will focus on resuscitation using intravenous fluids (a drip), oxygen and emergency drugs.
- A diagnosis will then be aimed for, to find out the cause of the collapse. Blood tests, X-rays and a variety of other tests may be called for.

Tip

Ill cats that are found in a collapsed state outside may be extremely cold (hypothermic) and warming up should be started. Wrapping in bubble wrap, blankets and the use of warm (not hot) water bottles should be used while the cat is being transported.

Related or similar conditions

- **Accident**
- **Breathing problems**
- **Choking**
- **Fits**
- **Heart disease**
- **Poisoning**

Conjunctivitis

The conjunctiva is a very, thin normally transparent membrane which lines the eyelids and surface of the eye. When this becomes inflamed (conjunctivitis) it becomes reddened and itchy or sore. Thus conjunctivitis often causes a red, itchy eye with an eye discharge. Sometimes the swelling can be so severe as to hide the eye itself almost completely, or the eyelids may become affected and swell up.

Conjunctivitis is seen frequently with **Cat flu**, but can arise from other causes too, e.g. irritation, **Allergy** and bacterial infection such as **Chlamydia infection**.

☎ Urgency

The urgency depends on the amount of discomfort being caused. Careful observation of the patient is needed.

A slightly red eye with mild discharge can be checked at a routine appointment. The cat will not be in significant discomfort and should be bright, eating and active. The eyelids are open as normal. The condition should not be deteriorating significantly and is probably due to mild infection or allergy. First aid will help greatly meantime.

A clear or cloudy discharge in a cat with a known tendency for **Cat flu**, and which has had previous bouts of this type of conjunctivitis, is also routine. Again, apply first aid and arrange a routine appointment.

A red eye which is causing severe pain which is depressing the cat or causing eyelid spasms or light sensitivity should be classed as an emergency. There may be something stuck in the eye or else severe internal inflammation of the eye could be in progress. Similarly, any change in the overall size of the eye must be checked quickly.

✚ First aid & nursing

Gentle bathing can be used to clear discharges, keep the eyelids moist and keep the eye open. Use water which has been boiled and allowed to cool or else sterile saline, available from chemists. Soak a cotton wool ball and squeeze out slightly before applying the wad gently to the eye and then wiping slowly towards the corner of the eye. Repeat 4–6 times daily.

Artificial tears (obtainable from chemists) can be applied, using a few drops every 2–3 hours. The human preparation 'Visco-Tears' is very suitable. This keeps the eye moist and comfortable.

Veterinary treatment

- Eye examinations usually involve several simple tests to check for ulceration of the cornea (the clear window that is the front of the eye) or damage to internal eye structures.
- A course of treatment will then be decided upon, most often a course of drops or ointment.
- Serious cases may be referred to ophthalmic specialists for assessment.

Tip

The eye is a sensitive organ and cannot withstand disease for long. All eye problems should be seen by a veterinary surgeon as serious conditions can sometimes mimick less dangerous ones. Prompt treatment may be needed to limit damage to the eye.

Related or similar conditions

- **Cat flu**
- **Chlamydia infection**
- **Eye problems – general**

Constipation

Constipation is difficulty in passing faeces, with consequent straining, abdominal discomfort and general malaise. Note that cats with diarrhoea will also strain, often to pass a small amount of liquid faeces. They will usually have passed larger quantities of semi-liquid faeces earlier but the irritation and discomfort caused by the underlying problem remains, creating the urge to pass more. In contrast to constipated cats, their bowels are completely empty.

Constipated cats only ever pass a small amount of hard faeces, if anything at all. It is a miserable condition, if severe, and some badly constipated cats may go for weeks without properly passing faeces. This very severe form of constipation is known as 'obstipation' and can lead on to dehydration and even toxaemia (blood poisoning).

The causes are various, from unsuitable diet, impaction with bones, feathers or fur in hunting cats, to problems within the bowel itself (the colon) whereby normal coordinated emptying movements do not occur. Cats which have had severe pelvic fractures may suffer from constipation due to physical narrowing of the pelvic canal by the healed fracture.

☎ Urgency

Constipation is rarely an urgent problem. First aid measures should be carried out and a routine appointment made. Quite often, in cats not prone to recurrent bouts, the first aid treatment alone will suffice.

✚ First aid & nursing

Encourage the cat to drink. Often adding some milk to the water bowl will be successful. Milk is a laxative in some cats (i.e. it tends to cause diarrhoea), so this otherwise undesirable effect can be helpful in constipated cats.

Giving some liquid paraffin (available from chemists) directly by mouth or mixed in to a small amount of food is often successful. No more than 5 mls should be given twice daily for a few days. If giving directly by mouth, use a syringe or table spoon. If the cat struggles, put the liquid into the food instead as there is a danger some of it could be inhaled. Liquid paraffin is tasteless and is usually readily accepted by cats.

Products obtainable from pet stores to help in the passage of hair balls (e.g. 'Katalax') are also suitable. These mostly contain liquid or soft paraffin wax or similar substances. They have the advantage that they are flavoured to appeal to many cats! If the cat will not take it directly, smearing a thick layer on to the forepaws will result in the cat grooming this off and swallowing the product.

Feeding oily based fish foods (e.g. sardines in oil) may also be helpful.

Various other stool softeners are available from chemists and veterinary practices but it is best to take veterinary advice before trying these.

Veterinary treatment

- Severely constipated cats often need to be anaesthetised for warm water and lubricating enemas to loosen, dissolve and remove the cement-like faeces. This process may need to be repeated several times in bad cases which have accumulated faeces over a number of weeks.
- Intravenous fluids (a drip) are often required in severe cases to rehydrate the animal and improve water balance within the body as seriously constipated cats typically go off their food and become dehydrated and toxic.
- Attention can then be focused on prevention, by manipulating the diet, adding supplements or stool softeners, etc. A close watch should be kept on the litter tray to detect recurrences early.
- The unpleasant condition of 'megacolon', encountered quite frequently in cats, is usually best treated by surgery to remove the block of inactive colon which accumulates the faeces without expelling them. This operation, though a major one, is often very successful. After the surgery, cats usually have loose faeces or diarrhoea for several weeks until the rest of the bowel compensates for the missing segment, when faeces then return to a normal state. There should be no further constipation after this procedure.

Tip

Be aware that it can sometimes be difficult to tell *why* a cat is straining. The problem may be in the urinary system, and cats with cystitis may sometimes appear as if constipated. In male cats, the potentially very serious condition of urethral obstruction (see under **Cystitis**) may also on occasion mimic constipation. Careful observation, together with reading the appropriate sections of this book, should help distinguish these problems. If there are any doubts, obtain telephone advice from a veterinary surgeon.

Related or similar conditions

- **Colic**
- **Cystitis**
- **Fur ball**
- **Key Gaskell syndrome**
- **Straining**

Cough

Coughing usually indicates disease of the respiratory system (lungs) or, less frequently in cats, the heart. It can however sometimes be difficult to distinguish coughing from the quite similar symptoms of retching, regurgitation and vomiting. Generally:

- *Retching* or *vomiting* result in the production of saliva, froth or semi-digested food material. Strong repeated contractions of the abdomen are accompanied by gagging sounds.
- *Regurgitation* results in the production of completely undigested food, often in a tubular shape. Regurgitation occurs

without any effort or strong abdominal contractions.

Retching and regurgitation are common symptoms in cats – commoner than true coughing – and usually follow grass eating, grooming (with production of hair balls/matts) or rapid eating.

- *Coughing* rarely results in the production of any fluid or mucus in animals and the terms 'productive' and 'non-productive' cough, as used in people, are not really relevant. Coughing can occur in bouts or singly; often, the breathing pattern is also abnormal, with a faster than normal breathing rate or increased effort being put into breathing – usually visible by extra effort used by the muscles of the abdomen (stomach area). Wheezes may be heard on close listening, especially in the cat suffering from asthma, one of the commoner causes of cough.

☎ Urgency

True coughing, if persistent, is viewed seriously in cats and usually requires investigation. If breathing difficulty or signs of general illness or lethargy are also present, advice should be sought urgently.

Short isolated bouts of coughing are incidental and usually harmless – they may be in response to minor irritation of the upper airways which quickly passes over within 5–15 minutes. The worst type of cough is quiet, moist cough in a subdued cat. This often indicates severe disease of the lungs and, even at rest, there may be evidence of breathing difficulty. Such cats must be handled extremely carefully, avoiding all stress, and assessed promptly by a veterinary surgeon.

Sneezing is a much commoner, and usually less serious, symptom in cats.

✚ First aid & nursing

The advice given under **Choking** and **Breathing problems** may be appropriate. Other than reducing stress and making sure that the cat is not subjected to dust, smoke or fumes, there is little suitable first aid for coughing. Take care that the cat with respiratory problems does not overheat in warm weather. Use cool air fans and bathe the paws and face area with cold water as necessary.

Veterinary treatment

- Coughing is encountered fairly infrequently in cats although, as mentioned above, various other symptoms may appear in a similar sort of way, especially to the inexperienced owner. Many cats with cat flu and hairball irritation may 'cough' at times. The task in diagnosis is to sort through these potential causes and unravel the precise nature of the symptoms. Careful observation by the owner can help greatly.
- A fairly common cause of cough in cats is asthma, sometimes called feline bronchitis. This is discussed separately and can usually be controlled successfully.
- More serious causes of cough include other chest diseases (e.g. feline infectious peritonitis, FIP; lung tumour) and heart problems. X-rays are important in the diagnosis, and blood tests are also often indicated. The outlook for these conditions is variable.

Related or similar conditions

- **Asthma**
- **Breathing problems**
- **Choking**
- **Heart disease**

Cystitis and feline lower urinary tract disease (FLUTD)

Cystitis is inflammation of the lining of the bladder, giving rise to symptoms of increased frequency of urination, blood in urine, straining to urinate, passing small quantities of urine, general discomfort and irritability. It is a relatively common problem in cats and, although many cases of cystitis are treated using antibiotics, the frequency of bacterial infection as being the main cause is actually thought to be quite low.

Many cases of cystitis are of idiopathic (unknown) cause or are attributed to a non-infectious condition termed 'feline idiopathic cystitis' (FIC) or 'feline lower urinary tract disease' (FLUTD). This condition describes a type of inflammation which is found in the lower urinary tract of cats, and leads on to typical symptoms of cystitis. The cause of the inflammation is not fully understood but stress is thought to play a role in susceptible cats. In simple cases, the symptoms pass over after several days, irrespective of what treatment (if any) is given, i.e. cats that are untreated recover in about the same time as those that are given antibiotics, for example. The condition is the subject of on-going research at present and it may be related to similar problems encountered in people. Several new ideas for treatment are under development.

Infectious causes of cystitis (caused by bacterial infection of the bladder) do occur in cats, but they are probably fairly infrequent. Cystitis may also be caused by the formation of bladder stones within the bladder. These irritate the bladder lining, giving rise to symptoms.

Many cats produce mineral crystals which are suspended in their urine without aggregating to form actual stones. The role of these crystals is currently under investigation. If very numerous, and of certain types, the crystals may also contribute to irritation of the bladder lining.

☎ Urgency

Cystitis is an unpleasant condition although, in its straightforward form, it is not particularly urgent – a routine appointment is usually fine. The problem arises when a potentially very serious form develops, and this is seen especially in male cats. This condition results in the production in the urine of a 'sludge' of inflammatory debris and deposit which can completely block the very slender diameter of the male urethra, leading on to the potentially fatal condition of urethral obstruction.

The urine in a 'blocked cat' cannot escape from the bladder, so the bladder swells to enormous proportions and back pressure causes the kidneys to malfunction. Serious metabolic complications then follow which can be fatal and the bladder itself may rupture.

This condition needs to be diagnosed rapidly because it is so serious. In the early stages, the symptoms can be just like cystitis, however the cat's condition worsens progressively and discomfort and straining become intense. Typically, no urine at all is produced despite all the straining.

Eventually, after 12–24 hours, collapse and sudden death may occur due to heart and metabolic complications.

+ First aid & nursing

As stress is thought to play a role, try to avoid stressful situations in susceptible cats. When a cat is experiencing simple cystitis, make sure there are sufficient litter trays around as the cat may wish to urinate much more frequently. Some cats also tend to pass urine in other places in the house, sometimes quite indiscriminately, and owners worry that they may be incontinent. This is not usually the case but restriction to one room may be practical.

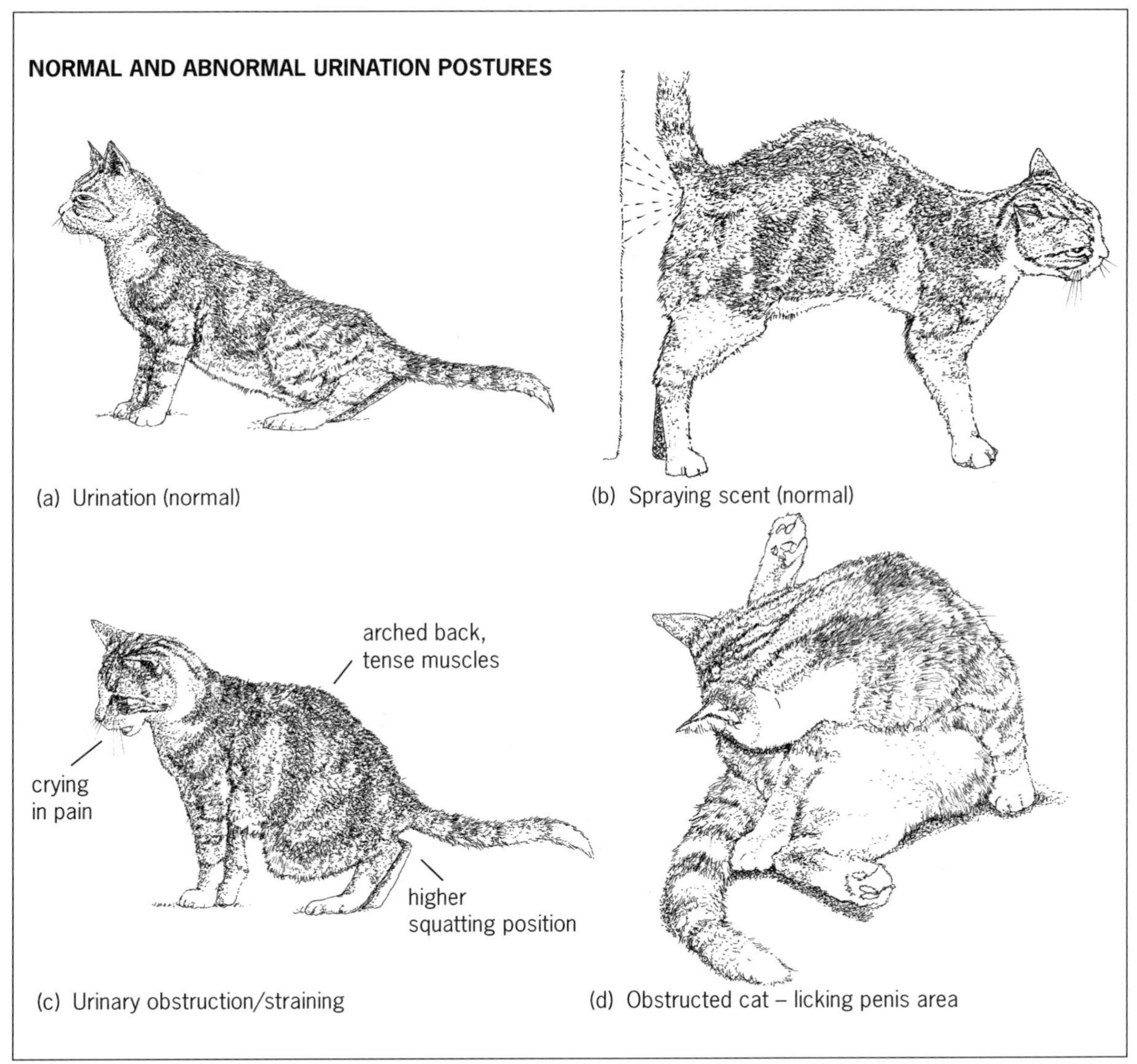

(a), (b): Normal urination and spraying positions. (c), (d): Positions adopted with possible urinary obstruction.

In cystitis, an increased throughput of water is beneficial. Encouraging water intake is not easy in cats, but several things can be tried:

- Some cats enjoy drinking from taps. If so, leave a tap dripping to encourage this.
- Some cats also seem to like licking ice cubes! Again, try this to see if your cat enjoys it. Ice cubes can also be flavoured with gravy, tinned fish juice, etc.
- Extra bowls of water can be put out around the house.
- For cats which seem to like milk, some can be added to flavour the drinking water. Milk causes diarrhoea in some cats, so look out for this.
- Extra water can be added into the food, especially easy if tinned food is being fed.
- Some cats prefer rain water – presumably their sensitive sense of smell picks up chemicals used to treat human drinking water. Collect rainwater and offer this to the cat.
- Water fountains are popular with many cats and are available from pet stores. The moving, aerated water encourages the cat to drink more.

There is no first aid for suspected urinary obstruction in a male cat – the patient needs to be taken to a vet as soon as possible.

How do I know if my cat has urinary obstruction?

Any sign of straining to urinate in male cats is of sufficient concern to merit a veterinary check up. Obstruction is much less likely in females.

If you feel your cat's abdomen and it is distended, tense and painful, do not delay. You have an emergency on your hands.

Veterinary treatment

- Usually, a urine sample is tested and a clinical examination, perhaps supported by X-rays, will be carried out.
- Stones in the bladder will need to be surgically removed or dissolved using special diets.
- Courses of tablets, e.g. antibiotics or other drugs, may be needed.
- Advice on preventing further attacks will usually be given.
- For urethral obstruction in male cats, emergency relief of the bladder obstruction is required, combined with intensive treatment and fluid therapy using a drip to correct the adverse effects of the obstruction. Usually, several days of hospitalisation are needed.

Tip

Cats prone to cystitis/lower urinary tract inflammation should be fed on tinned food rather than dry. The increased water content of the tinned food is beneficial in preventing future attacks.

Related or similar conditions

▶ **Constipation**
▶ **Straining**
▶ **Urination problems**

D

Dandruff

See **Skin problems**. Dandruff is usually caused by skin irritation, infection or allergy. Obese (overweight) cats are prone to dandruff and poor skin generally.

Deafness

Deafness can be a congenital problem (present at birth) in white cats with blue eyes. No treatment is available. The best medical test for deafness is a painless procedure which measures electrical signals occurring in the brain, but usually the problem can be diagnosed confidently by making loud noises when you are sure the cat is not able to see you making the sound or detecting air vibrations via the very sensitive whiskers. Obviously, deaf cats are at special risk out of doors since they will not hear approaching vehicles or dogs.

Ear problems can also cause impaired hearing or deafness and many elderly cats appear to have reduced hearing ability attributed to the ageing process.

Dehydration

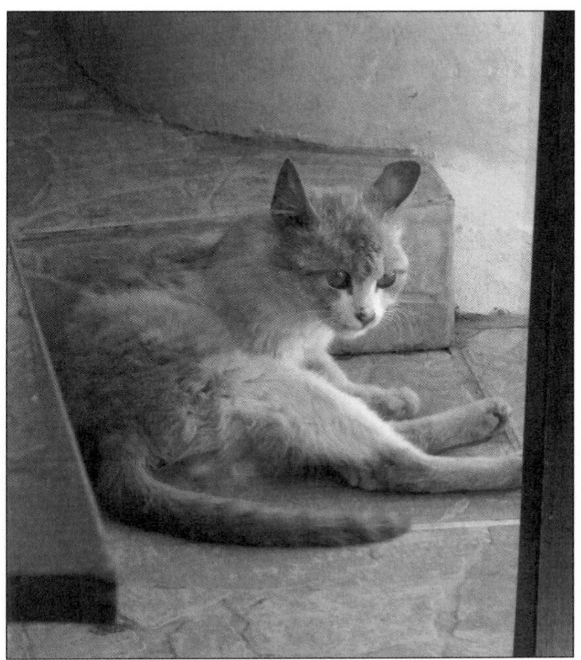

Dehydration is common in older cats with poor health.

Dehydration is the medical condition arising when the total water content of the body is reduced. It is a dangerous problem because dehydration puts many organs and tissues under strain; normal body function is disrupted and a vicious circle of adverse effects can be set up, leading ultimately to death after several days.

Cats, being small animals, are prone to the effects of dehydration quite quickly if they stop eating and drinking. Also, repeated vomiting and diarrhoea can rapidly bring about dehydration. Many diseases can lead onto the problem as a complication, e.g. **Diabetes, Kidney disease**, overactive **Thyroid gland**, infectious diseases. In fact, cats ill for almost any reason may show some degree of dehydration if they have stopped eating or if they have vomiting or diarrhoea. Overheating and stress can also cause dehydration.

Signs suggestive of severe dehydration

- Lethargic/depressed cat
- Reluctant to eat or drink
- Little urine output
- Sunken, lack-lustre eyes
- Skin remains tented up when pinched gently, instead of springing back down quickly
- Dry, tacky gums
- Frequent vomiting or diarrhoea

☎ Urgency

Mild dehydration is not urgent, and often resolves quickly if the underlying problem (e.g. a high temperature) is treated. Mild dehydration is probably only likely to be picked up by a veterinary surgeon after a clinical examination.

More severe dehydration is inevitable if there has been no food or fluid intake for 48 hours or if there is frequent vomiting and diarrhoea.

Severe dehydration must be corrected quickly if organ damage is to be avoided.

First aid & nursing

If the cat is vomiting frequently, seek immediate attention from the vet as it is likely that any attempts to encourage eating or drinking, or syringe feeding, will simply result in more vomiting. If vomiting is not present, or is infrequent, the dehydration can be prevented from worsening by encouraging fluid and food intake. Water or electrolyte replacement drinks are suitable, and tempting foods can be tried, e.g. warmed sardines in tomato juice, cooked chicken, etc.

If the cat will not eat or drink voluntarily, it may be possible to syringe feed with about 5mls of fluid every hour or so. The best solution to use is an animal electrolyte replacement drink, obtainable from veterinary practices or sometimes large pet stores. However glucose solution (1 teaspoon glucose powder to 1 pint [560 ml] water) and human rehydration drinks, such as Dioralyte, are also suitable in the first aid situation.

Veterinary treatment

- Severely dehydrated animals are treated using intravenous fluids to be supplied to the animal without the necessity for eating or drinking. This requires hospitalization and observation and observation and is often a life-saving procedure.
- At the same time as the animal is being rehydrated, tests will usually be carried out to discover why the dehydration has occurred in the first place, and then treatment for that problem started as well.
- If a dehydrated animal requires surgery, it is safest to correct at least part of the dehydration before embarking on major surgical operations, otherwise complications are likely. This may mean that the surgery is delayed slightly while the fluid balance of the cat is improved in preparation.

Related or similar conditions

- **Appetite (abnormal)**
- **Diarrhoea**
- **Kidney disease**
- **Vomiting**

Dermatitis

Cats are prone to several types of dermatitis (inflammation of the skin). The commonest one is caused by fleas, but other parasites and allergies can also be to blame. See under **Allergy**, **Fleas** and **Skin problems** for further details on dermatitis.

Diabetes

Diabetes mellitus (sugar diabetes) is a condition arising from insufficient insulin in the cat's body. Insulin is an important hormone, produced by the pancreas, which regulates blood glucose (sugar) levels. With there is not enough insulin, blood glucose increases to an unhealthy level and causes characteristic symptoms. The symptoms shown are usually one, or several, of:

- Weight loss
- Increased thirst and urination
- Normal or increased appetite
- Poor coat quality and general signs of ill health

  If uncorrected, symptoms progress over days or weeks to:
- Poor appetite
- Vomiting
- Dehydration
- Coma and death

In cats, diabetes is usually detected in middle aged or older patients, and is slightly more common in males. It is one of a number of conditions which lead to increased thirst and urination in cats, other common ones being overactive **Thyroid gland** and **Kidney disease**.

☎ Urgency

Diabetes develops over weeks or months and, in uncomplicated cases, is not an urgent condition. At the time of diagnosis, many cats will have been living with diabetes for some time and their metabolism has compensated somewhat for the problem.

However, if uncorrected, diabetes does worsen and a point comes when the condition presents as an emergency, life-threatening situation. In these cases, the cats have developed severe symptoms and complications arising from chronic high blood sugar levels. These cats may enter the dangerous phase of 'ketoacidosis', when they may enter a coma. Death is imminent at this point since many different organs become affected and malfunction as a result of the complications associated with the diabetes.

Danger signs to look out for

- Depression or extreme lethargy
- Reluctance to eat or drink
- Vomiting

✚ First aid & nursing

Never restrict access to water in a cat which has increased thirst, even if the cat is urinating to excess and wetting in the house. The cat is usually unable to control thirst, and deprivation of water will cause dehydration.

If possible, collect a urine sample to take along to the vets. Simple tests on this can usually rule out diabetes and help with other diagnoses as well.

In comatose cats, follow the advice given under **Collapse** and seek help immediately.

Veterinary treatment

- Unfortunately, most diabetic cats cannot be controlled with tablets (as some people suffering from certain types of diabetes can). Instead, daily insulin injections administered by the owner are required. Many cats do best when injected twice daily, but once daily injections are also possible and may suit owners better.
- There is no standard dose of insulin. Every cat is different and a routine is worked out for them by the veterinary practice concerned. Stabilisation is a gradual process and usually is stretched over several weeks.
- Diabetes makes high demands on cat owners since regular daily routines, careful attention to diet and weight, and regular blood tests carried out at the veterinary practice will be required. Some owners feel they cannot cope with the demands and, in these cases, if an alternative home cannot be found, euthanasia is usually the kindest option for the diabetic cat which requires treatment. Having said this, many owners (though daunted at first) soon pick up the techniques of injection, can manage to organise care of the cat successfully, and experience great satisfaction from returning their cat to better health.
- On-going expenses include blood testing, health checks and the costs of insulin, needles are other disposable items (e.g. urine test sticks) that may be used.
- Once the correct dose is arrived at, check ups can be reduced in number and owner and cat can settle into a predictable daily routine. Many cats go on to have a good quality of life, though their lifespan is likely to be reduced by their diabetes.

Some common problems in treating diabetes

In the initial stages, owners can encounter several problems regarding the care of their diabetic cat. In general, always approach the practice concerned with your cat but the following guidelines may be useful background information in these situations.

Problem 1. 'I think I may have 'missed' when giving the injection'

This is a common problem in the early stages, before owners have become fully proficient at giving the insulin injections. Some of the insulin may be lost on to the cat's coat, or else the very sharp needles may pass through two layers of skin without owner (or cat!) noticing.

What to do: If you are sure no insulin was received, repeat the injection. If there is any doubt, it is safer to wait until the next injection is due. The cat may be destabilised slightly, but this is unlikely to cause any serious problem. Overdosage could be more dangerous.

Problem 2. 'Too much insulin has accidentally been given'

Either the incorrect dose was withdrawn and injected or else, possibly, another person in the house could give the cat an injection without realising that this had already been done by someone else.

What to do: Always be clear who is treating the cat, and when! Careful filling-in of the diabetic treatment chart and keeping this in a prominent place should avoid accidental repetition of the injection. Make sure you understand how to read the markings on the insulin syringes and, if necessary, ask the veterinary staff to make a mark on a syringe to indicate the correct dose.

Assuming an error has occurred, or too much was given for another reason, the cat must be observed carefully during the following 24 hours. The danger is that blood glucose will fall dangerously low due to the excess insulin. As this begins to happen, most cats will become hungry, so food should be available at all times. Sources of sugar/glucose should also be kept to hand and if trembling or unconsciousness occurs, the sugar source should be put in the cat's mouth or rubbed on to the gums. This normally quickly corrects the condition unless a massive overdosage was given. Contact the veterinary practice in each case.

Problem 3: Cat is found collapsed/ trembling

In this situation, it may not be known whether overdosage or underdosage has occurred. The safest course of action is to treat for overdosage (i.e. give sugar/ glucose as above) and seek help immediately. In the cat under treatment for diabetes, overdosage is more likely unless there have been serious problems in giving insulin over the previous days.

Related or similar conditions

- **Fits**
- **Kidney disease**
- **Thyroid gland (overactive)**

Diarrhoea

Diarrhoea is a less frequent symptom in cats compared to dogs, but a variety of problems can cause it. Diarrhoea is usually termed either acute (lasting a few days) or chronic (lasting weeks or months, or else recurring frequently). Some cats are prone to repeated bouts of diarrhoea, with the intervals in between lasting anything from a few days to a few months.

Usually, cats with diarrhoea pass faeces much more frequently than normal and the faeces passed are semi-liquid or watery in consistency. Sometimes traces of blood or mucus (clear jelly-like substance) may be seen mixed among the faeces passed. Diarrhoea can lead to frequent straining, leading some owners to believe their cats are constipated. The straining arises from irritation/inflammation in the colon which creates the urge to pass faeces even although very little may be present.

In cats with diarrhoea, the unusual pattern of passing faeces may upset normal litter box training temporarily, and faeces may be passed outside of but close to the box or in other places. It is possible that cats may be 'caught short' and pass faeces in other areas of the house too. This usually stops once the diarrhoea is under control.

☎ Urgency

Diarrhoea without vomiting, when occurring in an otherwise healthy and alert cat, is not an urgent condition. It should be checked out during a routine appointment within 24–48 hours. In the meantime, first aid can be very helpful.

Severe diarrhoea with blood present, when combined with vomiting, or when the cat appears lethargic, is more urgent and should be attended to quickly as dehydration is a potential risk. As a general rule, if episodes of diarrhoea are occurring more than once every 3–6 hours, advice should be sought promptly.

Diarrhoea occurring in young kittens is viewed more seriously as they are more prone to the effects of dehydration and are susceptible to important infectious diseases. Again, seek advice early.

✚ First aid & nursing

Fluids should always be made available. The most suitable are plain water or electrolyte rehydration fluids designed for animals (obtainable from veterinary practices). Human fluid replacement drinks such as Dioralyte are also suitable, although it has got to be said that not all cats find these palatable. However, they may accept syringe feeding of small quantities (e.g. 5–10 mls) every hour. Do not offer cow's milk or prepared 'cat milk' products.

A 'light diet' is often helpful with diarrhoea. This consists of bland, easily digestible foods. The most suitable are:

1. Cooked chicken
2. Cooked fish
3. Scrambled egg (made with water not milk)

These can be mixed with a little boiled rice if the cat will eat this. Small meals should be offered every 4 hours or so. After several days, the normal diet is reintroduced but this should be done gradually, mixing only a small amount into the light diet at first, then increasing over the next 3–5 days.

The litter tray may require more frequent cleaning in cats with diarrhoea and in old or debilitated cats any soiled fur around the anal area should be carefully cleaned and dried. Long haired cats with diarrhoea may benefit from having hair clipped away from this region otherwise they can become extremely messy – ask at the veterinary practice if one of the nurses could clip the hair using electric clippers.

Veterinary treatment

- Vets view chronic diarrhoea very differently from acute, short-lasting episodes. Many of the latter cases can be dealt with successfully using simple treatment and diet regulation as mentioned under first aid above: after a few days, the cat is back to normal and no further bouts occur.
- Chronic or recurring diarrhoea may require a variety of different tests to establish a cause. These tend to be worked through in a sequence, so diagnosis is not always immediate for this type of problem. Common ones used include X-rays, blood tests, faeces examination and biopsies. Full investigation can therefore be expensive.
- Treatment may take the form of drugs (e.g. for inflammatory bowel disease), surgery (forms of tumour that are amenable to treatment) or dietary control.

Related or similar conditions

- ▶ **Constipation**
- ▶ **Feline enteritis**
- ▶ **Vomiting**

Drooling

See under **Salivation** for full details. This symptom can be caused by quite a variety of problems in cats, not all of them related to the mouth.

Drowning

Cats usually swim well but drowning or near-drowning can occur in turbulent water, if a cat gets stuck in a container of water (e.g. rainwater barrel) or when walking on thin ice on a river or lake. Unfortunately, malicious drowning of cats and kittens does occasionally occur.

A cat which has nearly drowned will be collapsed and inert and may have stopped breathing. The main concern is oxygen deprivation to the brain – this is the crucial factor which determines whether survival will be possible after resuscitation. There is evidence which suggests that near drowning in very cold water may be tolerated better because hypothermia causes the animal's metabolism to shut down to some degree, in order to protect the oxygen supply to the vital organs of brain, heart, liver, etc. This does not happen to the same extent in warmer water, and hence the vital oxygen supply contained in the body gets used up quicker, threatening the survival of the brain.

☎ Urgency

The situation is obviously a very urgent one and success depends on effective resuscitation and also the time that has elapsed between discovering the cat and starting attempts to resuscitate.

✚ First aid & nursing

The 'ABC' resuscitation routine described under **Accident** should be followed after an attempt has been made to clear the lungs of fluid, as described below.

Lift the cat by the hindlegs so that he adopts a head down position. Swing the cat from side to side several times in a wide pendulum motion to help displace water trapped in the lungs. Then place the cat in the recovery position and begin resuscitation.

If breathing starts, transport the cat to a clinic as quickly as possible. Monitor the breathing, assisting as necessary, and wrap the cat up to conserve heat.

Veterinary treatment

- Treatment will focus on resuscitation and supporting/protecting the respiratory system and brain, and also treating the adverse effects of shock.
- Success depends on the amount of oxygen starvation that has occurred. If this has been severe, survival may unfortunately not be possible even after successful initial resuscitation, because brain function will have been affected beyond that which can be coped with.

Related or similar conditions

- ▶ **Accident**
- ▶ **Collapse**
- ▶ **Shock**

E

Ear problems

Ear problems are common in cats and lead to typical signs of head shaking, scratching the ear or the side of the face, ear discharge or swelling of the ear flap. Severe problems can lead to head tilt or loss of balance as well. Ear pain is notoriously unpleasant and cats with severe diseases can be irritable and miserable.

The ear is made up of the ear tip and flap (pinna), the external ear, the ear drum and the middle and inner ears. Most problems arise in the external ear canal, which is a long narrow tube leading down to the ear drum. The ear drum is so called because it vibrates (like a drum) when sounds waves hit it; these vibrations are transmitted across the middle ear and then converted into nerve impulses which are relayed to the brain, creating the sensation of hearing.

The commonest ear problems in cats are:

- **Dermatitis** of the ear tip in white cats or cats which sun-bathe a lot, e.g. on window shelves. This 'solar dermatitis', caused by ultraviolet light, is considered

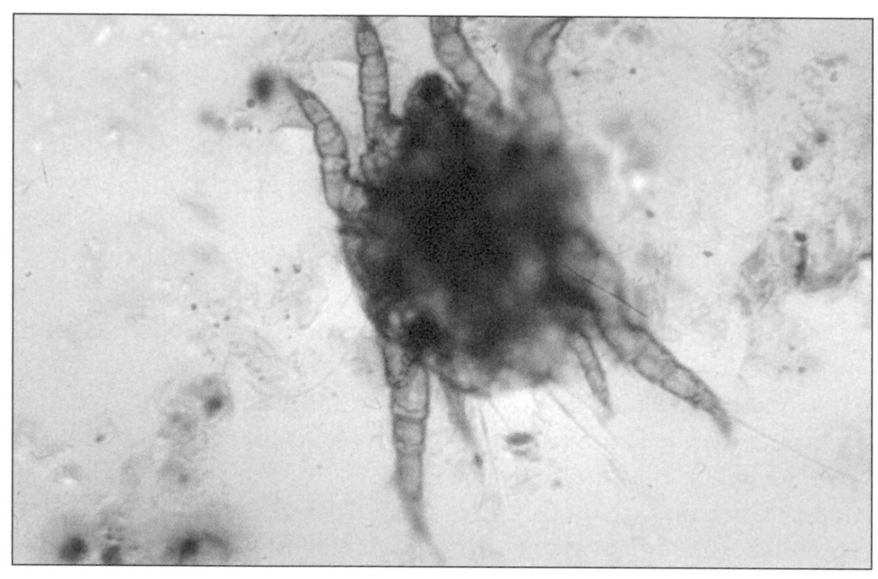

High powered photograph of the cat ear mite, *Otodectes cynotis*.

a pre-cancerous condition, which may progress to carcinoma of the ear tip, rather like skin cancer in people. If treated early, this malignant tumour can be cured by removal of most of the ear, but it is best prevented by limiting exposure to sun or applying sun block to exposed areas of skin.

- **Aural (ear) haematoma.** This common condition results in a soft swelling in the ear flap caused by excess head shaking. It is discussed in detail under **Blood blister** (haematoma). It nearly always arises as a result of another condition causing head shaking or ear itching, causing rupture of a small blood vessel and then bleeding between the layers of skin of the ear flap. It is a common problem after untreated ear mite infection.
- **Ear mites.** Ear mites are very small parasites, best visible under the microscope, which cause intense itch and excess wax production in the ear and sometimes dermatitis (skin irritation/inflammation) on the skin around the ear. They are easily infectious between cats and can also cause problems in dogs. Most cats probably carry a few ear mites but in certain situations they increase in numbers and cause symptoms.
- **Otitis externa.** This medical term means inflammation of the outer part of the ear, and is a common problem. Various things can cause otitis including wax build up, ear mites, irritation from foreign bodies (e.g. grass awns), allergy, infection and growths.
- **Growths/tumours.** These are possible in any part of the ear. They may be benign growths (polyps), usually arising as a result of chronic inflammation. Malignant ear tumours are also possible.
- **Vestibular syndrome.** This is a problem of the middle and inner ear, where the organs of balance are located. Any disease (e.g. infection, inflammation, tumours) affecting these deep parts of the ear may cause symptoms of imbalance, staggering and head tilt. 'Idiopathic' vestibular syndrome has an unknown cause, but usually resolves on its own after several days or weeks. See also **Balance (loss of)**.
- **Traumatic injuries.** The ear may be injured in fights or other accidents. Ear injuries tend to bleed readily, the problem usually being worsened by constant shaking of the head. Although major blood loss is unlikely, the mess can be considerable due to shaking.
- **Wax build-up.** In cats, this is usually a symptom of ear mites. The irritation caused by the tiny parasites causes excess wax to be produced. This clogs up the ear canal and becomes uncomfortable in

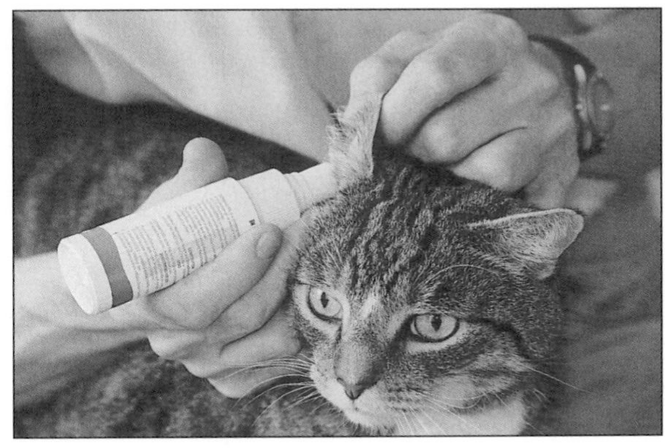

Use of a cat ear cleaner solution to shift excess wax and debris. Warming the solution to blood heat makes the process more bearable.

itself. A small amount of wax is normal and is part of the ear's self-cleaning process – the wax dries, flakes and then falls out of the ear.

☎ Urgency

Ear problems are rarely life-threatening but they are usually very unpleasant and an early routine appointment should always be obtained. The ear can only tolerate a limited amount of inflammation before permanent damage becomes likely. Untreated ears or persistent problems lead on to chronic changes in the ear which can then be very difficult to clear up completely.

✚ First aid & nursing

Examination and first aid of the ear is made easier if someone else holds the cat in a sitting position with the front legs controlled. Wrapping in a towel can help.

Any obvious foreign bodies (e.g. grass awns) that are seen near the top of the ear can be removed with fingers. However do not insert cotton buds or instruments like tweezers into the ear as you may cause more damage to the sensitive lining, as well as causing intense pain to the cat.

If there is an excessive build up of dark waxy material (a common symptom of ear mites), use of a wax loosener or ear cleaner will help disperse this prior to veterinary treatment. Gentle oil-based cleaners (available from veterinary practices) are best, but olive oil or almond oil is also very suitable. Apply about 1ml of warm oil into the ear and massage the base of the ear to disperse it. The oil should only be at body heat, no warmer. The cat will probably then shake its head, and waxy material may fly out. Check the other ear also. Cats with this problem often enjoy having the ear base massaged as it provides relief from itchy discomfort. The oil can be applied twice daily.

If the discharge from the ear is more liquid and a yellow or green colour, avoid putting anything into the ear, but the top part of the ear can be bathed clean with tepid saline or water to help shift the discharges and clear crusts and debris. If this is too painful, leave the ear alone until a veterinary surgeon has assessed the problem.

Cuts on the ear tip can be a problem because they tend to bleed excessively. The problem is that a blood clot does not get a chance to form due to excess shaking of the head. Keeping the cat quiet, perhaps by holding her, for 30 minutes or so may help, as may gentle pressure applied across the bleeding area using cotton wool. Leave the cotton wool wisps in position afterwards because they can help the blood clot to remain in place.

Veterinary treatment

- A diagnosis is important and this is usually possible by examining the ear with the naked eye and by using a magnified, illuminated torch (auroscope) to look into the ear canals. Quite often, the diseased ear is far too painful to allow close examination with an auroscope and in these cases, warm saline is used to clear discharges and debris and, if necessary, X-rays and biopsies can be taken.
- The commonest form of ear treatment is a course of ear drops, which must be applied correctly and for the full duration of treatment. If you are having problems applying the drops, or are not

sure if you are doing so effectively, ask the veterinary staff for guidance since the medication must reach the correct place for it to work. Tablets are frequently prescribed also – again, the full course (which may be lengthy) must be completed. Ear problems have a frustrating tendency to recur, especially if a full treatment course is not completed.

- Surgery is indicated for haematomas, chronically inflamed ears which are not responding to other treatments, and where polyps or tumours are present. The type of operation depends on exactly what is wrong: that for haematomas is a fairly simple operation, but the surgery for chronically inflamed ears, and for some tumours, is time-consuming and therefore liable to be more expensive. If successful, however, it can put an end to months of chronic ear pain and owners often remark how their cats seem 'years younger' afterwards.

Related or similar conditions

- ▶ **Balance (loss of)**
- ▶ **Blood blister (haematoma)**
- ▶ **Deafness**

Eczema

Eczema is a descriptive term which means inflammation within the top layers of the skin. It is not really a disease diagnosis in itself, rather the result of some other problem. Common symptoms of eczema are itch, redness, crusting, weeping areas and skin scales or flakes. Often, the coat has a 'grainy' feel when the fingers are run through it, especially along the back or around the neck area in cats. This condition, called **Miliary eczema** or miliary dermatitis, is quite common, and is often caused by fleas or other allergies.

For further details, see under **Skin problems**, **Fleas** and **Allergy**.

Electrocution

Cats are less likely to chew on electrical cables than dogs, however occasionally kittens will do this and some cats enjoy lying behind objects such as televisions, computers and hi-fi equipment where there may be cables.

Mild shocks will cause no lasting harm but a severe electric shock can result in a collapsed cat, possibly with burns at the point of contact. Lung complications are also possible.

☎ Urgency

If collapse has occurred, urgent treatment is necessary and the cat should be treated as an emergency. Apply first aid as below then transport to a veterinary practice as soon as possible.

✚ First aid & nursing

> **Note:** First ensure you are not in danger yourself!

Switch off the electricity supply at the mains and then move the cat away from the source of the shock using a wooden broom handle or similar. Begin resuscitation using the 'ABC' routine as described under **Accident** and seek help.

Veterinary treatment

- Resuscitation and treatment for electrical burns would be required. If first aid has been successful, the outlook is favourable but severe electric shocks can lead to lung complications, with fluid accumulating. This would require treatment in the veterinary hospital.

Related or similar conditions

- ▶ **Accident**
- ▶ **Burns**
- ▶ **Collapse**

Enteritis

Enteritis means inflammation of the lining of the intestines or bowel. Gastritis means inflammation of the lining of the stomach, and gastro-enteritis means inflammation of both stomach and intestine.

The inflammation of enteritis can be caused by infections (bacteria, viruses and protozoa), allergy or food intolerances as well as various inflammatory diseases which are probably at least partly associated with stress (e.g. colitis, inflammatory bowel disease). Often, cats ill with other diseases such as kidney disease and overactive thyroid gland will show bouts of enteritis. Parasites (worms) do not often cause enteritis unless they are present in huge numbers, or in kittens.

The most frequent symptoms of severe enteritis are diarrhoea and vomiting, both of which may contain traces of blood. Cats will also often appear miserable, be reluctant to eat or drink and may show signs of abdominal pain. Dehydration is a risk.

☎ Urgency

Severe symptoms mean that an urgent appointment is necessary, due to risks of dehydration and complicating problems. Cats which remain bright, interested and active despite having some diarrhoea should be watched carefully for deterioration and a routine next-day appointment made if symptoms are first noticed at night.

Vomiting is viewed more seriously than diarrhoea and any cat which is vomiting frequently (more than once every 2 hours) must be seen quickly. Similarly any cat which is unresponsive and lethargic is probably dehydrated or in severe pain: seek advice immediately.

Kittens can rapidly become dehydrated, so advice should always be sought at an early stage if there are persistent symptoms in cats less than 5 months of age.

✚ First aid & nursing

This is basically as for **Diarrhoea**. It consists of encouraging fluid intake (water, glucose or electrolyte replacement drinks), by syringe if necessary, keeping the cat warm, and observing closely for deterioration.

Cats with lots of diarrhoea must be kept clean and all contaminated bedding etc. disposed of hygienically.

Veterinary treatment

- This rests on finding a cause for the enteritis and then treating that. Dehydration, if present, will need corrected and various blood tests, X-rays or biopsies may be called for in chronic or persistent cases.
- Feline infectious enteritis, being a viral illness, has no specific cure – only general supportive treatment can be

given whilst, hopefully, waiting for the cat's own immune system to cope with the disease.

Related or similar conditions

- ▶ **Colic**
- ▶ **Dehydration**
- ▶ **Diarrhoea**
- ▶ **Vaccination**
- ▶ **Vomiting**

Epilepsy

Epilepsy is one cause of fits (also known as convulsions or seizures). This general symptom is considered in detail in the section on **Fits**. Attempts will usually be made to diagnose the cause of the fits in any affected cat, and many possibilities are present, including **Poisoning**, **Brain damage**, **Diabetes**, and various other body system or organ problems as well as epilepsy. The first step is usually a series of blood tests, followed perhaps by X-rays and even brain scans. If epilepsy is diagnosed, usually by the exclusion of other possibilities, continuous medication may be needed to keep the fits under control unless they are infrequent enough not to merit treatment.

Euthanasia

Euthanasia means bringing about death by painless means. In veterinary medicine, this is usually necessary because of pain and suffering caused by incurable diseases, or because of a poor overall quality of life with little prospect of improvement. Euthanasia is an important duty of the veterinary surgeon and it is one he or she must perform on an almost daily basis.

When is the right time?

Decisions are easier when there is clearly pain or distress that cannot be helped and when prospects of a cure are low. Harder decisions are those when quality of life is thought to be poor, but the cat seems to have 'good days and bad days'. This is often the situation with old cats suffering from chronic health problems such as **Kidney disease**. There may be additional age-related problems such as **Arthritis** and perhaps overactive **Thyroid gland** which also need to be taken into account and some kind of judgement needs to be made about when it is kindest to stop treatment.

Quality of life can be gauged in a straightforward way as follows, but ultimately a decision is often instinctively felt about what is the right time. Impartial advice from the veterinary surgeon can greatly help here. Never feel bad raising the subject of euthanasia as the best person to assess the cat's overall quality of life is usually the owner.

Good quality of life

- Fairly responsive and mobile, though may sleep more
- Recognises owner/companions
- Fairly reliable appetite and use of litter tray
- No major distressing symptoms

Poor quality of life

- Not responsive; reluctant to move most of the time Does not recognise owner/companions

- Appetite poor; incontinent
- Frequent unpleasant symptoms, e.g. vomiting, diarrhoea

Natural death

Owners would often prefer that their old or ill cat dies 'in his sleep', and this does occasionally occur, eliminating the need to make distressing decisions about euthanasia. Unfortunately, the main worry with avoiding euthanasia in this way is that there may be unpleasant symptoms, fear or anxiety before death. The end stages of some diseases may be distressing for both cat and owner and it is to avoid these that euthanasia is usually recommended. It is wise to discuss your thoughts on these points well in advance so that you are comfortable with the course of action being taken. Euthanasia should be seen as an act of kindness – the last thing an owner can do for their companion animal and one intended to avoid any distress or prolonged suffering at the end of a cat's life.

What happens during euthanasia?

Euthanasia is carried out by means of a large overdose of anaesthetic – the cat literally falls asleep, and the procedure is exactly the same as when administering a routine anaesthetic for other purposes, e.g. X-rays or operations. Usually, the anaesthetic solution is injected into the vein in the foreleg. Within seconds, consciousness is lost and death follows soon after. The experience is probably very similar to that which we experience when receiving a general anaesthetic – usually a sensation of gradually falling backwards that is not in itself unpleasant.

The technique of administering the injection requires skill on the part of the person administering it, and the assistant holding the cat. A certain amount of cooperation is required from the cat but most patients are not upset by the procedure when sympathetically and patiently handled. For those that are, perhaps because of pain, anxiety or fear, sedatives can be given beforehand. These are simpler injections which make the cat very drowsy, and thus easier to handle for the final anaesthetic injection into the vein. This process takes a little longer (a sedative usually requires about 15 minutes to take effect) but it may be necessary to reduce stress in certain situations.

Very sick cats may have poor blood pressure. In these patients, the injection may be given into the abdomen because of problems finding a suitable vein. Again, this takes longer than when it goes directly into the bloodstream, but is equally as effective.

Euthanasia at home

Many owners wish their cat to be 'put to sleep' at home. This is quite understandable and owners can gain comfort from the fact that their pet's last moments were in familiar surroundings. Home euthanasia requires a veterinary house visit and therefore is usually arranged in advance for a time when the vet can safely leave the practice or hospital. Often, an assistant will be brought to help support the cat. Home visits will be more expensive than clinic appointments but for some owners the peace of mind is worth any additional cost.

In certain situations, e.g. at night or in

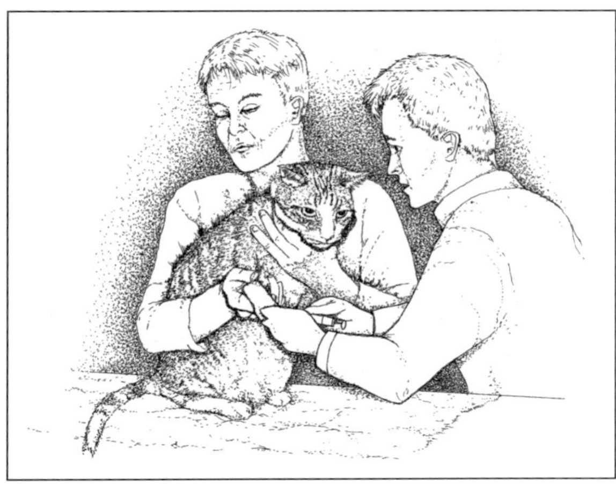

Receiving the injection: the cat literally 'falls asleep'.

busy animal welfare charity hospitals, it may be very difficult for a veterinary surgeon to leave hospital premises because of other emergencies being attended to. In this circumstance, you may be asked, if at all possible, to attend the clinic rather than have a house visit. This is to ensure that all sick or injured animals receive the optimum standard of care.

To stay or not

Most owners who witness euthanasia are reassured by the swift and painless procedure. Naturally, they are upset at losing their companion but, later on, can take comfort from the fact that no suffering was caused by euthanasia, that it was an easy way out for a much loved companion animal. Also, from the cat's point of view, having their owner nearby will obviously be reassuring. However if you cannot bring yourself to stay, the veterinary staff will undoubtedly make every effort to reassure the cat – they are pet owners themselves and know the trauma of pet loss from first hand experience.

After euthanasia

After the injection has been administered, the cat will gently collapse and lie down. It is normal for the body to give several small twitches at this stage. Often, too, there are a few deep gasps, which can be alarming if you are not prepared for them. This is a breathing reflex in the unconscious cat, and can continue for some minutes, especially in cats which have been poorly for some time or are very old. It is not a sign that the injection hasn't worked, it is simply the respiratory system shutting down. The eyes will remain open and urine may be passed as the bladder relaxes. All these events are normal.

The body can be taken home for burial in the garden afterwards, or else cremation can be arranged through the veterinary practice. Cremation is the option favoured by most owners. Ashes can be returned for scattering or burial, perhaps in a favourite or special place. Pet crematoriums operate to high standards and usually welcome visitors to their premises. Although they operate a collection service for veterinary practices, it is usually also possible for owners to transport the body to the crematorium themselves if they wish. Bodies left at practices will be kept in cold storage until collected by the crematorium.

Pet cemeteries are also available in some towns and cities. If you choose this option, you should ideally visit the cemetery beforehand to view the pet graveyard and find out about collection and burial arrangements.

Grief after pet loss

It is normal to cry and experience symptoms of grief for several days, or longer, after the death of a close animal companion. Veterinary staff will testify to the close relationships that exist between animals and their owners. The duration and intensity of the feelings felt depend on many factors, including the temperament of the owner, the closeness and duration of the bond between cat and owner, personal circumstances and support networks, and the nature of the death (whether sudden or expected).

After a few days, symptoms of acute grief usually give way to an acceptance of the situation and then, eventually, an ability to think and speak about the deceased cat without becoming unduly upset.

Some feelings of guilt are common and people will often think things like: 'I should have spotted he was ill sooner. Maybe he would still be alive if I had?', 'I didn't give her all the tablets. Was it my fault?', 'Maybe I should have got a second opinion?', and so on. These feelings should be recognised as a natural part of the bereavement process. Often, talking the situation over with friends or the veterinary staff will help dispel them. Note that few things are absolutely clear cut in medicine, whether animal or human, so relentless cross-examination of the circumstances leading up to a pet's death is rarely helpful after the event. It is difficult enough for vets to diagnose illnesses, let alone cat owners, so no guilt should be felt even if abnormalities were not recognised or treated early on.

Related or similar conditions

- ▶ **Bereavement**
- ▶ **Old age problems**

Eye problems – general

The eye is a sensitive organ which cannot tolerate injury or inflammation for long. All eye problems should be assessed promptly by a veterinary surgeon. Most cases will be simple, easily treatable conditions such as conjunctivitis but one of the difficulties with eye diseases is that serious, sight-threatening problems can, in the early stages, sometimes look very similar to fairly harmless ones. The safest course of action is always to get the eyes checked early on.

To test a cat's vision, follow the instructions given under **Blindness**.

Common cat eye problems are as follows:

- **Eyelid problems.** The commonest two are blepharitis (inflammation of eyelids), caused by allergy or infection, and growths on the eyelid.
- **Conjunctivitis.** This is inflammation of the conjunctiva – a very thin, normally transparent membrane which lines the eyelids and the front of the eye. When this membrane becomes inflamed, blood flow in it increases, giving a red eye. Conjunctivitis is usually caused by infection or allergy. It is a common problem with cat flu and results in a watery or discharging eye. In severe cases, the conjunctiva can swell up so much that it virtually obscures the eye – all you see is pink swollen tissue bulging forwards. See **Conjunctivitis**.
- **Corneal ulcers.** The cornea is the clear window at the front of the eye. It is a sensitive structure with many nerve endings and if it becomes damaged, painful

ulcers can result. Superficial (shallow) ulcers are commonplace, but deep ones can be very dangerous – the eyeball may rupture and collapse. All corneal ulcers are therefore taken seriously; they often result in eye pain and discharge.

- **Iritis/anterior uveitis.** This is a particularly unpleasant and painful condition resulting from inflammation occurring deep within the eye. Confusingly, it often looks just like conjunctivitis in the early stages, i.e. the eye appears red, but this condition is much more serious. Cats are often miserable and grumpy.
- **Glaucoma.** This condition results when pressure builds up within the eyeball. This may make the eye noticeably larger than its fellow eye. Glaucomatous eyes frequently become blind and removal of the eye is necessary to alleviate chronic pain.
- **Cataract.** This is a condition affecting the lens of the eye. The lens becomes cloudy or opaque, and vision is interfered with.
- **Watery eye.** This can result from overproduction of tears due to irritation or allergy or, more commonly, because of poor drainage of tears away from the eye due to a blocked duct. Duct blockage can result following viral infection, inflammation or injury. Sometimes it may be possible to clear the duct, otherwise the condition may need to be lived with. It is harmless although may cause staining of the hair on the face area.
- **Eye injuries.** These result from trauma. The eye withstands sharp trauma better than general blunt trauma, but even so, all eye injuries are potentially devastating because blindness can result.
- **Eye tumours.** Sometimes, cancer is first detected in the eye even although it is present elsewhere in the body as well. When a tumour is restricted to the eye, removal of the eye may completely cure the cancer. Cats cope very well with one eye and quality of life remains good.

☎ Urgency

Never ignore a red eye, a painful one or one with a discharge. If the cat seems subdued, holds the eyelids closed and seems to shy away from light, it is likely that a serious inflammatory condition is present. Urgent attention is needed.

Cats which are bright and alert with a mild discharge and no apparent pain are probably suffering from conjunctivitis: book a routine appointment but keep a close watch for any deterioration.

✚ First aid & nursing

An eye that is crusted with matter should be bathed gently in tepid saline or water. Use a wet pad of cotton wool and hold this against the eye and then wipe into the inside corner of the eye. Repeated until all debris has gone. In severe cases, do a little at a time until all the material has been loosened and shifted.

Many superficial eye problems can be helped a lot by applying artificial tears into the eye. This lubricates the eye surface to prevent dessication and also relieves discomfort and grittiness. 'Visco-Tears' or other similar human preparation is ideal and the drops can be applied 6–8 times daily. Do not use human prescription drops of any type as the antibiotics or other drugs contained in them may damage the cat's eye.

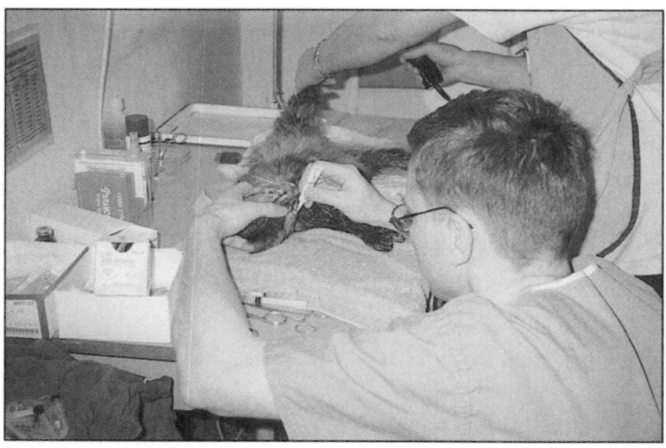
Treating the eyes of a feral cat at a cat welfare neutering clinic in Thessaloniki, Greece.

Severe trauma to the eye must be dealt with urgently. Hold the cat or apply an Elizabethan collar (see page 151) to prevent self-inflicted damage. If possible, apply a pad of damp cotton over the eye area to prevent drying out while you seek help. Cats in severe distress should be contained in a secure basket and taken urgently to a veterinary practice.

Veterinary treatment

- Most eye problems can be diagnosed in the awake cat, using various instruments and simple techniques to check the various parts of the eye and assess the damage and outlook.
- Treatment most often takes the form of prescription drops (which sometimes need to be applied very regularly) or surgery in suitable cases. Frequent reassessment of the eye is needed to see how it is responding to treatment, since changes (improvements as well as deteriorations) can occur quickly. In severe cases, hospitalisation is often of benefit.
- In sightless eyes or those which are causing relentless pain, removal is by far the kindest option since cats cope well with one eye and will be far happier when the source of deep discomfort is taken away. Such cats often resent having the sore eye examined/ treated at home, compounding the problem and causing difficulties and worries for the owner.

Tip

Cats have a third eyelid, normally seen at the inside corner of the eye. On occasions this eyelid can move across the eye, hiding part of the eye. Vets usually check the third eyelid. Foreign bodies (e.g. grass seeds) can sometimes get trapped behind it. Other illnesses may cause the third eyelid to become more prominent, creating a disconcerting appearance to the eye.

Related or similar conditions

- **Blindness**
- **Cat flu**
- **Chlamydia infection**
- **Conjunctivitis**

F

Falls

Falls from a height are a fairly common accident in urban cats. Many city cats spend time on window sills and on balconies. A sudden fright or falling asleep there may result in a momentary loss of balance and fall. The injuries depend on the height fallen from and the surface landed on. The term 'high rise syndrome' is used by vets for these types of accident as a characteristic pattern of injury is often seen. This may include fractures or dislocations in the front legs, mouth injuries, including fracture of the hard palate, and other serious internal problems.

Sometimes, the injuries are far fewer than would be expected from the height fallen and it can be truly amazing how lucky some cats seem to be after this type of accident. However, to be on the safe side, internal problems must also be considered and careful observation for 24–48 hours is required even for the apparently unaffected cat.

☎ Urgency

This is an urgent problem and all fallen cats should be treated as emergencies and advice sought from a veterinary surgeon. If there is apparently nothing wrong, the vet may just give telephone advice on what to look out for should complications start. Often, examination of the cat will be recommended, especially to check that the hard palate is intact and that breathing is normal.

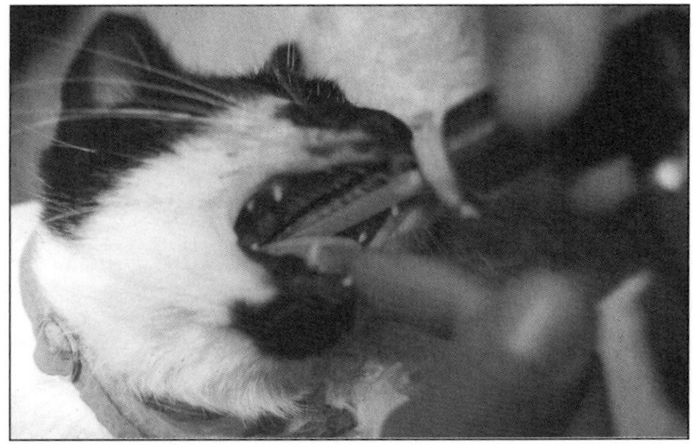

Falls may cause damage within the mouth, e.g. fractured hard palate.

+ First aid & nursing

This depends on the injuries incurred. The most serious cases will require resuscitation, as described under the **Accident** (ABC guide), and urgent transportation to a veterinary practice.

Cats that appear normal, can walk and are responsive, should be kept indoors and watched carefully for any signs of deterioration, e.g. breathing difficulty, pain, bleeding from the mouth or nose, whilst advice is sought from a veterinary surgeon.

After this type of accident, any lameness suggests a fracture or dislocation has occurred, although severe sprain/strain is also possible.

Veterinary treatment

- Initial treatment will be for shock and pain relief and will usually consist of intravenous fluids (a drip) in severe cases and strong painkillers.
- X-rays may well be advised to check for limb and internal injuries. If the hard palate is fractured, surgery may be needed to repair this and most cats benefit from having a temporary feeding tube placed in the neck area to rest the injured tissues of the mouth while they heal. Such feeding tubes are usually well tolerated and avoid complications due to poor nutrition during the recovery period (see p. 151).
- Despite the severity of some of these injuries, many cats go on to make a good recovery but treatment of severely injured cats can be lengthy and expensive.

Related or similar conditions

- ▶ **Accident**
- ▶ **Brain damage**
- ▶ **Collapse**
- ▶ **Fractures/dislocations**
- ▶ **Shock**

Fear

See **Anxiety/Fear**.

Feline calicivirus

This is one of the viruses that causes the respiratory symptoms typical of **Cat flu**. The virus is very common in the cat population and by itself usually causes slightly milder disease than the other flu virus (**Feline herpes virus** or feline rhino-tracheitis virus, see below). Feline calicivirus often causes ulcers in the tongue, palate or nose areas. Sneezing and eye discharges are also seen but they are of a milder nature than those caused by herpesvirus. Sometimes, more severe strains of calicivirus are encountered and these produce a high temperature and transient lameness.

Treatment is as described under **Cat flu**.

Feline enteritis

This serious disease, mainly of young cats, is also known as feline panleucopenia virus, and is related to an equally devastating disease (parvovirus) in dogs. The virus is extremely infectious and very resistant – it can easily survive for up to a year in the environment and it can withstand many common disinfectants. After infection through the mouth or nose, the virus targets rapidly dividing cells in the bone marrow and intestine, laying the cat open to serious secondary infections, since immunity is affected.

Typical symptoms are of extreme lethargy, high temperature, vomiting, diarrhoea and dehydration. Sudden death is possible. Milder forms also exist, when the symptoms may be difficult to detect or only of very short duration. In adult pregnant females, abortion can be caused (as it can with **Feline leukaemia virus**, discussed below).

☎ Urgency

Any kitten or young cat displaying signs similar to those above must be seen quickly, since this disease can be rapidly fatal in its severe form. If vaccination is known to have taken place (i.e. you have an up to date vaccination record card), then feline enteritis is very unlikely to be the cause, nevertheless such symptoms still merit attention as other serious illnesses can cause them.

✚ First aid & nursing

This consists of keeping the cat warm and, if they can be kept down, giving fluids by mouth. Water, glucose or electrolyte replacement drinks (obtainable from veterinary practices) can be used. Give approximately 5–8 mls every hour. The mouth, eyes and nose areas should be kept clean. Most very sick cats require a drip due to severe vomiting and diarrhoea initially, but if recovering can be transferred on to liquidised foods when the vomiting stops.

Thorough nursing hygiene must be practised. The cat should be isolated from others in a 'sick room'. Disposable gloves (and, ideally, apron and shoe covers) should be put on when entering the room and removed before leaving. All soiled bedding materials should be carefully disposed of. A disinfectant effective against parvovirus should be obtained from a veterinary practice and used to clean bowls, litter tray and surrounding areas. Any contaminated areas should be washed in detergent (e.g. washing up liquid), rinsed thoroughly and then have the disinfectant put on them as per the usage instructions. An alternative effective disinfectant is household bleach diluted 1 part bleach to 32 parts water – however note that this may affect some fabrics.

Close attention should be paid to any other unvaccinated cats at risk, and early attention sought if they become lethargic or develop a poor appetite.

Veterinary treatment

- Treatment is only supportive whilst, hopefully, waiting for the body to mount an effective immune response against the virus of feline enteritis. Antibiotics, vitamins and fluid therapy (a drip) are all important, as well as excellent nursing and psychological stimulation for the sick cat. When vomiting is severe, drugs can be given to suppress this.
- A major concern is the development of secondary infections due to the tendency of this virus to attack the bone marrow and white blood cells (the cells which protect the body against infections). This is the reason that antibiotics are often used – they will not eliminate the virus itself, but they can help against bacteria which take advantage of the poor immune defences.
- Very sick kittens with poor prospects may be more kindly put to sleep if recovery seems unlikely and suffering is intense.

🐾 Tip

This disease is easily preventable by vaccination. Vaccination has reduced the incidence of feline enteritis considerably.

However unvaccinated feral or stray kittens, or those from rescue catteries, may still be susceptible.

Related or similar conditions

- **Dehydration**
- **Diarrhoea**
- **Vomiting**

Feline herpes virus

This virus is also known as feline rhino-tracheitis virus, and is one of the viruses which causes the common signs of **Cat flu** (the other is **Feline calicivirus**, see above). The virus is common in the cat population. Herpes virus causes more severe signs than the other flu virus, and cats often show high temperatures, severe sneezing, eye discharges caused by conjunctivitis and a runny nose. Occasionally, problems in the cornea of eye are caused, with corneal ulcers developing.

Treatment is as described under **Cat flu**.

Feline immunodeficiency virus (FIV)

This disease is the cat form of HIV/AIDS although infected cats pose no risk to humans, only to other cats. Males are affected twice as frequently as females, and unneutered tom cats with access to the outdoors are in the highest risk category. Transmission is most commonly through bites and, since entire tom cats are frequently involved in territorial disputes, they are more likely to get bitten than neutered tom cats or females. If an infected cat lives with other cats, there is a risk that these other cats will also be carrying the virus even if they show no signs of illness at the time since cats can harbour this disease for a long period (several years) before any symptoms are seen. FIV is diagnosed most often in middle aged or older cats.

The disease shows itself in various ways. A common symptom is recurring mouth infections and gingivitis (gum inflammation). Other symptoms can include high temperature (fever), respiratory symptoms, depression, weight loss and less specific problems such as chronic diarrhoea. The disease can also affect the eye and brain and anemia is a common finding.

Diagnosis of FIV requires a blood test. In suspect cases, two tests may be taken some weeks apart for a more accurate result. Infected cats live with the virus for several years before becoming terminally ill with this disease. Before that, it is likely that there will be episodes of illness (e.g. high temperature, mouth problems) which require treatment to bring them under control again. At the time when the cat seems to stop responding to medication for these associated infections, and quality of life becomes poor, euthanasia is the kindest option.

☎ Urgency

FIV is not an urgent problem – in fact, a characteristic of the disease is its gradual onset with typical recurring problems which do not respond, or respond only poorly, to medical treatment.

Very ill cats with FIV can become emergencies if problems such as dehydration, respiratory infections or anaemia take hold.

Are my other cats at risk?

If you have a cat which has tested positive for FIV, the first thing to do is have the other cats in the house tested. If they are negative (sometimes confirmed with a repeat test 3 months later), then they are at theoretical risk from the infected cat, especially if any fighting occurs amongst the cats. If fighting does not occur, the risk will be smaller. A vaccine is available in some countries. This does not give total protection, owing to different strains of the virus, however evidence suggests it gives useful protection to cats at risk of the disease. If a vaccine is not available uninfected cats should not share the same food bowls as infected ones.

+ First aid & nursing

Good nursing is vital. Appetite must be tempted (see information given under **Appetite** (**Abnormal**)) and prescription medication given as directed. The mouth, eyes and nose area may need frequent bathing to be kept clean and the cat's demeanour encouraged by interaction with the owner, grooming and playing.

Because the disease is spread from cat-to-cat, an FIV-infected cat should not be allowed to roam outdoors as any fighting may infect other cats. It is fine for a cat to go into an enclosed garden or courtyard, preferably when supervised – indeed, this can be of psychological as well as physical benefit to a sick cat.

Veterinary treatment

- Treatment comprises dealing with secondary 'opportunistic' infections and associated problems. A course of antibiotics may be required, and steroid drugs are also used in many cases to help alleviate symptoms and improve quality of life. If dehydration occurs, fluid therapy in the form of a drip may be needed. Multivitamins may also be prescribed.
- Antiviral drugs such as AZT can be used but are expensive.
- During the later stages of the disease, when problems seem to follow with increasing frequency and appetite and demeanour is poor, consideration about humane **Euthanasia** should take place.

Related or similar conditions

- ▶ **Anemia**
- ▶ **Appetite (abnormal)**
- ▶ **Feline leukaemia virus (FeLV)**
- ▶ **Fever**
- ▶ **Fights**
- ▶ **Gingivitis/stomatitis**

Feline infectious anemia (FIA)

This is a disease caused by a microscopic parasite which enters and destroys red blood cells, the cells responsible for trapping and carrying oxygen around the body. A deficiency of red blood cells is called anemia. The parasite responsible for this infectious form of anemia is called *Mycoplasma haemofelis*. Signs of this disease include poor appetite, lethargy and pale gums. In long standing cases, weight loss may be seen.

Presence of this disease always raises suspicion that another problem affecting the immune system may be present, and in fact feline infectious anemia is commoner in cats suffering from **Feline leukaemia virus** infection. The stressed or deficient immune system of affected cats is unable to fend off the *Mycoplasma* parasite.

The disease is diagnosed by examining the cat and studying a blood sample to look for the tiny parasites inside the red blood cells.

☎ Urgency

This is quite often a chronic disease and cats may be ill for a week or two before diagnosis. However severe symptoms of weakness and collapse always require urgent attention if they were to occur, regardless of the cause.

✚ First aid & nursing

The cat should be kept warm, quiet and stress-free. The appetite should be tempted with appetising foods.

Veterinary treatment

- Antibiotics are given to kill the blood parasites. In severe cases, hospitalisation for a drip, oxygen and even blood transfusion may be required. During recovery, vitamins may be used.
- Additional tests to look for underlying illnesses that may have led on to this condition are often needed. The commonest one is feline leukaemia virus infection (FeLV).

Related or similar conditions

- ▶ **Anemia**
- ▶ **Appetite (abnormal)**
- ▶ **Feline leukaemia virus (FeLV)**

Feline infectious peritonitis (FIP)

This disease is caused by a virus which, in most cats and kittens, usually causes only slight illness, e.g. mild diarrhoea, which clears up after a few days. Feline infectious peritonitis (FIP) results when the infection is much more severe. The reason why some cats develop the illness in this severe way is not entirely clear, but may be related to the functioning of the cat's immune system and to the virulence of the particular virus infecting a cat. Some cats can become carriers of FIP without showing major symptoms themselves, but they may infect other cats who can go on to become very ill.

The disease is almost invariably a fatal one eventually, and results in fluid accumulating in body cavities, e.g. the chest and abdomen, or in granulomas (inflammatory nodules) in vital body organs. Symptoms start off being very vague – the only things shown may be poor appetite, a temperature and reluctance to move around as usual. 'Wet' FIP, with fluid accumulation in the abdomen, results in weight loss, abdominal swelling and progressive illness. Respiratory problems result if fluid accumulates in the chest.

'Dry' FIP – the form which involves granulomas in body organs – usually shows as symptoms relating to the liver, kidneys, brain or eyes. These cats often have recurrent high temperatures, poor appetite, weight loss and low energy levels. Paralysis, fits or incoordination may be caused if the brain is affected.

The diagnosis of this disease is extremely

difficult and usually relies on the presence of a number of suggestive abnormalities on blood and other tests. There is no specific test which can be used (unlike FIV and FeLV for example) so diagnosis usually ends up being a balance of probabilities.

☎ Urgency

As with FIV, this disease is a gradual and progressive one and does not usually result in an urgent situation developing. Most cat owners seek help before their cat deteriorates to the extent when there are breathing problems or life-threatening dehydration. However, brain involvement can result in fits, and in these cases emergency advice would be needed and in some cases the respiratory problems can come on or worsen very suddenly.

✚ First aid & nursing

Good nursing care, with promotion of the appetite, is vital for the cat suffering from suspected FIP. See the advice given under **Appetite** (**Abnormal**), to encourage eating.

A stress-free environment is important. Interaction with the owner, grooming and cleaning of the eyes and face, and gentle exercise or time spent outdoors in good weather can all help to boost morale. Prescription drugs should be given as advised. Make sure there is easy access to a litter tray and that the cat can rest in a comfortable room temperature (neither too hot nor cold).

Veterinary treatment

- This is a very difficult disease, both to diagnose and treat, and tends to pursue a relentless course in most cats. Symptomatic treatment involving antibiotics, steroid drugs and sometimes immune suppressant drugs can offset symptoms to some extent.
- In most cases, **Euthanasia** is required for humane reasons when symptoms become unpleasant.

Related or similar conditions

- ▶ **Appetite (abnormal)**
- ▶ **Breathing problems**
- ▶ **Feline immunodeficiency virus (FIV)**
- ▶ **Feline leukaemia virus (FeLV)**
- ▶ **Fever**
- ▶ **Fits**

Feline leukaemia virus (FeLV)

This is most often a disease of young adult cats and is thought to be the commonest infectious cause of death in this age group. The disease is spread mainly by saliva, though it is also present in urine, faeces and, in lactating cats, milk. The virus targets, and multiplies in, lymphoid tissue in the body, particularly the bone marrow.

Many cats successfully eliminate the virus through an immune response and make a complete recovery. It is the individuals who do not succeed in removing the virus from their body that develop one of a number of associated disease 'syndromes' (collections of symptoms which can vary slightly between cats). Cats or kittens in multi-cat households where FeLV is present can receive exposure to a very large amount of the virus, and infection and disease is much more likely than, say, the individual cat encountering the virus for a short time when outside.

Persistent infection in those cats whose immune systems do not eliminate the virus show several sorts of symptoms:

- **Cancers.** Lymphosarcoma is a form of cancer which has a high occurrence in cats infected with FeLV. There are various forms of this disease, affecting organs such as the thymus (in the chest), the bowel, other lymphoid organs and spleen, and the bone marrow. Symptoms often include weight loss, high temperatures, poor appetite, vomiting and anaemia.
- **Anemia.** This occurs frequently with FeLV, often in conjunction with other symptoms of the disease. Cats with FeLV are prone to **Feline infectious anemia** (see above).
- **Infertility.** FeLV causes loss of developing kittens about half way through pregnancy.
- **Immune system problems.** The virus interferes with the immune system, and makes the cat much more liable to other infections in the same way as FIV does. Infections of the gastrointestinal tract and respiratory system are common; abscesses can occur frequently and simple wounds may not heal well.

FeLV is diagnosed by blood or saliva test. If a positive result is obtained, the test is repeated after 12 weeks to see whether the cat's immune system has coped with the infection – if it has not, another positive result will be given. When two positives are obtained, the cat is persistently infected and at risk for developing associated problems mentioned above.

☎ Urgency

As with the other viral illnesses, FIV and FIP, this disease does not usually show as an urgent problem unless sudden deterioration in respiratory function occurs. Rather, cats will have vague signs of illness which will stretch over a period of a few days to a few weeks, or recurrent infections will be seen and these may take some time to clear up. Eventually, if the cat does not respond as well as expected to routine treatments, suspicion of FeLV may prompt a blood test.

✚ First aid & nursing

As with FIV and FIP, this relies on keeping the cat clean, comfortable, eating and with a positive demeanour. See the advice given under the above sections. Good nursing and home care can make a tremendous difference.

Veterinary treatment

- Supportive treatment is likely to include antibiotics for 'opportunistic' infections as they occur. Dehydrated cats may need fluid therapy (a drip) and other drugs, e.g. vitamins, may be given from time to time. Drugs to lower the temperature may also be used since cats with a fever are usually miserable and reluctant to eat.
- Some of the cancer syndromes can be kept at bay using chemotherapy, however this requires close supervision for potential side-effects and is not suitable in every case.

Tip

FeLV can be prevented by vaccination. First vaccination is usually at 9 weeks old; a second primary vaccine is given 3 weeks later, at 12 weeks, and then once yearly boosters are given after that. Adult cats can be vaccinated too, preferably after a blood test to make sure they are not already harbouring the virus. If the blood test is omitted, the small risk of the cat already being infected has to be accepted.

Related or similar conditions

- **Anemia**
- **Appetite (abnormal)**
- **Cancer**
- **Feline immunodeficiency virus (FIV)**
- **Feline infectious anemia (FIA)**
- **Feline infectious peritonitis (FIP)**
- **Fever**

Fever/high temperature

The body temperature of cats and all other warm blooded animals is kept within narrow limits, normal body temperature of a cat typically being between 38.0–39.2 °C. Complex control mechanisms in the brain and elsewhere maintain temperature at these precise levels. Slight elevations in temperature are not usually significant and can be caused by stress, such as travel or visiting the veterinary practice, but more severe elevations usually have a medical cause. The medical term for fever/high temperature is pyrexia. The opposite problem – that of too low a body temperature – is **Hypothermia**.

Fever can occur for a wide variety of reasons. It is an important and natural response to infections, as it allows aspects of the immune system to function more effectively, thereby helping to eliminate the cause of the fever in the first place. Fever also tends to enforce rest, which is beneficial when the body is fighting an infection. In this sense, fever should not be seen as an abnormality, but instead as a sign of the body coping with an infection in an entirely natural way. Fever does however become a problem when it is prolonged, because then other symptoms such as dehydration can develop.

In cats, common causes of fever include viral or bacterial infections, certain cancers, immune system problems and internal infections occurring in any body organ such as the kidney or bone.

Cats with a high temperature are usually subdued, irritable and have a poor appetite. They may lie still in one place and object to being moved. They probably feel much the same as we do when suffering from a nasty bout of flu, with aching limbs and unpleasant shivery sensations. Uncharacteristic aggression may be shown.

☎ Urgency

In most instances, a routine appointment can be made provided the cat has not gone without food or water intake for more than 24 hours. If other severe symptoms are present, e.g. vomiting, diarrhoea, breathing problems, then urgent advice should be sought. Owners usually do not know if the temperature is raised since measuring it requires the use of a clinical thermometer, and unless this technique has been demonstrated to you, it is best not to attempt to take the temperature of your cat. However the characteristic behavioural response of the cat, as described above, is often fairly accurate. Sometimes the cat may ‘feel hot’, but many cats with a high temperature do not feel at all hot, and cats that seem warm to the touch may in fact have a perfectly normal temperature – touch is generally not a very accurate guide to body temperature in animals.

Hyperthermia/heatstroke

Hyperthermia/heatstroke is when body temperature becomes dangerously high without any infection or other medical problem being present. The commonest cause is a cat trapped in an enclosed space where ambient temperature and humidity are high and from which the cat cannot escape, e.g. a car. Hyperthermia can also occur during prolonged fits, due to the internal heat generated by excessive muscular contractions.

First aid action involves cooling by pouring or spraying cold water on the cat and the use of cool air fans. The cat can be placed in a carrier/cage in which bags of frozen food are placed. Veterinary advice is needed because complications can arise after hyperthermia.

+ First aid & nursing

Quiet rest is important so let the cat settle in a suitable place. Water and glucose solution should be available and a small amount of tempting food can be left close by, but many cats with a high temperature refuse to eat for 24–48 hours. Ensure no disturbance from children or other animals. Bathing the forehead and paw areas with cold water can be comforting for the cat, but if any handling is resented, it is best to simply leave the patient alone. A cool air fan nearby may be appreciated. Leave a litter tray nearby also.

Veterinary treatment

- Measurement of the core body temperature using a clinical thermometer confirms whether there is a fever.
- Drugs may be given to help bring the temperature down. Antibiotics may be used when bacterial infection is suspected or to prevent bacterial complications of viral illnesses.
- Dehydrated animals with a fever will require fluid therapy (a drip) and hospitalisation.
- For cases of recurrent fever, a wide variety of tests may be needed to find out the cause. Many cases are caused by the feline viruses mentioned earlier in this section (FIV, FIP and FeLV), but other problems can also result in fever and a few cats are diagnosed with 'fever of unknown origin' when, despite tests, no underlying cause can be found.

Related or similar conditions

- ▶ **Abscess**
- ▶ **Aggression**
- ▶ **Cat flu**
- ▶ **Feline immunodeficiency virus (FIV)**
- ▶ **Feline infectious peritonitis (FIP)**
- ▶ **Feline leukaemia virus (FeLV)**

Fights

Cat fights occur frequently, especially in neighbourhoods where there are a number of feline residents roaming around at night. Undoubtedly, the worst culprits for fighting are unneutered tom cats, most of whom are constantly in scrapes and have many scars from fighting. However neutered males and females may also indulge in territorial disputes and when a new cat enters the neighbourhood, rearrangement of the pecking order may result in an outbreak of squabbles.

The injuries from fighting are mainly bite wounds, which can form abscesses. Painful inflammation of muscles (cellulitis) can also occur. Affected cats are likely to be miserable, grumpy, off their food and with a high temperature. Bitten areas of the body may be painful and swollen and lameness will occur if the legs were affected. Abscesses can burst and discharge pus to the surface.

More seriously, infectious diseases can be transmitted by bites, especially **Feline immunodeficiency virus** (FIV) and **Feline leukaemia virus** (FeLV), discussed above.

For more details see also under **Abscess** and **Bites**.

Fireworks

The bangs and hissing noises caused by fireworks can be terrifying to many cats. When possible, keep the cat indoors around Guy Fawkes night. This does not, however, escape the problem of fireworks being let off well before and after 5 November, or at other times of the year.

☎ Urgency

It is best for cats to remain in their home environment and vets are likely to give advice along the lines of that outlined below.

+ First aid & nursing

Allowing the cat to find a secure hiding place, reassurance, and playing television, radio or music can all help – as can the presence of another animal which is not bothered by the noises. Some cats benefit from owner interaction; others are best left alone.

Veterinary treatment

- There are not really any drugs which work reliably for this problem in cats.
- In dogs, this sort of fear anxiety can be successfully treated using audio CDs which gradually decondition the dog to the fear response. Veterinary input is also needed. This can also be tried for cats although cats seem more prone to take themselves off somewhere to hide and sit out the episodes.

Related or similar conditions

► **Anxiety/fear**

Fits

Fits may also be referred to as convulsions or seizures, which essentially describe the same thing. There is no doubt that any animal or human having a fit presents an alarming sight to the observer, especially the first time it is witnessed. When owners experience their pet having a fit, they are often in considerable distress and feel helpless. It is important to realise, however, that despite the appearance the animal is not in severe pain – rather, normal control and organisation of body movements is completely disrupted producing the chaotic state of a fit or convulsion. In most cases, the animal is probably unaware of what is going on.

The cause of these dramatic symptoms is

brain malfunction for any one of a number of reasons. The chemistry and electrical functioning of the brain is somehow disrupted and normal control mechanisms are lost – it is rather like a computer going awry, except the brain is much more complex then even the most powerful computer. Some common causes of fits include **Poisoning**, **Brain damage**, **Epilepsy**, heatstroke (see **Fever**), **Diabetes**, severe **Liver** or **Kidney disease** and **Infections**.

Cats having fits may show any or all of the following features:

- Disorientated appearance, restless pacing and apparent vision disturbances ('doesn't seem to be seeing properly')
- Incoordination and 'drunken' staggery gait
- Unable to stand upright, falling to one side or circling
- Loss of consciousness
- Rapid paddling movements of the legs while lying on the side
- Head drawn back on neck
- Salivation
- Severe body twitches and spasms ('throwing themselves around')
- Passing urine or faeces involuntarily.

Which of these symptoms are shown depends on the severity of the fit and its underlying cause.

Most fits stop after 5–10 minutes but those caused by certain problems (e.g. poisoning) may persist indefinitely and pose a threat to life.

☎ Urgency

Any protracted fit is an urgent situation since complications associated with oxygen deprivation to the brain can occur. Advice should be sought immediately and, even for very short fits which pass over quickly, advice is still required since the fit could recur or could reflect some underlying problem which needs diagnosis.

✚ First aid & nursing

It is important to stay calm. Additional noise, excitement or panic can prolong the fit by giving the cat more sensory stimulation. Take the following action:

1. Switch off television, radio or music and remove frightened children from the room.
2. Switch off or dim the room lights.
3. Note the time.
4. Observe the cat carefully to make sure he does not get caught up under furniture or roll towards fires, etc.
5. If the fit lasts for more than 15 minutes, call a vet for advice immediately.

After a fit it is normal for the cat to be disorientated and restless for several hours. Some cats immediately sleep; others may appear hungry. It is okay to give some food at this point.

If the cat has never had a fit before, seek advice from a vet. If the cat is known to have fits, record the date, time and duration in your 'fit diary' so that medication, etc. can be adjusted if needed after discussion with your vet.

Veterinary treatment

- It is important to try to find a cause for the fit, and this may entail a wide variety of tests such as blood tests, X-rays and scans. Poisonings are quite

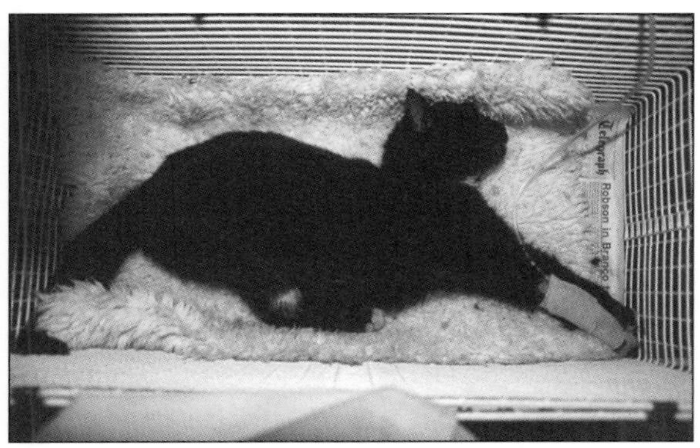

Cat recovering from fits in a padded cage.

common in cats, e.g. after overdosing with flea control products, and these are treated by heavy sedation, fluid therapy (a drip) and oxygen if needed.

- On-going fits can often be controlled by sedative medication; it may not be possible to eliminate the fits completely, but their frequency and severity may be able to be reduced.
- Overall, fits are much less common in cats compared to dogs.

Tip

Owners of young, unneutered female cats sometimes think their pet is having a fit when the cat displays signs of **Oestrus** (heat). When in season, female cats may roll around on their back, yowl and make strange arching movements with the back and legs. There is however no loss of consciousness and they can normally be diverted from the action – which is not possible with fits.

Related or similar conditions

- **Brain damage**
- **Oestrus**
- **Poisoning**

Fleas

Cat fleas are the commonest external parasite found on domestic cats. Many skin problems are caused or made worse by the presence of fleas. Fleas are just visible to the naked eye as small, brownish parasites that jump quickly.

The cat flea, *Ctenocephalides felis*, is very common on dogs too (more so than the dog flea, *Ctenocephalides canis*). Dogs may show more itchiness and scratching than cats. People can also be bitten by cat fleas (often around the ankles). The adult flea spends a lot of time on the host, but larval fleas are in the environment (the house), and modern, carpeted and centrally heated houses provide the ideal environment for year-round flea life cycles. This makes treating the house just as important as treating the animal when trying to get rid of fleas. Using good quality products, it should be easy to eliminate fleas from your cat, dog and house.

Although many cats tolerate a low number of fleas without problems it is generally recommended that treatment is carried out if any evidcence of fleas is seen on your cat. It is not always necessary to see live fleas on a cat in order to diagnose a flea problem. Flea dirt provides an equally convincing diagnosis, and one can say with absolute certainty that fleas are around if specks of flea dirt are found in the coat.

In those cats which are extremely sensitive to fleas – the condition of flea allergic dermatitis (FAD) or flea bite hypersensitivity (FBS) – it may not be possible even to find flea dirt, but often flea treatment is recommended for any skin problems since these patients are usually displaying a hypersensitive reaction to a miniscule allergic stimulus – just maybe one or two flea bites. This is analogous to people with peanut allergies and the like – tiny quantities of the substance can produce severe reactions in the body.

Fleas generally cause itching and hair loss. When severe, the itching can induce serious self-trauma to the skin, resulting in bald, sore and flaky skin, with secondary infections setting in. Sometimes, only the pet dog shows these signs – the cat appears fine. This confusing situation emphasises the need to treat *all* animals in the house. Some animals can act as a reservoir of infection, not showing many signs themselves, but continually reinfecting those other pets (dogs or cats) with more sensitive skins.

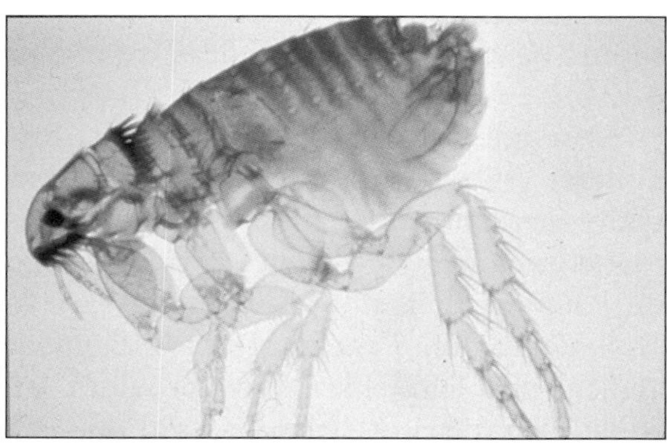

The ubiquitous cat flea, highly magnified.

☎ Urgency

The problem is a non-urgent one and a routine appointment should be obtained. Meanwhile, follow the guidance given under first aid below.

+ First aid & nursing

If you see fleas or flea dirt, or if this has been diagnosed, it is important to follow a thorough and safe procedure for ridding the house and animals of fleas. Although it is possible to buy products 'over the counter' in supermarkets, pet stores and other places, a clinic check by a vet or vet nurse is advisable. A veterinary examination also allows drugs to be prescribed for secondary skin infections and irritations, which will keep the cat comfortable whilst the flea control products are working.

Safety is an important issue. There is a temptation to repeat doses of products that do not seem to have been effective, or perhaps to try another type of product. Many cats suffer from cumulative toxicities when inappropriate doses or combinations of product have been applied in this way in far too short a space of time. Individually, the products are probably safe enough but, because they are sometimes not successful in removing fleas, owners may be inclined to try again. The worst cases are when owners try first with a shampoo, then flea powder and then perhaps a flea collar or 'spot-on' preparation, all in the space of a few days. Severe problems can arise due to absorption of these products into the body, resulting in toxicities and even fits.

The best first aid action for fleas is *not* to apply anything on to the cat. Do not wash the coat either – this could remove useful clues as to the skin disorder. Instead, vacuum the house, dispose of the vacuum bag, wash all pet bedding and use a proprietary house spray according to the instructions. Make a veterinary nurse check appointment for the cat and collect flea control products for all animals in the house at that time. Until that time, use of a flea comb is recommended.

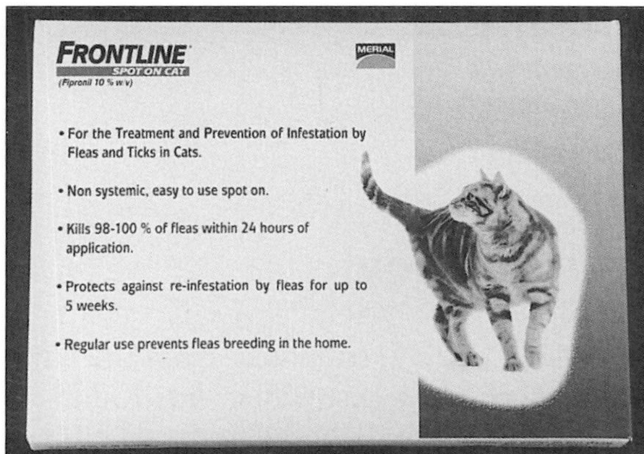

A wide variety of flea control products are available, with spot-on preparations being very popular. Flea powders and aerosol sprays are not recommended for cats

Veterinary treatment

- Flea control uses prescription products which are either sprayed (pump-action, not aerosol) on to the cat, applied on to the skin by dropper from a plastic vial, injected under the skin or given by mouth in tablet form. It is very important that the correct dose is given (often, the cat must be weighed), that this is repeated only at stated intervals, and that no other flea control product is used in conjunction (e.g. flea collars, shampoos). Environmental (house) treatment is also required.
- Skin problems caused by the intense itch and scratching may also need attended to. Antibiotics and/or short course of anti-inflammatory steroid drugs are often used to alleviate the discomfort.
- Shampoos may be soothing but most cats do not enjoy being bathed. If shampooing is used, a mild hypoallergenic shampoo should be used (not a flea shampoo), and this should be carried out before the application of any products on to the cat's skin.

Tip: Checking for flea dirt

This is easiest on white cats or on white patches of coat. Using a flea comb or your fingers, part the hair so that you can see down to the skin surface. The best place to look is along the back towards the tail area. Flea dirt consists of small dark specks of granular material near the skin. Pick some up and place on moistened cotton wool or white paper. If the black material blots out a reddish colour, you have the diagnosis. The red colour is because the dirt consists of digested blood from your cat.

Related or similar conditions

- **Mange mites**
- **Ringworm**
- **Skin problems**
- **Tapeworm**

Food allergy

Food allergies tend to show as skin or digestive system symptoms, sometimes both. The cat may have an itchy skin or localised rashes. Digestive symptoms include diarrhoea and, less frequently, vomiting. Overall, food allergies are not common and other causes of these symptoms tend to be investigated first.

Food allergies are usually to proteins in the diet and, unfortunately, it can be extremely difficult to isolate which protein or proteins are causing the problem. Commercial pet foods contain a wide variety of protein sources and flavours labelled as 'chicken', 'tuna', 'duck' etc. also contain other protein sources as well, so it is probably impossible to prove a food allergy using commercially prepared foods.

The diagnostic technique used is exacting and involves use of a specific exclusion diet which must be fed for a prolonged period of time (e.g. several months). If the symptoms improve during this time, then recur when the cat is switched back on to normal food, and are then corrected again by a further return to the exclusion diet, a food allergy can be assumed. Identifying the specific foods involved requires further detective work.

☎ Urgency

This is not an urgent problem. Investigating it takes, literally, months. Many owners find it difficult and frustrating, however it can be worth all the effort if a true allergy is operating.

✚ First aid & nursing

The principles of an exclusion diet, outlined above, must be understood and followed by everyone in the household. One person giving treats could spoil the whole test! Exclusion diets should only be carried out on veterinary advice.

Veterinary treatment

- Exclusion diets are described in principle above. It is best if no other medication is given at this time, otherwise one is never sure what is contributing to any positive effects seen. Sometimes, in severe cases of itching, antihistamines may be prescribed; these are fairly innocuous compared to other drugs.

Related or similar conditions

- ▶ **Allergy**
- ▶ **Diarrhoea**
- ▶ **Skin problems**
- ▶ **Vomiting**

Foreign body

A 'foreign body' is an object from the environment or elsewhere which has found its way into the cat's body and, usually, is causing some problems. Common examples of foreign bodies encountered in cats are:

- **Needles** that have been swallowed after cats have been playing with wool or thread. If unattached to the thread, these often (surprisingly) pass right through the digestive system without causing any problems, although monitoring of their progress by X-ray is advised and a short anaesthetic may be needed for safe removal at the end of their journey at the anal area. If the thread or wool is still attached, it becomes a much more serious prospect: surgery is often needed as the linear nature of the thread or wool can cause major bowel damage due to the bowel adopting a 'concertina' effect over the strand.
- **Airgun pellets** from cats that have been shot (see **Airgun injury**).
- **Other swallowed objects** – these can be many and various, from stones to wedding rings. Most need to be removed surgically.

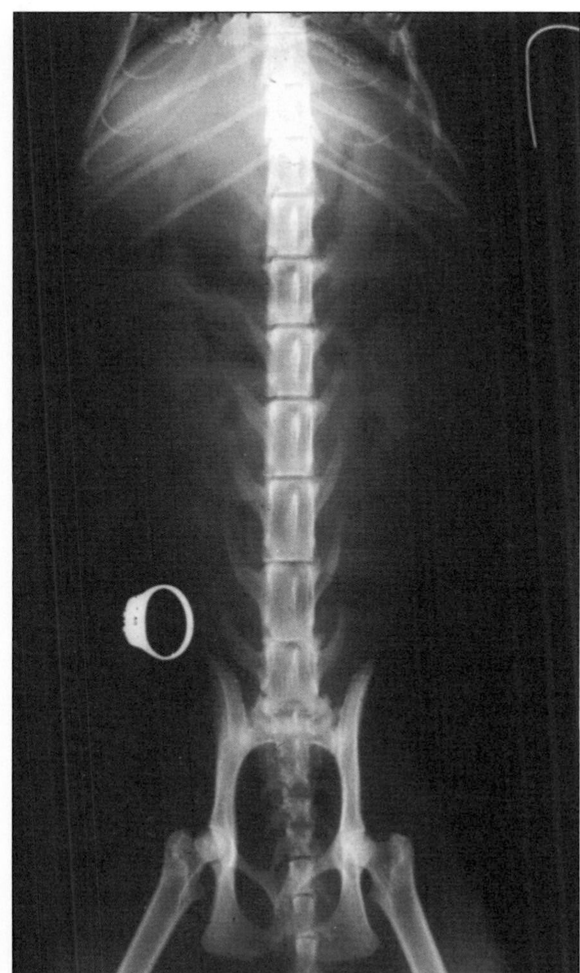

This cat swallowed a ring which was partly obstructing the small intestine.

- **Grass seeds** – these may be found in the ear, nose or throat areas where they cause intense irritation. Anaesthesia is often needed to allow removal.
- **Tooth fragments** – a problem in fighting cats, especially unneutered males. They may be found in wounds or under the skin surface and can occasionally cause chronic discharging wounds.
- **Pieces of glass, wood, etc.** – occasionally in the paws, though not nearly so commonly as in dogs. These can be troublesome to find because they may be very small, yet can be responsible for quite severe lameness and pain.

☎ Urgency

Foreign bodies can be the cause of sudden, severe signs (e.g. an airgun injury affecting important organs, a grass seed becoming stuck in the ear) or else grumbling chronic ones (e.g. tiny fragment of glass lodged in foot pad). Foreign bodies affecting the bowel can lead on to severe vomiting, causing dehydration and upsets in body chemistry. In severe cases, bowel rupture and life-threatening peritonitis can occur. The urgency therefore depends on the symptoms shown, and on the degree of distress exhibited by the cat. Breathing irregularities, persistent vomiting or severe pain all merit immediate attention.

+ First aid & nursing

It is tempting to try to remove foreign bodies if you can see them. Certainly, if you see a grass seed protruding from the ear or nose, or spot a fragment of glass in a foot pad, there is no harm in gently trying to release it if the cat will tolerate this.

However if thread or wool is spotted protruding from the mouth or anus, on no account should this be pulled, however tempting it may be to do so. Severe internal damage can quite easily result. Instead, seek help immediately as a general anaesthetic is likely. A vet will assess the situation and decide on the safest means of removal of the object without risking internal organ damage.

Persistently discharging wounds can be

bathed with tepid salty water (1 teaspoon to a pint [560 ml]) until attended to. Quite often, the reason for a chronic discharge like this is a foreign body embedded in the wound, preventing normal healing.

Veterinary treatment

- Anaesthesia and surgery are quite often needed for foreign body removal, no matter where they are. Provided removal can be accomplished safely, and organ damage is not severe, most cats recover well.
- A serious form of obstruction is caused by linear foreign bodies (string, wool, fishing line, cassette tape, etc). This is quite common in cats, who often like to play with these things. When swallowed, the linear object may become trapped around the base of the tongue at one end. The other end passes on down the digestive system into the bowel, which then tends to 'creep up' the line in a concertina fashion because of the natural bowel undulations and movements. A cheesewire effect can then occur as the material tightens, with severe bowel damage resulting. Most linear foreign bodies of this type require major surgery for safe removal.

Related or similar conditions

- ▶ **Airgun injury**
- ▶ **Appetite (abnormal)**
- ▶ **Vomiting**

Fractures/dislocations

Most bone fractures are caused by traumatic accidents such as road traffic

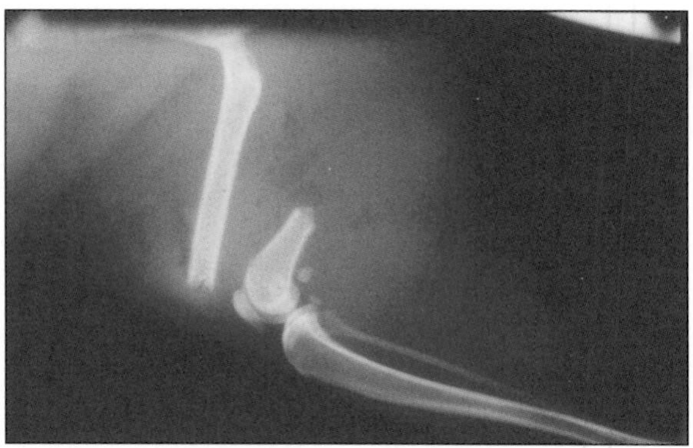

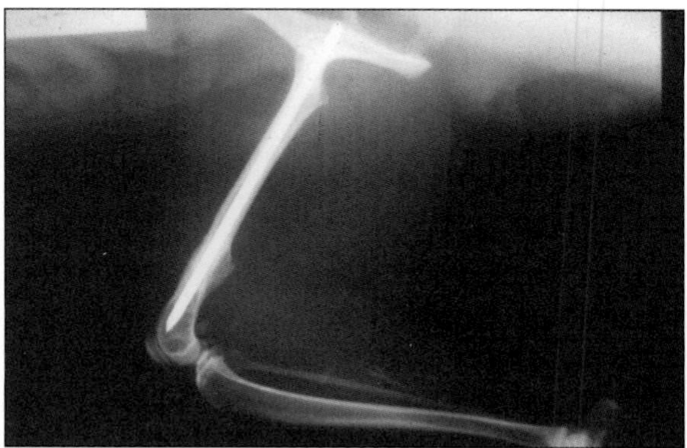

X-rays of a cat's hind leg showing fracture of the femur (thigh bone) and repair using a metal bone pin. The cat had been hit by a car.

accidents and falls. Bones will also break when badly diseased by infection or bone tumours – these, though, are much rarer than other types of fracture. Bone is remarkably strong for its weight and fracture requires considerable force. Depending on the stresses put on the bone, the fracture may be simple (two pieces) or complex (many fragments). If the bone breaks through the skin surface (an open or compound fracture), risks of infection are superimposed on the problem of the fracture itself.

Common bones that are fractured in cats

are the femur (leg bone), tibia (shin bone), humerus (arm bone) and radius/ ulna (forearm bones). The pelvis is very commonly fractured in cats that have been in road accidents. Fractures of any of the other bones, such as the skull or vertebrae, are also possible, but these are seen less commonly than the above.

Dislocation refers to the problem that occurs when a joint becomes distorted such that the normal arrangement of the bones of the joint is lost. Like fractures, the usual cause is severe trauma or incoordinated movement. Dislocations are often accompanied by ligament rupture and, sometimes, fractures of adjacent bones. Common dislocations in the cat are of the hip joint and the tail bones, but any other joint, e.g. elbow, shoulder, could also be dislocated if appropriate forces are put across it

Signs of a fracture or dislocation include reluctance or inability to walk, lameness of varying degree (from slight limp to complete carrying of the leg) and abnormal angulation of the affected limb. When the injured bone or joint is felt, it may show crepitus –abnormal grating of the displaced bone ends. Cats with fractures or dislocations are also often in pain and may protect or guard the injured area and show aggression.

☎ Urgency

If you suspect a fracture, the cat should be assessed urgently. The reason is that any injury sufficient to cause a bone fracture could also easily have led to hidden internal damage of the chest and abdomen – and this is more serious and immediately life-threatening than the fracture itself. Cats involved in road accidents or other trauma are also susceptible to shock – a serious and life-threatening medical problem. Relief of pain caused by the fracture should also be started as soon as possible.

Quite often, very lame cats turn out to have bite injuries and cellulitis (muscle/ tissue inflammation) rather than bone fractures. However, in the first aid situation there is no way of knowing this unless you see actual bite marks near the injured area. The lameness in each case can appear just the same.

✚ First aid & nursing

Follow the advice given under **Accident** if the cat is collapsed and needs resuscitation after a serious accident.

For the fracture itself, it is usually best not to attempt to apply any form of splint or bandage. Any manipulation of the leg will be extremely sore and a splint improperly applied can lead to the leg being fixed in a very uncomfortable position. Instead, allow the cat to adopt a posture which brings it most comfort. Quite often, cats will choose to lie on the fractured leg – this itself splints the leg against the firmer surface below and can bring considerable relief from pain, so do not be worried if you see this happening.

Put the cat into a well padded cat carrier or cage for transportation to the veterinary practice. If lifting or moving the cat is difficult, wear stout gloves or wrap the cat (including head) in a thick blanket and lift firmly. Small wounds are not important at this stage but larger, heavily bleeding wounds must be attended to. See **Bleeding**.

Veterinary treatment

- Initial treatment may be for shock, and

treatment of the fracture or dislocation itself will be a lower priority, as this is not life-threatening. Hospitalisation, fluid therapy (a drip), oxygen and, if needed, surgery for such internal problems as ruptured bladder may be required. It is not unusual for fracture treatment to be deferred for several days after a serious accident, to allow the cat's system to recuperate before major surgery is embarked upon.

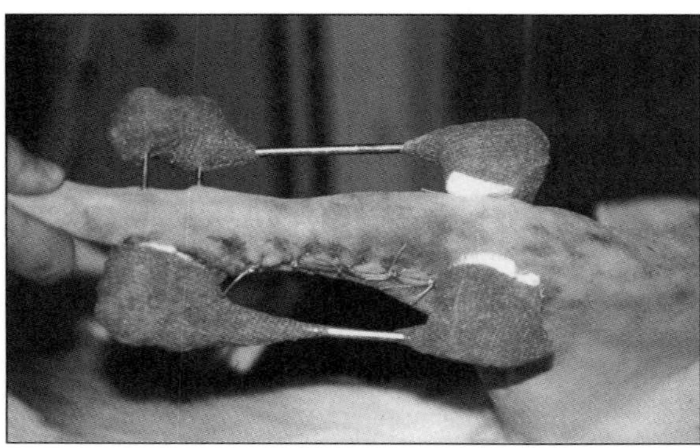

Serious leg fracture being treated using an external fixator frame.

- Fracture treatment depends on the location and type of fracture. Most pelvic fractures respond well to cage rest for 6–8 weeks, coupled with pain relief and good nursing. Fractures of limb bones are often treated using surgery, when metal devices such as pins or external fixation frames hold the bone ends together while they heal. Plaster of Paris casts are now used less frequently in animals since other methods often prove more satisfactory for various reasons.
- Fracture healing depends on the age of animal, complexity of the fracture and success of the repair technique. Most fractures have shown good signs of healing by 12 weeks unless there are complications.
- Dislocations may be able to be replaced under general anaesthesia. If instability is a problem, surgery can be needed to improve the function of the joint.

Related or similar conditions

- ▶ **Accident**
- ▶ **Bleeding**
- ▶ **Pain**
- ▶ **Shock**

Fur ball

Fur ball or hair ball is the accumulation of hair in the stomach following grooming, when the hair is swallowed by the cat. It can sometimes result in symptoms of mild gastritis (inflammation/irritation of the stomach lining) with poorish appetite and intermittent vomiting until the hair is regurgitated or passes on through the digestive system. Colic symptoms and irritability are also sometimes seen. Usually the hair is eventually brought up in a tangled matt of hair mixed with saliva and deposited on the carpet.

It can be a problem with certain skin disorders, especially fleas, when the cat licks or grooms itself excessively, and so swallows large amounts of hair. Long haired cats may be more prone to it, as may cats that indulge in overgrooming for nervous/behavioural reasons.

☎ Urgency

Fur ball is a non-urgent condition. It often resolves by itself or after simple treatment (see below). However you shouldn't assume that vomiting in a cat is automatically due to fur ball. Vomiting is a common, and sometimes serious, symptom of many diseases.

If your cat has had fur ball in the past, is bright and alert and otherwise his normal self and is only vomiting once or twice daily, then it is likely to be the same thing again. Keep a watch for any worsening or other symptoms and arrange a routine check up if worried.

✚ First aid & nursing

Symptoms usually stop once the hair has been regurgitated. Giving proprietary hair ball treatments (e.g. 'Katalax') or small amounts of liquid paraffin (1–2 mls) daily for several days often helps in removal or passage of the hair ball. It does tend to recur, but not usually for several months. Grooming the cat more will reduce the quantities of loose hair that are actually swallowed.

Some cats have mild colicky symptoms which are associated with the stomach irritation – they may resent their abdomen being touched or palpated and may be generally grumpy.

Veterinary treatment

- Only rarely is surgery needed for this problem, when perhaps very large accumulations of hair are causing persistent problems. Most cats succeed in getting rid of the hair 'little and often' by regurgitating it.

Related or similar conditions

- ▶ **Appetite (abnormal)**
- ▶ **Colic**
- ▶ **Vomiting**

Fur mite

This is a parasite, much less common than fleas, that typically produces a dry scaly coat with copious quantities of dandruff. The condition is often called 'walking dandruff' because if the cat is brushed on to a dark sheet of paper, some of the dandruff/scale may appear to 'walk'! Actually, these moving objects are the mites themselves which live and feed on the skin surface.

Symptoms are usually fairly mild, although a few cats react more severely and some people are sensitive to them and develop a rash on the arms.

Treatment is along the same lines as for **Fleas**.

G

Gangrene

Gangrene is a very serious form of infection which is a potential problem whenever there is major tissue damage, especially near the extremities of the body, e.g. tail tip, feet and toes. It results when blood circulation is impaired so that body tissue dies off and then becomes susceptible to a progressive bacterial infection. This infection spreads to affect adjacent tissue, causing a worsening pain and fever. Affected skin areas are usually dark and with an unpleasant odour. The cat may appear seriously ill.

Common situations which can lead to tissue death and gangrene involve things such as accidental (by young children) or even malicious placement of elastic bands or ties around cats' legs or tails, cutting off the circulation of blood. Any trapping of an extremity such that circulation is cut off for a prolonged period of time (e.g. in a trap or snare) has the same effect. Neglected or soaked bandages which tighten up and constrict the leg are also potential causes, and is one of the reasons why cats with bandaged limbs or limbs in plaster or resin casts should *always* be kept indoors for supervision.

Neglected wounds may also on occasion develop gangrene, especially in debilitated cats.

☎ Urgency

The situation is an urgent one and emergency attention should be sought. This is necessary not only to try to save as much tissue as possible, but also to limit the general effects of the gangrene on the whole body of the cat, since toxaemia (blood poisoning) is a life-threatening risk.

✚ First aid & nursing

In most cases, attention to the wound and attempted removal of any constricting material (e.g. rubber band) is best not attempted, unless it is very obvious that this can be achieved easily and safely, as emergency attention should be given and removal is best carried out under controlled circumstances (e.g. under anaesthetic).

If the cat is trapped in wire, netting or other material, cut enough to free the cat in order to allow lifting and transportation. Removal of the rest of the material is again best probably done under professional supervision unless interference with breathing is being caused.

Veterinary treatment

- This involves wound treatment, surgical excision of damaged and dead tissue, and antibiotics and nursing care. The extent of the damaged tissue may be larger than it first appears.

Related or similar conditions

- ▶ **Accident**
- ▶ **Pain**
- ▶ **Wounds**

Gastritis

Gastritis means inflammation of the lining of the stomach. This is a very common condition in dogs, slightly less so in cats. The stomach lining can be irritated by unsuitable foods, scavenging and, particularly in cats, physical irritation from feathers, fur balls etc. The usual symptom is vomiting in the absence of other major signs of illness.

Gastritis can occasionally be present in association with other more serious diseases such as **Kidney disease**, **Poisoning** and inflammatory bowel disease. Usually, other symptoms would also be present.

☎ Urgency

Simple gastritis causes infrequent vomiting in an otherwise healthy and alert cat. A routine appointment should be obtained. If the vomiting worsens and is more frequent (more than 4 times daily) seek advice sooner.

✚ First aid & nursing

Feed a light diet (e.g. cooked chicken/rice; cooked fish/rice) to allow the stomach to settle. If your cat is prone to fur/hair ball, giving a **Fur Ball** treatment or liquid paraffin can help.

Veterinary treatment

- For simple gastritis, no treatment may be needed other than that outlined above. If the gastritis is thought to be related to another problem, then additional tests may be called for.
- Frequent or chronic vomiting is always viewed seriously as it usually means a more serious condition is present.

Related or similar conditions

- ▶ **Enteritis**
- ▶ **Fur ball**
- ▶ **Vomiting**

Gingivitis/stomatitis

Gingivitis (gum inflammation) and stomatitis (mouth inflammation) are major problems in cats, and have a variety of causes. The simplest one is bad teeth caused by accumulation of plaque or loosening of decayed teeth – this can usually be cleared up quickly with appropriate dental treatment under general anaesthetic. See under **Mouth problems**.

However, gingivitis can also be a symptom of other diseases in cats. It is commonly seen in cats suffering from **Feline immunodeficiency virus** (FIV) and some other viral diseases, especially **Feline leukaemia virus** (FeLV) and **Feline calicivirus**. In fact, it is an important marker for the first two diseases. Many other general diseases, such as **Kidney disease**, can cause mouth/gum inflammation and ulceration, and cats can also show this symptom in the absence of any other diagnosed diseases, i.e. cause unknown. There is no doubt that it can be a frustrating disease to treat and a painful one for the cat to experience.

Cats also suffer from a severe inflammatory condition of the mouth called chronic feline gingivo-stomatitis. The cause is not fully understood and various treatments may be tried. In severe cases, removal of all the teeth may be necessary. This sounds drastic but the disease is highly unpleasant. After tooth removal, cats do very well and have a good quality of life. Other treatments, such as interferon, may be used, though can be expensive.

Common symptoms of gingivitis/stomatitis are poor appetite, pawing at the mouth, drooling and irritability. Poor grooming can also be a symptom, and many cats suffering from gingivitis/stomatitis have bad breath. Examination of the mouth reveals reddened gums with, in severe cases, ulcers and open sores. Such very inflamed gums may bleed easily when touched. Cats may not allow the head area to be handled at all.

☎ Urgency

This is an unpleasant but not life-threatening problem. Seek an early routine appointment since a very sore mouth can lead to dehydration due to lack of food and water intake, and this can be serious in older cats.

✚ First aid & nursing

When the mouth is sore, offer small meals of soft and tempting food, e.g. sardines, chicken, etc. Warming and mashing this up may help stimulate the appetite. Keep the external lip areas clean by bathing gently with warm salty water (1 teaspoon salt to 1 pint [560 ml] warm water) if the cat will tolerate it.

After veterinary treatment, mouth rinses, gels or pastes may be supplied to help treat any underlying problems.

Veterinary treatment

- Efforts will be made to try to establish a cause for the gum or mouth inflammation. This may involve dental examination including X-rays, blood tests (for cat viruses such as FIV and FeLV) and biopsies. In order to examine the mouth and teeth properly, a general anaesthetic is required.
- At its worst, gingivitis/stomatitis is an unpleasant and difficult disease which may be best treated by extensive tooth removal. It is thought that some cats develop an immune reaction to plaque and that removal of this, permanently, is only achievable by tooth extractions. Domestic cats can cope well with no or very few teeth. They may require softer food and help with grooming.

Tip

When starting to use any mouth treatment (including brushing teeth), begin very gradually, spending only a minute or two at a time. Regular short application/ treatment is better then occasional lengthy struggles!

Grooming can help improve demeanour since many of these cats will have stopped grooming themselves due to mouth pain and cats often seem to become depressed when unable to keep themselves clean as normal.

Related or similar conditions

- ► **Feline immunodeficiency virus (FIV)**
- ► **Feline leukaemia virus (FeLV)**
- ► **Mouth problems**

Glands

A gland is a general term which describes a collection of cells which exist to secrete or store a substance. There are many different glands in the body, e.g. those associated with digestion and the hormonal system. Two common ones encountered in everyday cat problems are the anal glands and the lymph glands or (more correctly termed) lymph *nodes*. During routine examination, vets often check the lymph nodes. Easily located nodes appear in the throat area, in front of the shoulders and in the hamstring area of the back legs. Enlargement of lymph nodes usually indicates infection in a nearby area; if many lymph nodes are enlarged a form of spreading cancer may be suspected. Health problems in cats which may involve glands include: **Anal glands**, **Cancer**, and **Diabetes**.

Glaucoma

Glaucoma is a serious condition that usually results in blindness and is a common cause for removing an eye. It results when pressure builds up in the eye, destroying the internal structures of vision and causing severe pain. In animals, glaucoma tends to be diagnosed much later on in the course of the disease than in people (since pets cannot report the subtle early symptoms of the disease to us), hence the problem is often very advanced at the time of diagnosis.

Cats cope very well with one eye and it is more humane to remove a chronically painful eye than leave it in place. See also **Eye problems**.

Granulomas

A granuloma is an area of inflammation. In cats, the term is often used to describe red, moist and angry-looking hairless patches on the lips or skin surface. Various terms are used, including eosinophilic granuloma, indolent ulcer and rodent ulcer, to describe these patches. Ulcers usually occur on the lip areas, whereas patches or plaques can occur anywhere on the skin surface. The skin plaques tend to be itchy and can be quite extensive and unsightly.

The cause of these problems is not fully understood. In some cases, allergy (to fleas, food constituents or pollens) may be involved.

☎ Urgency

The problem is not an urgent one, but does tend to progress over the course of several weeks. In cats that have had them before, early treatment can help reduce the severity of recurrences.

✚ First aid & nursing

Flea treatment should be carried out (see under **Fleas**), as this may be important in those cats with granulomas on the skin surface. If the cat is making the situation worse by excessive licking or scratching, a 'buster' collar should be fitted until treatment is received.

Veterinary treatment

- Prescription flea treatment is important in all cases as this can help to reduce the 'allergic load' in cats that are perhaps suffering from multiple hypersensitivities.
- Cats prone to pollen allergies could be

kept indoors during months when plants are in flower. This is obviously not a very satisfactory solution and should only be used when a pollen allergy has been definitely proven by specialised skin tests, otherwise the cat's quality of life could be adversely affected.

- Food allergies are also difficult to prove but, if present, may be important in these conditions.
- The main line of treatment involves using drugs, surgery or other techniques to suppress the inflammatory lesions. This often means the use of steroid drugs, although patches on the lips may respond to cryotherapy (freezing), laser treatment or conventional surgery to remove the inflammatory area. If used, the aim is always to get on to the minimum effective dose of steroids to keep symptoms at bay whilst avoiding side effects.

Related or similar conditions

- ▶ **Fleas**
- ▶ **Food allergy**
- ▶ **Skin problems**

Grass eating

Grass eating is entirely normal in cats, and sometimes leads on to retching or vomiting, often resulting in the production of a fur ball. Take care however that houseplants are not eaten – as well as being bad for the plants, some of these may be toxic (e.g. leopard lilly). If your cat seems to want to eat lots of plants, buying and growing 'kitty grass' from a pet store, and leaving this out for the cat, should provide a more palatable option.

Grazes

Grazes are superficial skin injuries in which the top layer of the skin is removed, causing bleeding. They often occur in association with more severe injuries of a road traffic accident, so you should observe your cat carefully for anything else that may be worrying if you do notice a graze anywhere.

Although they are not deep, grazes can be painful as there are sensitive nerve endings in the top layers of the skin.

☎ Urgency

By themselves, grazes are not urgent. Blood loss is minor and soon stops.

✚ First aid & nursing

Bathing can help, though it is not usually necessary to apply any form of dressing or wound covering unless the graze exposes underlying bone (in which case veterinary attention should be sought). Bathe in saline (1 teaspoon salt to 1 pint [560 ml] water).

Grazes heal quickly by granulation, i.e. a scab covering forms and then flakes off when the skin underneath has regenerated.

Veterinary treatment

- Grazes do not usually require much treatment unless there is infection or exposure of underlying bone. Dressings may occasionally be used for the deeper grazes. If licking by the cat is intense, a 'buster' collar may be recommended.

Related or similar conditions

- **Accident**
- **Bleeding**
- **Wounds**

Grief

See under **Bereavement**.

Grooming (poor)

Poor grooming results in an unkempt coat, with mats often appearing on the surface hair. In long haired cats these mats can become enormous and very thick, causing severe skin problems underneath due to build up of heat and humidity. In the perineal area (under the tail) matted hair is dangerous due to the contamination that is possible from faeces and urine, and consequent risks of infection and even fly strike in summer months (when flies lay eggs in the area, which hatch into larvae which can then eat the flesh causing horrendous damage).

Most healthy cats groom themselves adequately. If grooming is not occurring, there may be a reason. Common ones are:

- **Pain** from **Arthritis** of the spine or other joints. Often, the area of the central back is not groomed as it is too painful for the cat to reach round here. This is common in elderly cats. Pain from bad teeth or severe gum inflammation or mouth ulcers may also stop grooming.
- **Obesity.** Overweight cats do not groom properly due to physical problems reaching all their skin surface area. Their skin and general coat health is also likely to be poor.
- **Other diseases.** Cats chronically ill for various reasons may give up grooming. Regular gentle grooming of the sick cat is an important part of nursing care, with physical and psychological benefits.
- **Intolerance in long haired cats.** It is very important to begin grooming long haired cats when they are kittens, and to do this in a calm and gentle way so that they do not develop an aversion to grooming. Otherwise, severe matting can occur, requiring frequent and expensive anaesthetics to de-matt the cat.

Tip

Do not attempt to cut out severe matts, you may accidentally cut the skin. Take the cat to the veterinary practice where clippers can be used and a sedative given if necessary. After clipping, groom regularly with a soft brush and then, when the hair is long enough, a cat comb or your fingers.

Related or similar conditions

For discussion of underlying medical problems often relating to poor grooming, see especially:

- **Arthritis**
- **Gingivitis/stomatitis**
- **Kidney disease**
- **Mouth problems**
- **Obesity**

Growths

Growths are abnormal lumps or bumps appearing on the skin surface, or occurring

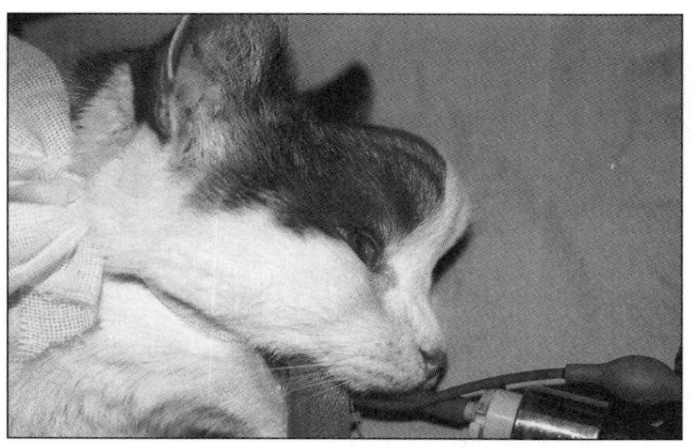

A growth on the head of an older cat. It was benign and did not come back after removal.

underneath the skin but which can be felt through it. They can occur on any part of the body from the nose to tail, and can vary widely in appearance.

It is always safest to have abnormal lumps or bumps checked out by a vet, since obviously they could indicate a tumour or cancer. Many turn out to be harmless but removal is still sometimes needed if they get in the way or get traumatised. For fuller details, see under **Cancer**.

H

Haematoma

Haematoma is the medical term for bleeding that has occurred into a space in the body or into tissue (especially muscle), where, if near the skin surface, it shows as bruising. See under **Blood blister** for full details of the common sites for haematomas in cats. The commonest one is in the ear flap.

Haematuria

Haematuria is the medical term for blood in the urine. This arises because of inflammation, infection or tumours. The commonest causes are inflammation and infection. 'Feline idiopathic cystitis (FIC)', also known as 'feline lower urinary tract disease (FLUTD)' is a very common cause of blood in urine in cats. See under **Cystitis**.

Haemobartonella felis

This is the parasite which causes **Feline infectious anemia**, discussed on page 87. The parasite enters red blood cells, in the process destroying them, and is passed between cats by fleas or other blood-sucking parasites. Many cats with this disease also turn out to have another problem, such as Feline Leukaemia (FeLV), which has weakened the immune system and allowed *Haemobartonella felis* to become established in the first place. (The causing organism is now referred to as *Mycoplasma haemofelis*.)

Haemorrhage

See under **Bleeding**.

Hair ball

See under its other common name, **Fur ball**.

Harvest mites

Harvest mites (*Trombicula autumnalis*), also known as berry bugs, are tiny parasitic larvae, just visible to the naked eye as orange dots. They are a common cause of skin problems and itchiness in late summer and autumn and are often to be found between the toes or in the folds of skin at the sides of the cat's ears (use a magnifying glass). They can cause an intense itch and skin reaction in some cats. Owners are often bothered by them too, especially after a period in the garden when itchiness can occur around the legs or waist.

Treatment is by using mild washes to remove the bugs physically and by applying flea control products under veterinary advice. Some cats with very intense reactions may require antiinflammatory drugs to ease the discomfort. The parasites disappear after the first frosts, which kill them. See also **Skin problems**.

Head tilt

Head tilt is a symptom that can be seen for several reasons, sometimes with additional problems such as incoordination, falling to one side, circling or even inability to stand being present as well as the head tilt.

One relatively simple cause of head tilt is cats in ear irritation or pain, e.g. from ear inflammation (otitis) caused by allergy, infection or ear mites. Something lodged in the ear, such as a grass seed or a growing polyp, will also cause sufficient irritation and discomfort to result in a head tilt, sometimes coupled with frantic shaking of the head and scratching/pawing at the ear. See under **Ear problems** for more details.

Head tilt can also be caused by various problems affecting the brain and nervous system, since the organs and mechanisms of balance can be interfered with, producing the symptoms. A variety of conditions can have this effect, including infections, trauma, poisonings or toxicities and tumours.

Perhaps the commonest cause is 'feline idiopathic vestibular syndrome' – a condition of unknown cause which can affect cats of any age. Symptoms can be severe, with rolling, falling, head tilts and rapid flickering eye movements, all of which come on very suddenly. It can be an alarming condition to witness. However the outlook for recovery is good, with most cats improving after several days and getting back to normal after several weeks. No treatment seems particularly effective, though sometimes sedative drugs may be used. Tests to rule out other problems may be needed.

☎ Urgency

A cat that seems in pain and distress should be assessed urgently as there may be an uncomfortable cause for the problem, e.g. something lodged in the ear. Cats that are very incoordinated usually also receive rapid attention since other problems could be occurring, e.g. fits, which need treated. Most owners find symptoms of imbalance and incoordination alarming in their pets and seek advice quickly.

A slight head tilt and no apparent pain or distress could be checked during a routine appointment.

✚ First aid & nursing

This entails ensuring the cat cannot damage itself when imbalanced by stumbling into fires or down stairs etc. Affected cats are best restricted to one room or even to a cat carrier, cage or box. They are best kept in a quiet place away from too much stimulation in the form of noise, movement or lights.

Do not attempt close examination of the inside of the ear or insert anything into the ear canal. Proper inspection of the ear usually requires an anaesthetic.

Veterinary treatment

- Attempts will be made to find out the

cause of the head tilt by examining the ears, using X-rays and perhaps performing blood tests. For suspected tumours, brain scans (if available) may also be used.

- Treatment depends on what is found. The commonest cause, feline idiopathic vestibular syndrome, does not have a specific line of treatment – the cat is just given time to recover from this condition.

Related or similar conditions

- **Balance (loss of)**
- **Brain damage**
- **Ear problems**
- **Fits**

Heart disease

Overall, heart and circulatory disease is less common in cats than it is in dogs. However cats do have several important heart-related disorders and these are being recognised more frequently as diagnostic methods improve. The problems can start in the heart and go on to affect other body organs or systems (primary heart disease), or else the heart can be affected after disease elsewhere in the body has become established (secondary heart disease).

In cats, symptoms of heart disease are often very vague and can mainly include things such as lethargy, reluctance to go out or play, poor appetite and other non-specific signs of 'being unwell'. Their independent lifestyles mean than heart symptoms do tend to be harder to pick up in cats compared to dogs. Cats are able to regulate their exercise better than dogs and often the amount they take is not really noticed by owners. Early symptoms of cardiac disease may simply mean that the cat sleeps more. More serious signs can include mouth breathing, rapid or forceful breathing and bluish gums.

Whilst coughing may be a sign of heart disease, probably more often in cats it reflects problems in the respiratory system (see **Breathing problems**). However the heart is nearly always examined too in these situations.

- **Arterial thromboembolism (iliac thrombosis)** is an important circulatory disease of cats with heart problems. Put simply, a clot forms in one of the heart chambers; this clot then moves out into the circulation to the arterial supply of the hind limbs, where it forms a blockage (thrombosis) in the blood supply known as the iliac artery. The thrombosis causes severe pain and hind limb muscle paralysis, with cool limbs and paws and an absence of normal pulses. The same process can also affect the front limbs, but this is not so common. This disease usually follows on from heart muscle disease (cardiomyopathy), discussed below.
- **Cardiomyopathy** is the main heart disease affecting cats and exists in two forms. 'Dilated' cardiomyopathy occurs when the heart enlarges and becomes distorted in shape and less efficient as a blood pump. What causes this is not fully understood. Young or middle aged cats are affected more, as are cats of the Siamese, Burmese and Abyssinian breeds. A deficiency of the amino acid taurine in the diet is thought to be one of a

number of possible factors which seem to act together in causing this problem. Since the discovery of taurine's role, most commercially made cat foods have been supplemented with taurine so no further addition to the diet is needed.

- 'Hypertrophic' cardiomyopathy, the commonest form of this condition, occurs either by itself or as a consequence of other diseases, especially overactive **Thyroid gland**. When the disease is the only problem present, it is seen more often in young to middle aged male cats. When in association with overactive thyroid gland, it is older cats (over 10 years) that are affected most. In this problem the heart thickens up abnormally, narrowing the size of its internal chambers and making the heart less elastic. The result, again, is that the heart ceases to function effectively as a blood pump. The heart has to work harder (beat faster) to maintain the circulation, and this can cause problems with the heart muscle itself being starved of oxygen.
- A parasite known as **heartworm** can invade and live in the heart chambers and major blood vessels of the chest. It is spread by biting insects in warm climates (e.g. southern Europe, the USA, Australia) and is not found in the United Kingdom. Symptoms may not always be shown but severe cases can occur, when illness is seen. In 'high risk' areas, preventive medication is usually administered by vets.

☎ Urgency

Mouth breathing, respiratory distress and noisy breathing all indicate severe problems in cats and urgent attention is required. Cats seem to cope with mild to moderate heart problems without showing major symptoms, so when noticeable signs do appear, it tends to mean that the situation is deteriorating.

✚ First aid & nursing

The over-riding concern is to avoid further stress if at all possible, as this can tip the balance and send the cat into a precipitous decline. Handle the cat slowly and quietly and stop if it becomes at all agitated. Some cats appreciate cool air fans, others seem to become upset by them. Place the cat in its box in readiness for any journey to the veterinary practice.

In cats already under treatment for heart disease, stress reduction is also important. Sources of stress (children, other animals, etc) should be avoided or limited. All medication needs to be given as directed and a careful watch kept for signs of deterioration, especially as these may be very vague, e.g. poor appetite, the cat being 'quieter' than normal, etc.

For resuscitation of the collapsed cat see **Collapse**.

Veterinary treatment

- Initial emphasis is on stabilising the patient, improving breathing and easing the work load on the heart. Oxygen therapy is often used as well as various heart drugs given by injection.
- Once fit enough, a series of diagnostic tests will be worked through to find out the precise nature of the problem. These often include X-rays, ECG tracings (measurements of the electrical activity going on in the heart) and ultrasound

scans.

- Medication can then be worked out for the individual cat. In many cases, a combination of drugs are used. This can occasionally cause problems in administration if the cat is not an easy one to give tablets to, as some of the drugs may need to be given twice daily. The last thing cats with heart problems need is additional stress caused by struggles while attempting to get them to take multiple tablets. In these difficult situations, discussion with the veterinary surgeon is needed to find out how best to get the treatment into the cat, or to prioritise which drugs are the most important ones. Sometimes, drugs can be combined into a single gelatin capsule, so that only one dosing is needed daily – this can often help considerably.

Tip: Check your cat's heart rate

Cats are often stressed in veterinary clinics and, for treatment purposes, it can be very helpful to know what the unstressed cat's resting heart rate is at home. This is fairly easily done in most cats. When your cat is lying or sitting beside you, place the flat of your hand on the chest wall, just behind the elbow on the left hand side (or place one hand on each side of the chest wall). Feel carefully for the vibration caused by the heart as it beats (you may need to move your fingers around a bit to get the right spot). Count the number of beats felt in one minute. Do this several times then take an average and note this down for the vet. The resting heart rate should be no more than 180 beats per minute. Taking the resting breathing rate (as described under **Breathing problems**) is also useful.

In fat cats, it can be impossible to feel the heart rate in this way – in this case your vet or nurse may show you how to take the pulse. However taking the pulse in cats requires considerable practice as it may be very difficult to find, especially in cats with heart problems.

Related or similar conditions

- **Breathing problems**
- **Collapse**
- **Thyroid gland (overactive)**
- **Blood pressure (high)**

Heatstroke (hyperthermia)

Cats are left unattended in cars far less frequently than dogs, so this common cause of heatstroke is not seen nearly so often. However cats have their own tendencies and may become trapped in greenhouses, enclosed porches or conservatories, etc. where temperature and humidity can rapidly escalate.

Signs of heatstroke including panting, collapse and, in extreme cases, fits which can prove fatal. If heatstroke is suspected, the guidance given under **Fever/high temperature** should be followed as quickly as possible as it is imperative to prevent the temperature from remaining dangerously high. Seek veterinary advice as well since prolonged high temperature can damage organs and tissues.

Hepatitis

Hepatitis means inflammation of the liver. This can arise as a result of infections, toxicities (from drugs or poisons) and several other causes, e.g. tumours. Cats also suffer from several specific liver diseases; their liver is generally much more susceptible to damage than that of dogs. More details are given under **Liver disease**.

Hernia

A hernia results when a body part becomes displaced into an abnormal location. This can occur after accidents, as in the serious condition of diaphragmatic hernia, when the contents of the abdomen are displaced through a ruptured diaphragm into the chest, where they cause breathing problems. Other traumatic hernias can occur on the body wall, if muscle gets badly damaged. Various organs and tissues may protrude through the hernia and, in doing so, their blood supply may become cut off, leading to serious and even life-threatening problems.

Other hernias are much less serious, e.g. many cats are born with congenital umbilical hernias. These usually consist of small pads of fat which result in a soft swelling in the mid-line on the underside of the abdomen. Most of these cause no problems at all and may be left alone or else conveniently repaired when the cat is being neutered.

☎ Urgency

The commonest hernia you are likely to encounter is the small congenital umbilical hernia mentioned above. These are soft, stay the same size (though the protruding fat can sometimes be 'popped' back into the abdomen by pressing on it) and generally cause no problems. They are not urgent though you may wish to get reassurance that this is what you are seeing and feeling, as skin lumps can sometimes look rather similar. Larger umbilical hernias may occasionally cause trapping of a piece of bowel; this is fairly rare and if your veterinary surgeon is concerned that this could happen, surgical repair of the hernia may be suggested.

Diaphragmatic hernias are always suspected in any cat that has experienced a traumatic accident and is showing breathing problems. Urgent attention is needed, though surgical repair of the hernia is normally postponed for at least 24 hours. Now and again, cats are discovered with chronic diaphragmatic hernias. They have lived with the problem for some time without any obvious symptoms. Decisions about treatment are hard to make, as the surgery is not without risk, but leaving the hernia is also risky as complications due to trapping of organs could occur even a long time after the initial injury.

✚ First aid & nursing

Umbilical hernias require no first aid or nursing. With suspected diaphragmatic hernia, advice should be sought. If collapse or severe breathing difficulty occurs, guidance given under **Collapse** should be followed.

Veterinary treatment

- Small umbilical hernias may not require any treatment.
- Larger hernias usually require surgical correction due to the risks of organ trapping. Diaphragmatic hernia requires major surgery, with attendant risks.

Related or similar conditions
- ▶ **Accident**
- ▶ **Breathing problems**
- ▶ **Surgery**

Horner's syndrome

Horner's syndrome is a collection of eye symptoms which result from nerve damage; this may arise due to various causes. The characteristic appearance of Horner's syndrome in an affected cat is:

- A small (constricted) pupil in one eye when compared with the fellow eye.
- Drooping of the eyelid in the affected eye.
- Prominence of the cat's 'third eyelid' in the corner of the affected eye; this partly covers the eye.
- Apparent withdrawal of the eye into the socket.

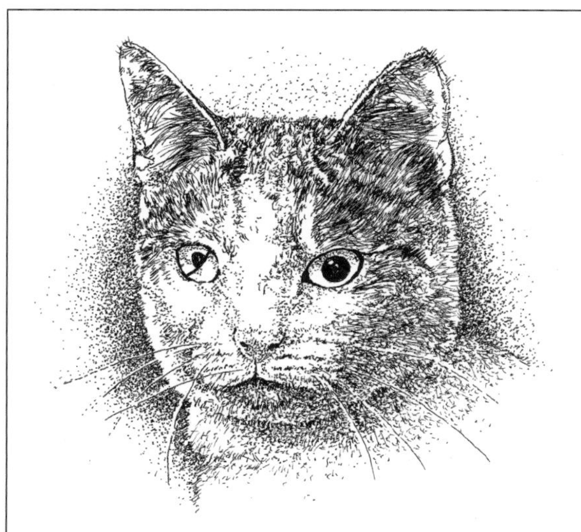

Horner's syndrome in the cat's right eye.

Ear disease can give rise to Horner's syndrome, as can nerve damage arising from trauma, infections or tumours.

☎ Urgency
Whenever you see Horner's syndrome, an early appointment should be obtained in order to find out the cause in your cat.

✚ First aid & nursing
Little first aid is appropriate, but the cat should be kept indoors and observed for any other symptoms, e.g. ear pain, lameness (which can sometimes occur with nerve damage).

Veterinary treatment
- Tests will be performed to check the ears, the function of other nerves and the general health of the cat, in order to try to find out what is causing the Horner's syndrome.
- Treatment (if any is needed) can then be decided on.

Related or similar conditions
- ▶ **Eye problems**
- ▶ **Head tilt**

Hyperactivity

The commonest cause of hyperactivity in older cats is an overactive **Thyroid gland**. In younger cats, **Behaviour problems** or, occasionally, **Fits** may be the cause. See the appropriate sections.

Hyperthyroidism

See **Thyroid gland** (**overactive**)

Hypothermia

Hypothermia means a dangerously low body temperature which, if persisting, can lead on to coma and death. In cats, hypothermia can occur in ill cats that become trapped outdoors or in young kittens, which have a poor ability to regulate body temperature. The normal body temperature of a cat, measured by a veterinary surgeon, nurse or experienced owner is around 38.6°C. Very low body temperature may not even register on a clinical thermometer.

Symptoms of hypothermia include a cold, immobile cat with breathing patterns that may be barely perceptible. The cat may be difficult or impossible to rouse into full consciousness.

☎ Urgency

Urgent treatment should be sought, but first aid is most important initially.

✚ First aid & nursing

If the cat is wet, dry with towels and, ideally, a hair dryer. The cat should then be wrapped in several layers of dry and warmed up covering, e.g. towels, jerseys, etc. Bubble packing is also an ideal thing to use as this has very good insulating properties – a 'jacket' can be made out of this to cover the cat's body and legs and then towels or other material placed on top. Thick socks can be put over the legs and tail.

Warm (not hot) water bottles should be placed around the cat. Don't put these in direct contact with the cat's body as severe skin burns can be caused (the cat is unable to move itself away from excessive heat applied to the skin). Instead, use the warm bottles outside the wrapping layers. Keep the cat in a warm environment and arrange for veterinary attention.

If resuscitation is needed, follow the advice given under **Accident.**

Veterinary treatment

- This will be very similar to the treatment outlined above with, in addition, warmed drip fluids being given into the bloodstream.
- It can take some time for the body temperature to reach normal levels again, though improvements are usually seen within 1–3 hours.

Related or similar conditions

- ▶ **Collapse**
- ▶ **Shock**

I

Iliac thrombosis

This is a circulatory disease of cats with heart problems, in which a blood clot (thrombus) forms and lodges in the arteries supplying the hind limbs. It is a very painful condition and results in weakness, paralysis and cold limbs. The condition is discussed under **Heart Disease**.

Incontinence

Incontinence is the passage of urine and/ or faeces without the cat being aware that this is happening. Cats are normally very clean animals and will not usually mess in the house or their bed areas unless there are medical problems of one type or another.

Sometimes, it can be difficult to distinguish true incontinence from other problems which result in the cat passing urine or faeces outside the litter tray. Common situations which might initially resemble incontinence are:

- **Cystitis**, which usually results in frequent attempts at urination, sometimes in unusual places. Cats with cystitis usually pass small amounts of urine at a time, often with straining, whereas true incontinence has no straining: the cat is unaware of urine dribbling or leaking. See under **Cystitis**.
- **Urethral obstruction** in male cats can sometimes resemble incontinence, as affected cats may strain frequently, passing small amounts of urine indiscriminately. See under **Cystitis**.
- **Behaviour problems**, resulting in inappropriate urination or marking of surfaces with urine (or sometimes faeces). This, again, is quite different from incontinence. The cat is aware of what is going on. The urine or faeces are passed normally but in inconvenient places.
- **Diarrhoea/colitis**, which can result in faeces being passed in unusual places owing to the cat being 'caught short'. Straining is usually present, whereas true incontinence with faeces has no straining. See under **Diarrhoea**.

Incontinence may be associated with senility (old age), other disease conditions or nerve damage. The bladder and its nerve supply is always at risk after pelvic fracture (a common injury in road traffic accidents) and urinary incontinence can result from this. This type of incontinence may be temporary or permanent. Spinal injury also carries the risk of incontinence.

☎ Urgency
This problem should always be assessed promptly, mainly because of the seriousness of urethral obstruction which can result in similar symptoms and has to be ruled out very quickly. Incontinence of faeces, although not life-threatening, is usually sufficiently distressing for cat and owner to merit rapid examination.

✚ First aid & nursing
Little in the way of practical first aid is appropriate, apart from restricting the cat to a small area and keeping the cat clean and dry.

Veterinary treatment
- Initial emphasis will be to establish the cause of the incontinence and see whether that is treatable by any means. In general, urinary incontinence is encountered far less frequently in cats than in dogs, where it is quite common in older, spayed bitches. Incontinence of faeces is a difficult problem to manage by any means.

Related or similar conditions
- ▶ **Cystitis**
- ▶ **Diarrhoea**

Incoordination

Incoordination can result from problems affecting the limbs and joints (e.g. **Fractures**, **Dislocations** and severe **Sprains/strains**), from diseases affecting the nervous system (the brain and spinal cord), from severe **Ear problems** and as a result of general weakness from other serious diseases such as **Diabetes**, **Fits** or **Feline infectious peritonitis**. Poisonings will also often result in an incoordinated cat since many poisons interfere with proper functioning of the nervous system, and any problems with vision may initially show as apparent incoordination.

Incoordination often results in lameness or a swaying or wobbly gait (the medical term is ataxia). Circling, falling to one side or a head tilt may be seen. Sometimes the changes are fairly slight and require close observation of the moving cat, and are possibly only detectable to the trained eye of the veterinary surgeon.

☎ Urgency
Because of the wide variety of possible causes, and the serious nature of some of them, early advice should be sought for the incoordinated cat.

✚ First aid & nursing
It is important to ensure the cat cannot damage himself by falling or staggering downstairs, into fires, or getting stuck or lost outside. Keep the cat indoors, in one room or in a cat box or carrier if necessary. Gentle reassurance and holding the cat may help. Keep the surroundings quiet and dimly lit to reduce extra stimulation, which may worsen any feelings of panic the cat may be experiencing, especially if the onset of symptoms was sudden.

Make some brief checks for any apparent injuries (e.g. to the limbs, back or head area) and inspect the eyes for normal appearance. Can the cat see as normal? (Perform a vision test, if required, as described on page 35). Is hearing and sound recognition apparently normal? This information will be of use to your vet.

Observe closely and try to describe the nature of the incoordination, e.g. 'He seems unable to position the left front leg properly.' 'She looks blind and keeps circling to the left.'

Veterinary treatment

- Examination and tests should point towards possible causes of the incoordination. This will then allow treatment to be started. A wide variety of causes exists but it is usually possible for the veterinary surgeon to narrow these down quite quickly after initial examination. A definite diagnosis may require more extensive tests in some cases.

Related or similar conditions

- ► **Balance (loss of)**
- ► **Brain damage**
- ► **Bone/joint problems**
- ► **Fits**
- ► **Head tilt**

Indigestion

This is a difficult problem to detect in cats and, while it probably does exist, the symptoms we are able to see are likely to be such things as intermittent vomiting, grumpiness, poorish appetite, tenderness of the abdomen and such like. Cats suffering from fur ball probably experience some symptoms of indigestion, as do those which have overindulged in unsuitable or rich food.

In general, the advice given under **Fur ball** and **Vomiting** should be followed.

Infections (general)

For specific infections of cats, see under the relevant headings of the individual infectious diseases of cats. These are listed under Related or Similar Conditions, at the end of this section, and are dealt with fully elsewhere in the book.

Infections are diseases caused in animals by the presence of other life-forms, much smaller than the infected animal, invading the body. Bacteria, viruses, protozoa, fungi, and various external or internal parasites (fleas, worms, mites, etc.) can all cause infections in cats. Most of the time, however, when vets talk about 'an infection', they mean a bacterial or viral illness. Bacteria and viruses are invisible to the naked eye, are present everywhere and are constantly 'challenging' the immune defences of all living animals. Fortunately, most of them are very successfully resisted or eliminated by the elaborate defences of the healthy immune system.

Infections cause symptoms by directly damaging organs or tissues and by activating the immune system itself, which attempts to (and usually succeeds in) eliminating the infection within a few days to a week. However infections do vary in severity and some may be so serious as to threaten life or result in permanent organ or tissue damage (**Rabies** is a good example, also **Feline enteritis**). If the cat's immune system is somehow damaged (e.g. by other diseases such as **Feline immunodeficiency virus** (FIV)) then infections which are normally very mild can become much more serious and even fatal. Similarly, very young and very old cats are more susceptible to the serious effects of some infections as their immune systems are less developed or effective.

Bacterial infections are usually present as 'secondary' infections in cats already suffering from a viral illness (e.g. cat flu or FIV), or as a result of bite infections – a very common cause – or other types of contamination of a wound or tissues. Bacterial infections can be treated using antibiotics, whereas viruses are not sensitive to these drugs.

☎ Urgency

Infections tend to follow a predetermined timecourse but this does vary somewhat depending on severity. Generally, by the time symptoms are shown, infection is well advanced. The urgency of the problem then depends on the nature of the symptoms and the degree of incapacity they are causing.

Mild sneezing of **Cat flu**, for example, is not urgent, but severe respiratory distress, possibly indicating pneumonia, definitely is. Occasional **Diarrhoea** perhaps caused by a protozoan infection (especially *Giardia*, which is quite common in cats) usually does not make the cat seem particularly unwell – appetite, activity and demeanour are all much as normal. However, the profound diarrhoea and vomiting caused by **Feline enteritis** can rapidly result in collapse, shock and death.

The best rule is, if in doubt, phone for advice and listen carefully to the veterinary surgeon's recommendations which will be made after a number of questions have been asked.

+ First aid & nursing

General nursing for the cat with an infection involves keeping the cat indoors, in quiet surroundings at a comfortable room temperature. Ensure a litter tray, supply of clean drinking water and soft bedding are to hand.

Sick cats often have poor appetites so offer small meals of tempting food, e.g. cooked chicken/fish, sardines in tomato juice, or anything you know your cat particularly enjoys. Most cats like cooked ham, prawns, etc. These are useful in small quantities to get the appetite going, before switching to cat food. Try not to surround the cat with plates full of uneaten food – remove them and offer again later.

Contact with the owner is important and many cats will start to eat when encouraged. Also short periods of grooming and bathing the mouth, nose and eyes often seem to improve demeanour. This is especially important when there are nose or eye discharges, e.g. in cat flu.

Keep a 'nursing sheet' and note things such as amount of food and water drunk, frequency of vomiting and diarrhoea and when urine or normal faeces is passed.

Veterinary treatment

- Attention is focused on diagnosing the infection and then treating it, if possible. Virus infections cannot be cured directly but the body can be supported using (if required) fluid drips, antibiotics for secondary infections and assisted feeding, while the immune system is working.
- Preventative vaccination is important for those diseases that can be controlled this way. Boosters are required after an initial vaccination course in the kitten.

Tip: Vaccination

Certain important infections in cats are preventable by vaccination. Vaccination 'prepares' the immune system in advance for an infection, without actually causing major symptoms of the disease itself. When a vaccinated cat is exposed to an infection, the virus is rapidly destroyed before major problems can be caused. Vaccination gives the cat immunity to a disease; the only other way to acquire immunity is to experience the disease once (and recover from it). However, with very serious diseases recovery may not always occur – the cat could die from the disease. Diseases routinely prevented by vaccination in cats are:

- Upper respiratory diseases (feline influenza or **Cat flu**)
- Feline panleucopaenia (**Feline enteritis**)
- **Feline leukaemia virus** (FeLV)
- **Chlamydia infection** (less commonly given than the above three)
- **Rabies** (in travelling cats only)

Certain important diseases cannot currently be vaccinated against or else vaccines are not widely available or regularly used – **Feline immunodeficiency virus** (FIV) and **Feline infectious peritonitis** (FIP) are examples.

Related or similar conditions

- ▶ **Abscess**
- ▶ **Bites**
- ▶ **Cat flu**
- ▶ **Chlamydia infection**
- ▶ **Feline enteritis**
- ▶ **Feline infectious peritonitis (FIP)**
- ▶ **Feline immunodeficiency virus (FIV)**
- ▶ **Feline leukaemia virus (FeLV)**

Infertility

Most pet female cats will have been neutered (spayed) at an early age, an operation which removes the ovaries and uterus and thus prevents reproductive cycling behaviour and pregnancy. On balance, spaying is generally recommended by vets for all companion female cats (and similarly castration is recommended for all companion tom cats) in order to prevent unwanted kittens and the welfare problems this can cause. Infertility is thus only seen in breeding females (queens), usually kept by professional cat breeders.

Infertility can be a complex problem and investigation may require several tests. One common cause would be a serious viral illness such as **Feline immunodeficiency virus** (FIV) or **Feline leukaemia** (FeLV), but many other infections and conditions may also cause infertility in cats. See also under **Abortion**.

Inflammation

Inflammation is part of the body's natural reaction to injury and infection and is an important initial phase of the healing response. Inflammatory conditions can affect a wide variety of organs and tissues and can be recognised by the presence of the suffix '*itis*' tagged on to the end of medical words, for example:

- **Arthritis** – inflammation of the joints
- **Dermatitis** – inflammation of the skin
- **Otitis** – inflammation of the ear
- **Iritis** – inflammation of the iris (eye)
- **Gastroenteritis** – inflammation of the stomach and intestines

- **Colitis** – inflammation of the colon
- **Rhinitis** – inflammation of the nose
- **Stomatitis** – inflammation of the mouth

and so on.

Inflammation gives several characteristic signs. These are: heat, pain, redness and swelling – the so-called 'cardinal signs of inflammation' in medical terminology. These symptoms are easiest seen after most types of skin injury, e.g. a scratch or a burn. The symptoms mainly arise through a hugely increased blood flow to the region, and it is this blood flow which transports inflammatory and immune cells to the area to help the animal fight the underlying cause of the injury or infection.

Inflammation is therefore a natural phenomenon, but it can also cause problems, especially when the underlying cause of the inflammation is difficult to identify or remove completely. In these situations, the inflammatory response can persist, creating discomfort or irritation for the animal. Medical treatment may be needed to alleviate this.

☎ Urgency

One form of inflammation which can cause a real life-threatening emergency is that affecting the throat area, when breathing can be interfered with. This may occur after a sting following a cat catching a bee or wasp, or sometimes in severe allergic reactions or after caustic burns to the mouth or throat area. Severe inflammation of the eye, showing only as a reddened, painful eye, should also be seen urgently.

Most other forms of inflammation are more gradual in onset and should be checked out during a routine appointment.

✚ First aid & nursing

For collapse from respiratory obstruction due to inflammation, see under **Accident**, for the resuscitation technique to follow. This is not a frequent occurrence in cats.

With any area of inflamed skin, great care should be taken regarding applying products or solutions to this. Antiseptics may be irritant and painful and in general the best advice is to prevent the cat making the problem worse (e.g. by fitting a protective collar) and to use very mild solutions to bathe the area, such as salt and water, Calamine lotion or, for stings, antihistamine cream.

Veterinary treatment

- The aim is always to treat the cause of the inflammation whenever possible. Remember that inflammation is usually only a symptom of some other problem. There would be little point in treated a very inflamed skin if the cause of the inflammation (e.g. fleas) was not also tackled at the same time.
- However, in quite a large number of inflammatory diseases, the cause cannot be adequately identified or treated (this is often the case in diseases of an allergic nature and in inflammatory bowel diseases, asthma, etc.) and in this situation the inflammation may need to be suppressed using potent anti-inflammatory drugs.
- Anti-inflammatory drugs are of two main types: those related to aspirin (a drug to which cats are extremely sensitive), the so-called non-steroidal anti-inflammatories. A wide variety of these exist in human and animal medicine, where they are generally used for

their pain relieving properties. However never be tempted to dose a cat with a human product or to give extra doses of a veterinary one – the consequences could be severe and result in permanent organ damage or even death. The other form of anti-inflammatories are the steroid drugs (also known as corticosteroids or glucocorticoids). These are very effective at reducing or eliminating inflammation. However with long-term use, side effects can be seen and the intention is always to use them for as short a period as possible or, if long term use is needed, to use the very lowest effective dose to keep symptoms controllable.

- Anti-histamines are a further drug type which have some anti-inflammatory properties. In general, they are not nearly so effective as the above two but as they have very few side effects, they may be tried out in suitable cases.

Related or similar conditions

- ▶ **Arthritis**
- ▶ **Asthma**
- ▶ **Enteritis/gastroenteritis**
- ▶ **Skin problems**

Influenza

See under **Cat Flu**.

Injury

Injury can affect cats physically and psychologically and the effects may be of short or long duration. Specific injuries are discussed fully elsewhere in the book but several important principles apply to the first aid of injury in general.

☎ Urgency

An injured cat should be assessed for life-threatening problems: breathing difficulty, severe bleeding, pale or white gums and lack of responsiveness or ability to move. Repeated observation is required even in apparently unaffected cats since some problems take time to show themselves. Advice should always be sought if in any doubt.

✚ First aid & nursing

Injured cats can be in pain and react aggressively so handle them with care. Try to find out where the injuries are and how severe they seem to be. Turn to the appropriate sections of this book to find out about bleeding, fractures, bites, eye injuries, etc. and what to do in these situations.

Most injured cats prefer to be allowed to rest quietly. They should not be let outdoors since they may tend to seek a secluded place to hide and are then in danger of hypothermia or dehydration if the injuries are incapacitating.

If the cat can walk well, is breathing normally and has no obvious wounds, the situation is probably not highly serious but the nature of the injuries should still be investigated by a vet.

Veterinary treatment

- Examination and tests such as X-rays, if needed, should reveal the nature of the problem.
- Internal injuries can be much more serious than external ones, and are often

harder to pick up. Problems such as internal bleeding, lung damage, bladder rupture, etc. are an ever present threat after any severe trauma. This is why an injured cat needs to be monitored closely for 24–48 hours – in case delayed symptoms start to emerge as a result of hidden injuries.

Related or similar conditions

- ▶ **Accident**
- ▶ **Bites**
- ▶ **Fractures/dislocations**
- ▶ **Sprains/strains**

Intussusception

This is a serious bowel disease that usually requires emergency surgery to treat. One segment of bowel becomes telescoped inside another, and produces a life-threatening bowel obstruction. Severe symptoms of vomiting, abdominal pain and, often, straining and scanty diarrhoea result. The condition can arise in any age group but is commoner in kittens and younger cats and may follow an episode of **Enteritis** (including feline infectious enteritis), diarrhoea or a heavy worm burden. Without treatment, peritonitis and death from shock can quickly follow.

☎ Urgency

Diagnosis of intussusception is not possible by owners, however the severe symptoms of vomiting, abdominal pain and worsening condition should always prompt emergency treatment. Even so, the condition can be hard to recognise at times, and death can occur despite treatment or even before treatment can be started, especially in very young kittens.

✚ First aid & nursing

For the severely vomiting cat, no practical first aid is appropriate. If a cat vomits soon after any food or water is taken, and this continues with signs of pain and depression/lethargy, it usually means a severe problem is present and professional attention is urgently needed.

Veterinary treatment

- X-rays or ultrasound scans may be used to confirm the diagnosis. Fluid therapy (a drip) will almost certainly be needed and surgery will be performed as soon as the cat seems strong enough to withstand a general anaesthetic.
- The outlook always has to be cautious for this serious condition, but excellent recoveries are possible.

Related or similar conditions

- ▶ **Diarrhoea**
- ▶ **Enteritis**
- ▶ **Vomiting**
- ▶ **Worms**

Irritability

Sick cats or those in pain are often irritable, and maybe even aggressive, and care should always be taken on handling them (see the useful advice given for handling nervous or fearful cats on page xvii). Some of the commonest medical situations leading to irritability in cats are given at the end of this section and these specific problems are dealt with elsewhere in the book.

You may be able to guess what might be going on by careful observation. For example, a cat with ear pain may paw or rub at the ear or hold the head to one side; there may be a bad smell or a discharge coming from the ear. Mouth pain can result in 'head shyness' or growling while attempting to eat or else chewing on one side of the mouth only or chewing very carefully; in severe cases, the cat may not be eating at all. Arthritic cats are painful on moving, especially after rest, and may resent grooming or their backs being touched. Cats with a high temperature often want to hide away, they are immobile and resent any interference at all; appetite is usually poor.

☎ Urgency

It does depend on what is causing the problem, and what other symptoms are present as to how urgent the situation is. In general terms, a mildly irritable cat is likely to be suffering from a non-life threatening but nevertheless uncomfortable condition. It may be safest to seek telephone advice from the vet as to what to do since it can be impossible to assess the situation without a full clinical examination.

Any irritable male cat with difficulties urinating should always be considered an emergency due to the potential problem of urethral obstruction.

✚ First aid & nursing

See under individual conditions. In general, irritable cats are best left alone in a quiet place. Provide food, water and a litter tray and observe them every hour or so to check there is no deterioration.

Veterinary treatment

- Examination and tests should reveal the cause of the problem and allow appropriate treatment. Many older irritable cats have problems like sore mouths and overactive thyroid gland.

Related or similar conditions

- ▶ **Abscess**
- ▶ **Arthritis**
- ▶ **Cystitis**
- ▶ **Ear problems**
- ▶ **Fever/high temperature**
- ▶ **Mouth problems**
- ▶ **Thyroid gland (overactive)**

Itching

Itching (the medical term is pruritis) arises from irritation in or on the skin. It is a very common symptom and the vast majority of cases are caused by cat **Fleas** or the intense allergy associated with this. However other parasites can also be responsible, e.g. **Mange**, **Mites**, **Lice**, **Ringworm**, **Harvest mites**, **Ticks**. Also, nonparasitic causes, though less common, may be present. These include food allergies, contact allergies (e.g. caused by the cat's bedding or even the detergent used to wash the bedding), allergies to pollens in the atmosphere (the medical condition of atopic dermatitis or atopy) and behavioural causes. See also under **Skin problems** and the individual conditions mentioned for full details of all these specific conditions.

☎ Urgency

Itching is not an urgent medical problem but do not leave treatment too long, otherwise severe skin damage from self-trauma can result, making the whole problem much more difficult (and expensive) to cure.

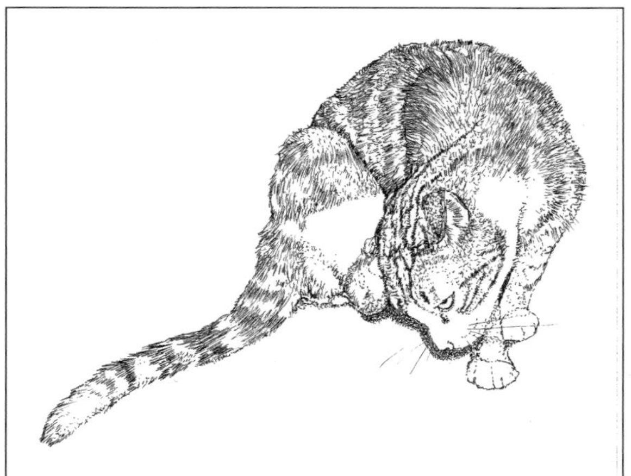

The itch-scratch cycle worsens the problem.

+ First aid & nursing

In general, avoid applying anything to the coat before seeking veterinary attention. If you have put anything on, explain this clearly to the vet and take the packaging along with you, as some products can be toxic if repeated too soon, if given with other drugs or if given in inappropriate dosages.

If you suspect fleas, vacuum and treat the house and wash all the cat's bedding but it is best to leave the cat untreated until after a veterinary examination.

Veterinary treatment

- The skilled examination by a vet is vital for skin diseases. If there is a parasitic problem, and this is not picked up, the skin problems are likely to persist and cause frustration for all concerned. Various tests are used to help diagnose the cause of itching, e.g. skin scrapes, biopsies, and so on. Most problems are quite readily diagnosed.

Related or similar conditions

- **Allergy**
- **Behaviour problems**
- **Dermatitis**
- **Fleas**
- **Harvest mites**
- **Lice**
- **Mange mites**
- **Ringworm**
- **Skin problems**

J

Jaundice

Jaundice is a medical term which describes a yellowish discolouration of body tissues caused by the accumulation of a blood pigment that is normally removed and processed by the liver. When the liver is diseased and not functioning well, the pigment accumulates in the body and discolours the skin, the white of the eye and the gums with a yellow tinge. In animals, jaundice is most easily seen in the white of the eye (the sclera) or in the gums because the hair coat masks any discolouration of the skin. Jaundice is a serious symptom and should always be investigated promptly. See **Liver Disease** for more details.

Jealousy

The behavioural problem of jealousy can be directed towards any other animal or human in a household, and can be a serious thing if it is associated with aggression. Behavioural problems in cats are complex and it is important not to attribute human emotions to feline behaviours; hence what we perceive as 'jealousy' may have elements of other behaviours as well, e.g. fear, which can cloud the picture. A detailed and objective analysis of the problem is needed and often the best person to perform this is someone from outside the immediate situation, such as a vet or cat behaviour specialist. It helps greatly if they can witness the situation at first hand via a home visit. Failing this, video footage combined with a detailed diary of where, when and why the problem seems to occur, is needed, as it is very unlikely that the cat would exhibit the behaviour problem outwith the home environment (e.g. in a clinic) in a way that would provide meaningful information for the therapist.

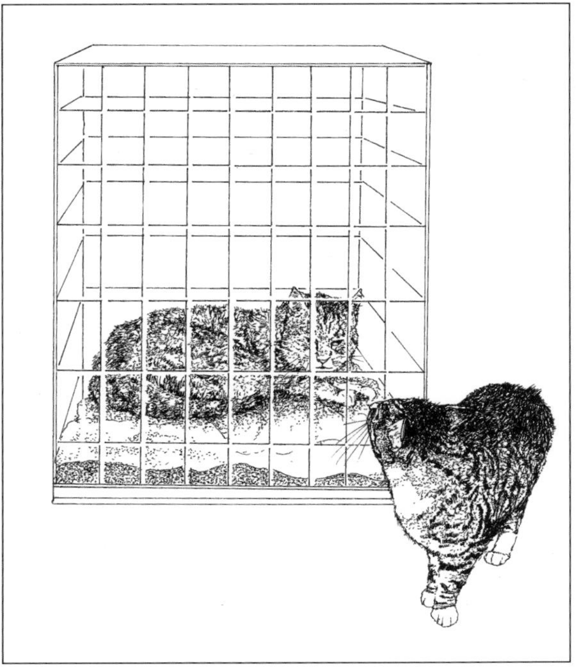

Introducing a new cat using an indoor kennel or cage.

☎ Urgency

Jealousy is not an urgent situation unless actual physical harm is done to another pet or human being, in which case medical attention should be sought. Cat bites can result in extremely serious infections in people, and medical help should always be obtained if you are bitten.

✚ First aid & nursing

Separate the fighting cats safely, if this is occurring, and try to fathom out what may be triggering the jealous type behaviour. Be as objective as possible. Punishment is usually futile, and may make the situation worse. In extreme cases, e.g. following the introduction of a cat (or dog) to the household, separation may need to be total for a while, before gradually introducing the unfamiliar pets to each other. Be alert to potential conflict situations such as access to food and resting areas. Introductions are sometimes better performed in neutral territory if this can be arranged. Between cats, a certain amount of interaction is natural and involves the cats establishing a hierarchical relationship to each other. However, true jealousy tends to be an on-going and persistent problem.

Remember to give your cat time to get accustomed to another cat or dog. 2–4 weeks is a reasonable estimate before concluding that you have a potential problem on your hands. There is no doubt that some cats never really get on with either other cats or dogs – the most that can be hoped for is an easy truce of toleration!

Be especially careful with rabbits, which may be viewed as prey animals by some cats.

> **Note** that cats are naturally more solitary animals than dogs.

Veterinary treatment

- Behaviour problems of all types are of growing interest in veterinary medicine. More and more vets are trained and interested in this area, or can refer you to someone who is. This type of problem is best approached with skilled advice since it is so easy to misread the situation and, by your actions, inadvertantly make it worse.

Related or similar conditions

▶ **Aggression**
▶ **Behaviour problems**

K

Keratitis

Keratitis is the medical term for inflammation of the cornea – the clear 'window' at the front of the eye. This inflammation may be superficial or deep and can be caused by a wide variety of infections or trauma; allergy is another potential cause. Typical signs are pain, squinting, blinking, discharge from the eye, a reddened eye and changes in the surface appearance of the eye. Deep ulceration of the cornea carries the risk of eye rupture. See under **Eye problems**.

Key Gaskell syndrome

This disease of cats, also known as feline dysautonomia, was common in the 1980s and then became much rarer. Recently, there has been some evidence that it may be increasing in frequency again. It is an illness with a variety of symptoms, most cats showing some of the following:

- Swallowing problems and regurgitation
- Dilated pupils
- Prominent third eyelids (the extra eyelid which cats have and which is normally only slightly visible in the inside corner of the eye)
- Dry mucous membranes (eyes, nose and mouth)
- Constipation
- Dehydration
- Abnormally slow heart rate.

☎ Urgency

The condition does not usually show as an urgent problem since the symptoms tend to be rather vague and insidious.

✚ First aid & nursing

Affected cats should be kept quiet and stress-free. If the pupils are dilated, cats should remain in areas of subdued lighting. First aid treatment for **Constipation** and **Dehydration** can be given if needed, and if the eyes are very dry artificial tears (from chemists and veterinary surgeons) can be applied to protect the surface of the cornea. Lubricating ointments are also available for this purpose (e.g. Lacrilube) and have the advantage of needing to be applied less frequently than drops. The **Appetite** should be tempted – see page xxii for advice. Good nursing is very important in this debilitating disease.

Veterinary treatment

- The cause of this disease is unknown and treatment has to be 'symptomatic', i.e. the main problems as they appear in individual cats are tackled. Common treatments include intravenous fluid therapy (a drip) for dehydration, drugs to improve the function of the bowel and relieve constipation, antibiotics for any supervening infections.

- Recovery is possible but overall the outlook can be poor for this disease. At present, it is not known whether recent cases are isolated outbreaks or the start of a new wave of Key Gaskell syndrome in cats, nor whether the disease will be as severe as when it was first discovered 15–20 years ago.

Related or similar conditions

- **Appetite (abnormal)**
- **Constipation**
- **Dehydration**
- **Vomiting**

Kidney disease

Kidney disease is common in cats and the most frequent diagnosis is a condition called chronic kidney disease (sometimes abbreviated to CKD). This disease is a slow, progressive loss in kidney function, often associated with advancing age. It is a disease that tends to creep up on old cats, with symptoms appearing and worsening over a period of a few months. However it can also occur in younger cats if their kidneys have been seriously damaged by injury, infection or poisoning.

Another kidney disease – acute renal failure – is a much more abrupt loss of kidney function. This usually occurs in response to severe infections, poisoning, trauma or blood loss. An important cause of acute renal failure is urethral obstruction in male cats unable to pass urine because of a blockage (see **Cystitis** section). If the underlying problem is treated promptly, recovery from acute renal failure is possible, but some affected cats go on to develop chronic renal failure afterwards – it all depends on how much damage was caused to the kidneys initially. The kidneys do have a remarkable ability to recover from mild to moderate damage, though this can take several weeks or months.

Kidney disease of any type is serious because the two, paired kidneys are vital body organs, responsible for a host of important functions. They receive a huge blood supply and are constantly fine-tuning the composition of the vital body fluids that keep all cells healthy. The production of urine is only one part of their function.

Mammals only require one kidney for survival, hence a kidney can be removed if necessary without lasting effects on health – provided the remaining one is healthy. Nature seems to have provided an extra one, just in case. Indications for removal of a kidney could be such things as tumour or severe disruption of one kidney after an accident.

Kidneys that are not working well are unable to clear toxic products from the bloodstream, and many of the effects of chronic kidney failure are related to the build up of these toxins, which affect other organs and tissues. One problem with kidney disease is that the kidneys cope extremely well with mild to moderate damage over a prolonged period of time, and few if any symptoms will be noticed. However once damage goes beyond a certain level (once more than about 60% of kidney function is lost), symptoms start to appear. Often, by this time, full recovery of kidney function is no longer possible and the emphasis has to be on preserving what kidney function remains for as long as possible. Kidney transplants are infrequently performed in cats. This may change in the future as the veterinary profession debates the ethics of this treatment.

Typical symptoms of the common form of kidney disease – chronic renal failure – are weight loss, poor appetite, drinking to excess and urinating to excess, vomiting, poor coat, bad breath and mouth problems, and dehydration. Symptoms can progress to collapse and fits before death, if untreated.

☎ Urgency

It is fairly unusual for kidney disease to show as an urgent problem except in the case of male cats with a blocked urethra. Much more common is the slow onset of symptoms characterised by chronic renal failure. Over a period of weeks to months owners may notice that their cat is drinking more, passing more urine, and has a variable or poor appetite. Weight loss, poor coat and bad breath may be seen. Intermittent vomiting is common. A routine appointment is usually made for these initial rather vague symptoms.

+ First aid & nursing

Even although affected cats may pass urine more frequently, their water intake should never be restricted as this can lead to dehydration and worsening of the kidney condition. In fact, water intake should be encouraged. Drinking replaces the water which is being lost in the very dilute urine which affected cats must pass (their kidneys are unable to concentrate the urine as normal due to poor function).

Appetite should be tempted as much as possible. It is likely that, during bad spells, affected cats feel nauseous and thus reluctant to eat. However this compounds the problem by leading to dehydration and a negative energy balance. Try tempting with small meals of white meat, fish, scrambled eggs, etc. Warming the food often helps and many cats like sardines in tomato sauce, which is also a good source of potassium. Although red meats are generally advised against in kidney disease, small amounts may help to get the appetite started again if the cat particularly likes this. Vitamin supplements may be prescribed by the veterinary surgeon and well as periodic use of other drugs, e.g. antibiotics.

Good nursing and grooming, gentle cleaning of the nose and eyes, etc. and communication with the cat can do wonders to improve demeanour and make a significant contribution to overall wellbeing. Try to avoid stressful situations if possible. Entering catteries may be associated with a deterioration in condition – whenever possible, cats with chronic renal failure should be looked after at home when the owners are away.

Veterinary treatment

- Kidney disease is diagnosed after blood and urine tests and its progress is monitored by repeat tests to check how effectively the kidneys are removing body toxins from the bloodstream.
- Initial treatment may involve intravenous fluids (a drip) to correct problems with body fluid balance, and this treatment may need to be repeated during bouts of illness to 'rescue' the failing kidneys.

- Other drugs that may be used include antibiotics, vitamins, drugs to promote blood flow to the kidneys, to control vomiting and several others. Advice on the diet is usually also given, particularly with respect to the type of protein that is fed. It is most important that kidney patients are kept eating, as this can often be the first sign of deterioration.
- The long-term trend is always downwards with chronic renal failure, however many cats can maintain a good quality of life for some time with appropriate treatment. Euthanasia is required when quality of life is poor, since appetite then tends to disappear, the cat becomes very subdued and may have distressing symptoms such as severe vomiting or even fits.

Related or similar conditions

- ▶ **Dehydration**
- ▶ **Thirst**
- ▶ **Thyroid gland (overactive)**
- ▶ **Vomiting**
- ▶ **Blood pressure (high)**

Kittens' problems

Most kittens are born healthy and develop normally. Litter size in cats is usually 4–6 kittens and most female cats make very good mothers if not unduly disturbed. It is important that a secure, safe nest area is available, that this is kept at a comfortable room temperature and that food, water and litter tray are within easy reach of the mother cat. Her food requirements increase considerably during pregnancy and lactation, and food should be constantly available when she is feeding kittens.

Ensure that kittens cannot become trapped behind any projections or in gaps, as they will soon start to move around and investigate their space. The best type of bedding is several layers of newspaper with a cotton sheet or 'Vetbed' on top, as this is easily changed/washed. Kittens can become trapped in the sleeves of old jerseys, etc.

Kittens' eyes open at around 2 weeks of age. At this age, they can be handled for short spells by all members of the family (washing the hands afterwards). This is an important early part of the socialisation process and should help to ensure that the cats are well adjusted with people. By age 6 weeks they should be lapping fluids and soft food well. They should be fully weaned by around 8 weeks, eating kitten food. At this age, healthy kittens are active, exploring and interested in their surroundings.

Signs that all may not be well include:

- Kittens that seem either unusually quiet or unusually noisy when compared to the rest of the litter. They may not be feeding well owing to a birth defect or health problem.
- Milk running down the nose after suckling. This can indicate a cleft palate.
- Swollen abdomen. This can indicate internal problems or lack of a normal anal opening. If caught early (within a few days of birth) this problem can be treated.
- Eye or nose discharges.
- Abnormally shaped limbs.
- Infection/discharge at the umbilicus. If you notice any of these problems, have all the kittens checked over by a vet.

☎ Urgency

Medical problems in kittens should be dealt with promptly as they have fewer reserves than adult cats and their condition can change (both deteriorate and improve) quickly. They are prone to **Dehydration** and, when very young, **Hypothermia**. Their immune systems are not fully functional and, in general, they exhibit fewer symptoms than adults so it can be harder to pick up that something is wrong.

+ First aid & nursing

Sick kittens must be kept warm since they are unable to regulate body temperature well and illness makes them prone to hypothermia. The background heat in the room should be that which a person would find warm (around 20–25°C or 70–80°F). Additional heat can then be supplied by wrapped warm (not hot) water bottles or warm packs. 'Bubble wrap' has good insulating properties and jackets can be made out of this to fit around sick kittens to preserve warmth.

Food and fluid intake must be kept up owing to the high metabolic rate of kittens. If the sick kitten is not suckling she will need to be hand-fed with an approved milk replacement product. These are available from pet stores and veterinary practices; do not use cow's milk or human infant milk products. If a milk replacer is not available, glucose solution can be used temporarily. Feeding should be frequent (every hour in young kittens less than 4 weeks old) but with small amounts, e.g. 2–4 ml at a time. Food or liquid should be warmed to body heat before giving and it is easiest if a syringe or dropper is used. Take care that the fluid enters the mouth slowly to avoid choking and inadvertent inhalation of the liquid into the chest.

Kittens do not empty their bladder and bowels voluntarily. Instead, this must be encouraged after every meal by gently rubbing the perineal area (under the tail) with a warm, damp towel to mimic the mother cat's tongue. Dry the area afterwards.

Veterinary treatment

- Examination of the kitten often reveals clues as to health problems, and other tests such as X-ray may also be utilised in the same way as in adult cats.

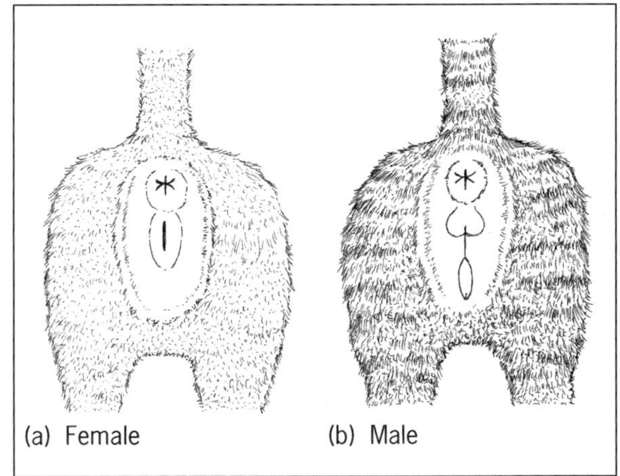

Telling the sex of kittens (see Tip below).

- Kittens may not be able to receive some of the drugs used in adult cats, however in most instances a safe alternative is available.
- Good nursing is vital to success of any treatment, especially in unweaned kittens.

Tip: Telling the sex of kittens

You may need help to do this as the differences are not so easy to spot in kittens as in adult cats. The kitten is held so that the tail can be raised. Locate the anal opening. In females, the vulva is very close to the anus. In males, the penile opening is much smaller and lower down. Between it and the anus is a raised area which will develop into the scrotum and testicles. It is often easier to sex kittens when you can compare several, rather than trying to decide on one individual seen alone!

Related or similar conditions

- **Abortion**
- **Birth**
- **Cat flu**
- **Intussusception**
- **Vaccination**
- **Worms**

L

Labour

See under **Birth**.

Lameness/limp

A very obvious lameness or limp is easy to spot as the cat will carry the leg most if not all of the time. With less intense pain, the cat puts reduced weight on the affected leg. On the front legs, the cat seems to collapse down on to the good leg while walking, in order to spare the sore one, which may be just touched to the ground and no more. On the back legs, most weight is again taken on the good leg, giving the impression of the cat leaning on to this side as it walks or hops along. Lameness on more than one leg can be harder to spot and may lead to the cat not wanting to move at all or else moving with a stilted, 'clockwork' gait.

Lameness is usually caused by one of the following:

- **Problems in the paw or foot area.** The commonest conditions here are torn nail, bites to the paw or foot area, foreign bodies (e.g. glass, thorns) in the paw pads or between the toes, infection between the toes, and broken toes.
- **Problems further up the leg.** Again, bites are a very common cause of lameness caused by painful muscle infection in the leg muscle groups. Fractures and dislocations can also occur, as can severe sprains and strains. Bone tumours are a much rarer cause of lameness but have to be considered in certain cases.

By far the majority of lameness in cats is caused by **Bite** injuries, causing an **Abscess** or cellulitis (muscle inflammation and pain), and traumatic **Fractures/dislocations**. Pelvic fractures are particularly common after road accidents in cats.

☎ Urgency

The urgency depends on the amount of pain that is being exhibited by the cat. You can gain a good impression of this by observing the cat carefully and cautiously examining the leg to see where it seems tender. If there is severe pain, it is best to seek advice promptly. Mild lameness (when the cat is able to touch the sore leg down while walking) can be checked out at a routine appointment.

✚ First aid & nursing

Keep the cat indoors and restrict activity to one room. Do not give any form of human painkiller or anti-inflammatory drug as toxicities (and even death) are common in cats given human painkillers. Most cats prefer to be left in peace but if an area seems hot and swollen, cold compresses can be tried. If the foot is swollen and infected, warm salt water bathing can help. If any part of the limb seems distorted in shape or cannot be moved by the cat, call the vet for advice as this suggests a fracture or dislocation. Cats with pelvic fractures will be very reluctant or unable to move and, usually, in severe pain. An emergency appointment is needed.

In cats thought to have been involved in road accidents or other trauma, observe carefully for breathing problems, e.g. irregular breathing, breathing that seems either abnormally fast, slow or requires more effort than normal, or abnormal noises during breathing.

Veterinary treatment

- Examination, possibly with X-rays, is used to diagnose the cause of the lameness and then appropriate treatment, e.g. antibiotics, painkillers, surgery if needed, can be given.
- Usually indoor room rest is needed for a period after this type of problem to allow the injured structures to heal.

Related or similar conditions

- ▶ **Accident**
- ▶ **Bites**
- ▶ **Bone/joint problems**
- ▶ **Fractures/dislocations**

Leukaemia

Leukaemia is a form of cancer affecting the bone marrow, resulting in large numbers of abnormal white blood cells being produced, as well as disease of other important organs such as the liver and spleen. Cats are susceptible to a viral form of leukaemia (see Feline leukaemia virus, FeLV).

Lice

Lice are small parasites, visible under a magnifying glass, which live on the skin surface and coat of cats. They are far less common than fleas, but are occasionally diagnosed in debilitated or neglected cats or kittens, when a heavy infestation may cause severe anemia. Long-haired breeds of cats can harbour lice infestations more easily than short haired breeds, especially if areas of matted hair are found on the body or back. Spread of lice occurs by direct contact between animals or use of shared grooming utensils, bedding, etc.

Lice are very 'host specific' parasites (unlike fleas) and rarely infest other species, i.e. the cat louse sticks to the cat and the dog louse sticks to the dog. Fleas are far less choosy about what animal they infest! Lice cement their eggs (known as nits) on to the hair shafts of their host. Skin irritation can be quite severe, with constant itching and hair loss, which is itself debilitating.

☎ Urgency

Lice infestation, though unpleasant, is not an urgent problem but should be checked out at an early routine appointment. In many cases, there is some other underlying disease present which has laid the cat open to infestation by lice since it is rare to find evidence of lice in healthy cats.

✚ First aid & nursing

Since cats with lice may be suffering from other disease problems, it is best not to apply anything at all to their coat, nor wash them, until a veterinary surgeon has seen your pet. Sick cats are more prone to the toxic effects of certain insecticides and bathing could be stressful (as well as ineffective) for the infested cat. Instead, keep the cat warm and quiet and tempt the appetite. Using a fine toothed comb can help physically remove nits from hair follicles. Infestation of human beings does not occur with cat lice.

Veterinary treatment

- Veterinary-approved anti-parasitic products are very effective at removing lice, but tests may be required to find out what has caused the infestation in the first place, i.e. is there an underlying disease that has debilitated the cat or kitten? Various blood tests may be called for.
- Severe anemia, when present, may need treated by good nursing, supplemental feeding or even in severe cases blood transfusion, though this is unusual.

Related or similar conditions

- ▶ **Baldness**
- ▶ **Fleas**
- ▶ **Mange mites**
- ▶ **Ringworm**
- ▶ **Skin problems**

Lipoma

A lipoma is a benign tumour of fat cells that may appear anywhere on the body surface. Lipomas are harmless in the sense that they do not spread like malignant cancers and affect other organs and tissues, however they can grow to be quite large and may cause 'local' problems such as skin irritation, ulceration or interference with nearby structures such as the eyelids.

Lipomas are characteristically soft, moveable and slow-growing. Feeling them does not usually cause any pain or discomfort to the cat and they can often be 'picked up' through the skin surface as they are not well attached to surrounding tissues. The problem can sometimes be one of making sure an unidentified lump is indeed a lipoma (or another form of benign tumour) and not something more sinister. To a large extent, this depends on experience and clinical knowledge, and your vet is the best person to make this sort of decision. Even so, the only way to be 100% certain of any lump is to take a biopsy or remove the lump completely and have it analysed by a pathologist.

☎ Urgency

Although it is undoubtedly worrying when you discover a lump anywhere on your cat, the problem is not an emergency one, but should be investigated during an early routine appointment. This small delay will not affect the outcome of the condition and reassurance may well be the only treatment needed.

✚ First aid & nursing

No first aid is necessary unless the lump is ulcerating or **Bleeding**, in which case the advice given in that section should be followed. Light bandaging across the body (e.g. using an old stocking stretched over the cat's body with holes for the legs) is very successful in stopping seepage from ulcerated lumps or those that have been knocked and are bleeding.

Veterinary treatment

- Biopsy or removal will give a definite answer as to what the nature of the lump or lipoma is, and any further treatment can be planned accordingly. Checking over the cat regularly for other lumps is always a good idea, also check for recurrence at the original site of removal.

Tip: Be advised by your vet

A small lipoma that is not causing any problems may simply be monitored over a period of a few weeks to a few months.

Removal or biopsy could be carried out if it appears to be changing or growing rapidly. Careful observation is often the course of action followed in older cats, or when an anaesthetic is not desirable for other reasons, e.g. heart problems.

Sometimes, however, even a small lipoma may have to be removed surgically if it is near an important structure (especially the eyelids) or if letting it grow too large would then cause problems for future removal because of a shortage of surrounding loose skin to close the wound afterwards – this is often the case on the lower part of the limbs or on the tail.

Related or similar conditions

- **Abscess**
- **Cancer**
- **Mammary (breast) problems**

Liver disease

The liver is the central organ of digestion and metabolism and is positioned in the front of the abdomen, surrounded by the last part of the rib cage. It is the largest body organ and receives a huge blood supply. It has many important functions in the body, including manufacture of proteins, regulation of blood glucose, storage of minerals, detoxifying poisons (and drugs) and dealing with the body's natural waste products.

It is a remarkable organ because of its ability to withstand damage and repair itself. About 80% of the liver can be damaged with very few adverse effects being seen. Unfortunately this does mean that when symptoms of liver disease do eventually appear, the damage is likely to be very severe. The liver of cats is different from dogs; they contain fewer detoxifying enzymes, which make cats much more sensitive to the adverse effects of some drugs, such as aspirin and paracetamol. For this reason, cats should never be given human painkillers or anti-inflammatory drugs as severe poisoning and death can be caused.

Liver disease causes fairly vague symptoms of illness and they can sometimes be quite difficult to pinpoint. Some or all of the following may be shown:

- Poor energy levels
- Weight loss and poor appetite
- Drinking to excess and urinating to excess
- Vomiting and/or diarrhoea
- Abdominal swelling due to fluid accumulation (known as ascites)
- High temperature

- Incoordination, disorientation, fits or apparent blindness
- Jaundice (yellowish discolouration of the whites of the eyes and gums)

The problem with liver symptoms is that most of the above problems are seen with several other diseases as well. This causes difficulties with diagnosis. The main diseases affecting the cat liver are:

- **Congenital shunts** in kittens and young cats, where blood by-passes the liver due to faulty circulation. This means that toxins are not removed by the liver as normal and so the cat is effectively 'poisoned' by its own blood. Symptoms of poor growth, lethargy, illness and incoordination/ fits are seen, and symptoms are often worse after eating. Many affected animals can appear blind and 'spaced out'.
- **Inflammatory conditions.** These diseases affect the bile ducts, gall bladder and liver and are termed cholangitis and cholangiohepatitis. The diseases produce symptoms of general illness and malaise, e.g. poor appetite, weight loss, vomiting. In acute inflammation, fever may be seen and some cats appear jaundiced. Chronic forms of the disease also occur.
- **Liver tumours.** Typical symptoms here would include weight loss and abdominal swelling due to fluid accumulation. Vomiting and a poor appetite are also likely.
- **Fatty infiltration.** Infiltration of the liver with fat (the condition of feline hepatic lipidosis) can occur, again producing vague general symptoms of poor appetite, no energy and occasional vomiting. This disease is commoner in obese cats which, for some reason, suddenly stop eating. This may be due to stress or another illness. The lack of food intake stimulates changes in the metabolism which can be life-threatening.
- **'Secondary' liver diseases** can occur in cats suffering from diseases such as overactive **Thyroid gland** and **Feline infectious peritonitis**.

☎ Urgency

Because of the characteristically vague nature of liver symptoms, the problem is not usually an emergency one. Most cats will have appeared slightly unwell for some time, with waxing and waning symptoms that may partly appear to respond to other treatments. Symptoms will probably get gradually worse, prompting further veterinary investigation.

✚ First aid & nursing

Cats that seem generally unwell with vague symptoms should be kept indoors as any deterioration that occurs while outside could be serious, especially if the cat is taken ill in cold weather.

The **Appetite** should be tempted and a careful note made of daily water intake, together with the frequency of other symptoms such as vomiting and diarrhoea. Checking the body weight every 3–4 days is also very helpful, especially as an aid to assessing response to treatment.

Most cats with liver disease are lethargic and need to rest a great deal. Comfortable surroundings in a quiet and stress-free area should be provided. Interaction with the owner and grooming helps to keep up demeanour.

Veterinary treatment

- Usually, liver problems are suggested by the cat's medical history followed by clinical examination. Blood tests are then needed to confirm that the liver is indeed not working effectively.
- Although blood tests can point to the liver as the source of the problem, they cannot usually tell what is actually wrong with the liver. This requires a range of further tests, usually X-rays, ultrasound and liver biopsy, which may entail major surgery.
- Liver problems are not always life-threatening. Several can be effectively treated: congenital shunts may be able to be corrected surgically, with a good outcome; cholangitis and cholangiohepatitis can be treated using drugs; infiltration with fat can be treated using drugs and intensive nursing; and secondary liver diseases caused by overactive **Thyroid gland** will improve when the underlying problem is dealt with.

Related or similar conditions

- ▶ **Appetite (abnormal)**
- ▶ **Diarrhoea**
- ▶ **Feline infectious peritonitis**
- ▶ **Fits**
- ▶ **Jaundice**
- ▶ **Thyroid gland (overactive)**
- ▶ **Vomiting**
- ▶ **Weight loss**

Loneliness

Cats are individuals and some individuals are more sociable than others, preferring company when others would shun it.

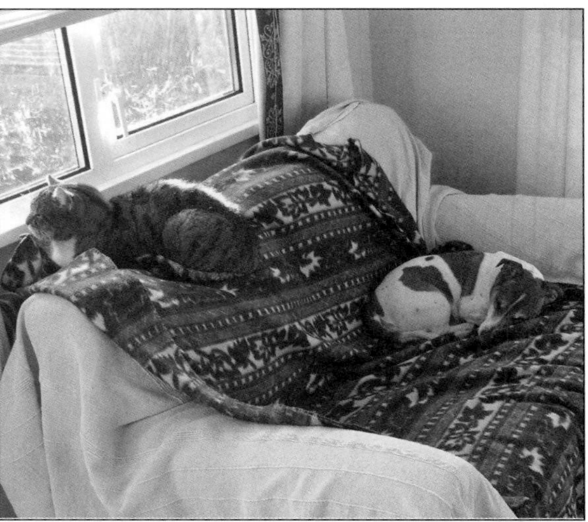

Although often solitary, some cats do seem to appreciate the company of other animals.

Although cats are considered quite solitary animals, loneliness can and does occur and is seen most often when pet cats have lost a companion cat, dog, other pet or human. Changed patterns of living can also result in loneliness, e.g. the house cat whose owner changes from part-time to full-time work; children growing up and leaving home, etc.

Symptoms of loneliness can be difficult to define; many individuals just 'seem unhappy' or withdrawn, but physical symptoms can also appear such as over-grooming, behavioural problems, poor appetite and the appearance or worsening of other health problems which had previously been under control.

☎ Urgency

The problem is not an urgent medical one and, sometimes, given time, the cat will adjust to the new situation. If not, then practical steps should be taken to try to counter the cat's problem.

+ First aid & nursing

When you are around, giving the cat more 'quality time' spent playing, grooming or speaking to the cat can help. When the cat has to be left alone, try leaving on a radio and lights to create the idea of the house being occupied. Perhaps a neighbour or friend could call in if lengthy spells of time are involved.

Acquiring another pet can often help with sociable cats, though time must be given for the new arrival to settle in and be accepted. This is often the most practical solution if handled properly.

Veterinary treatment

- There is no specific veterinary treatment for loneliness unless physical symptoms are associated with the problem, e.g. breakdown in urination behaviour, sores caused by over-grooming.

Tip: Stress-free introductions

If another cat is being acquired, try to choose a temperament that will compliment your existing cat's. The cat being introduced should be a relaxed and sociable animal if at all possible. Start off carefully, possibly leaving the new arrival in a basket for an hour or two to allow for safe introductions through the wire mesh! Indoor pens are useful, since a litter tray and bed can be put in here, allowing you to leave the house knowing that no major disagreements can occur. The cats, though able to see, hear and smell each other, will be physically separated, with the new cat secure in his or her pen.

Bear in mind it will take several weeks for normal relationships to establish, and do expect a few squabbles at the start. Adopt a quiet and relaxed approach when the cats are interacting and do not interfere too much. Kittens or older cats can both be accepted; fights are far less likely with kittens, which tend to be accepted more readily, but still make sure you supervise the introductions for the first few days (see p. 129).

Related or similar conditions

- **Anxiety/fear**
- **Behaviour problems**
- **Bereavement**

Lumps

Lumps can appear anywhere on the body surface (as well as internally) and should always be checked out by a veterinary surgeon. Many lumps appearing suddenly in cats that go outside turn out to be **Abscesses**, but **Lipomas** (fatty growths), **Blood blisters** (haematomas), **Stings**, **Allergy** and **Cancer/tumours** are also possible. See the appropriate sections for more details.

Lung worm

This is not a common problem but, when it occurs, symptoms may be shown in kittens which are carrying many **Roundworms**. A chronic cough is caused due to migration of worm larvae through the lung tissue. Treatment is by using medication from the veterinary surgeon to eliminate the worms.

Luxation

Luxation is the medical term for dislocation of a joint, and subluxation describes a partial dislocation. Usually, severe traumatic injury is the cause, e.g. road traffic accident, getting a leg caught while jumping, etc. The hip joint is the most commonly affected one, but any joint can be disrupted. Luxations produce severe **Lameness** (like a fracture) and subluxations produce varying lameness and instability. The shape or angulation of the leg may be altered.

☎ Urgency

These are serious injuries and should be treated promptly as this carries the best chance of full recovery of function of the joint. Additionally, any trauma severe enough to dislocate a joint could easily have also caused important internal injuries in the chest and abdomen which need to be looked out for.

✚ First aid & nursing

Restrict activity in a well-padded cage or basket until veterinary attention is sought. It is usually best not to attempt to apply any dressings, splints etc. This is difficult to do in the cat in pain and if improperly applied could make the discomfort worse. Most cats will find a posture that alleviates discomfort quite quickly.

Veterinary treatment

- X-rays are used to confirm the dislocation. Under anaesthetic, it may be possible to replace the joint and apply support dressings while the torn ligaments, joint capsule, etc heal (usually several weeks). Function should return largely to normal.
- Some dislocations cannot be kept in place; in these situations, surgery may be needed to secure the joint or modify the shape of the joint to allow a return to function.

Related or similar conditions

- ▶ **Accident**
- ▶ **Bone/joint problems**
- ▶ **Lameness**

Lymphoma/lymphosarcoma

This is a form of cancer which can involve various organs and tissues. It affects the lymphoid system – a network of vessels and nodes spread throughout the body. Lymph, a milky fluid containing white blood cells, flows through the vessels and is filtered by the nodes, where any signs of infection are detected by the immune system and acted upon.

Cancer of the lymphoid system produces symptoms which depend on the organ affected: if the organs of the chest are involved then breathing difficulty may be seen; if it is the abdomen, then vomiting, diarrhoea and poor appetite can be caused. Other organs can be affected too, e.g. the eye. Weight loss is usually present in patients with this problem. In cats, this form of cancer may be associated with **Feline leukaemia virus**, FeLV. See also **Cancer** for more general information.

M

Mammary gland (breast) problems

Mammary gland problems are encountered less often in queen (female) cats than in bitches, however several problems occur. In most of these, the mammary glands become swollen or thickened so it is important to have the cat checked by a veterinary surgeon to determine what exactly is going on. The commonest mammary gland problems are:

- **Swelling** of the glands in a female cat that has been feeding kittens. This happens especially at the time of weaning or, more commonly, if the kittens should die for any reason while milk production is still active. The glands may be swollen and firm, but the cat does not appear ill, as she would with mastitis (below).
- **Mastitis** – bacterial infection of the mammary glands during lactation. This is not common in queens but when it does occur it shows as a sick, lethargic cat with a high temperature and swollen, painful mammary glands. Suckling will be resented and there may be a foul discharge from the glands. The cat is likely to be off her food and thoroughly miserable.
- **Hyperplasia** of the mammary glands. In this condition, the mammary glands can enlarge enormously and a brownish fluid may leak from the nipples. This condition is seen around the time of oestrus (heat) in young female cats, and does tend to recur at subsequent oestrus cycles if the cat is not spayed. It can resemble mammary (breast) cancer, however cancer of the mammary gland is rare in young cats.
- **Mammary (breast) cancer.** This is unfortunately often a malignant disease in cats – usually around 80% of tumours are malignant ones (compared to only 50% in female dogs), and recurrence and spread of the tumour is likely. The cancer is found much more frequently in entire queens, i.e. those that have not been spayed, and in older cats.
- **Fat pads.** Cats often develop pendulous fat pads underneath the abdomen, running up between the hind legs. There is no pain from these loose folds of skin, which sometimes become so large that they swing slightly as the cat walks. They are harmless.

☎ Urgency

This depends on the overall condition of the cat. Mastitis can be a severe illness, endangering the life of not only the mother cat but also the kittens (who will probably not be feeding), so it should be treated urgently.

The other problems above are less immediately urgent, but should nevertheless be checked out promptly, especially if a tumour is suspected.

✚ First aid & nursing

Sick cats should be encouraged to eat and their **Appetite** tempted – this will be most likely with mastitis. Poulticing of inflamed mammary glands with warm cloth compresses can be very beneficial but, as the area will be tender, start off gradually and build up confidence with the cat: 5–10 minute sessions 4 or 6 times daily are best. However, some cats will not tolerate this at all.

Veterinary treatment

- This rests on making a diagnosis as to what is causing the mammary gland swelling. This is usually straightforward but, on occasion, may require biopsy to differentiate between hyperplasia and tumours, for example.
- For swelling due to milk accumulation, no treatment is necessary. The condition disappears as milk production ceases. Warm compresses and massage can help.
- Mastitis is treated using antibiotics and, if necessary, fluid therapy (a drip). If abscesses form, surgical treatment may be needed to deal with the tissue damage caused.
- Mammary hyperplasia is treated with drugs to reduce the swelling (usually diuretics and steroid drugs). Neutering (spaying) is performed to prevent recurrences at the next oestrus.
- Mammary tumours require careful assessment in cats, since many are malignant. If spread has already occurred elsewhere in the body, surgery to remove the primary tumour will not bring about a cure of the disease; the cancer could reappear elsewhere. Even if spread has not *apparently* occurred, there is always some risk that in fact it has, but has simply not been detected (since X-rays, ultrasound, etc. are never 100 per cent certain in this area of medicine). The outlook always has to be a very cautious one.
- For malignant tumours, any treatment given is palliative, i.e. symptoms are controlled to maintain quality of life, whilst accepting that euthanasia will ultimately be required due to the effects of cancer. This may not be necessary for some time however as tumours may progress quite slowly in some cases.
- Benign tumours that are completely removed will not reoccur and a complete cure from the disease is therefore possible. Deciding on whether a tumour is benign or malignant requires tests such as X-ray and, often, biopsy for the best chance of accuracy.

Related or similar conditions

▶ **Abscess**
▶ **Cancer**
▶ **Lipoma**

Mange mites

Mange is the term for a skin disease caused by microscopic parasitic mites, which live in or on the top layers of the skin – some mites burrow into the skin and others do not, staying on the surface. Mange is far less common than **Fleas** in cats and is not diagnosed nearly as often in routine veterinary practice.

Notoedric mange (caused by the mange mite *Notoedres cati*) is commoner than sarcoptic mange (scabies, caused by *Sarcoptes scabei*) in cats, but even so it is still a fairly rare disease. It causes intense itchiness, especially about the face and ears, with dry and crusty skin patches developing. It is highly contagious and can rapidly spread though a litter of kittens.

Another species of mite, this time affecting the ears, is commoner in cats; in fact most cats will be carrying this mite (called *Otodectes cynotis*, the cat ear mite). In many cases, little or no irritation is caused and cat and mite seem to tolerate each other reasonably well. However problems can occur, and the mite is a common cause of otitis (ear inflammation) in cats, when the irritation results in thick black wax and crusts in the ear, as well as intense itching. **Blood blisters** (haematomas) are often caused by ear mites in cats, due to the repeated head shaking and scratching at the ear that affected cats perform. The cat ear mite can also affect dogs and sometimes causes problems on the hair coat generally, away from the ears.

Two other mange mites affecting cats are the **Harvest mite** or berry bug, and a mite called *Cheyletiella*, which is sometimes given the imaginative name of 'walking dandruff'. Harvest mites tend only to be a problem in late summer and early autumn and cats seem to vary in their sensitivity to this parasite.

Walking dandruff mites are just visible to the naked eye. They cause fairly mild signs of itchiness but are very contagious. They result in a lot of skin flakes or dandruff being produced (hence the name), and this mite can also cause symptoms in people – indeed a persistent rash is common in owners of affected cats and this can be quite severe – much more severe than the symptoms produced in the cat! The human rash clears up once the cat is treated.

☎ Urgency

Skin problems caused by mites or other parasites are not urgent conditions, but do not leave it too long before seeking help because considerable skin damage can arise from self-trauma due to the 'itch-scratch-itch' cycle that is set up. This can then require lengthy courses of treatment to clear up.

✚ First aid & nursing

Do not apply anything to the skin or wash the cat before visiting the veterinary surgeon. Cats are easily poisoned by inappropriate use of insecticidal products and the best course of action is always to receive a professional diagnosis first. If you wash the cat, you may be washing away vital clues as to the nature of the problem.

If ears are very crusty, dry and waxy, applying a small amount of warm almond or olive oil and massaging the base of the ear will help to loosen debris and make the cat more comfortable whilst awaiting treatment. The cat is almost bound to shake the head afterwards so beware of flying oil droplets and pieces of wax!

Veterinary treatment

- Mange is diagnosed by examining skin scrapes or samples under a microscope.

Once the type of mange is known, prescription treatment can be given, together with any additional treatment for 'secondary' skin infections and intense irritation. Make sure all treatment courses are followed to the letter as otherwise incomplete cures may be obtained. Also always let the veterinary surgeon know if other animals or people are affected by any skin conditions because some parasites affect both animals and people.

- Ear mites can occasionally be frustrating to treat as the problem can grumble on, especially if applying drops is difficult in individual cats. Sometimes an anaesthetic is needed to thoroughly flush the ears free of accumulated wax and debris. Treatment will then be successful afterwards.
- Sometimes it is necessary to examine and treat other cats in the household who may be acting as a reservoir of infection, even although they exhibit no major symptoms themselves.

Related or similar conditions

▶ **Fleas**
▶ **Harvest mites**
▶ **Lice**
▶ **Ringworm**
▶ **Skin problems**

Miliary eczema

Miliary eczema or miliary dermatitis is an itchy skin condition in which tiny 'granules' are felt throughout the cat's coat, often along the back area or round the neck. These granules are small patches of scab or crusts sitting near the skin surface, but they are often easier to feel than see.

Most cats with this problem have an allergy to **Fleas**. There may be no fleas visible on the cat, and other cats in the house may have no problems either, but fleas are usually the cause nevertheless. This is an allergic condition, and only a very few fleas may trigger the hypersensitivity response (think how severe a reaction can be caused by traces of peanut when people who are allergic to them accidentally eat foods containing miniscule quantities).

☎ Urgency

This is a non-urgent condition and a routine appointment should be sought.

✚ First aid & nursing

It is best not to apply anything to the cat's coat, nor to wash the cat, before seeking veterinary advice. The vet will want to see the cat's coat as it is in order to assess what level of treatment is required.

If the cat has suffered from the problem before, then repeating prescription flea treatment (obtained from your veterinary practice) can be carried out, after confirming that the interval from last flea treatment is long enough to avoid any risk of toxicity. Remember to treat the house and all other dogs and cats present in it as well regardless of whether they are showing symptoms.

Veterinary treatment

- This is largely as for fleas. However if fleas have definitely been ruled out (by a rigorous flea control programme) then other causes may have to be investigated, since these are possible in a minority of cats. Hypersensitivities to other parasites (e.g. ear mites), foods and pollens can occasionally be the cause.

- In most cats the problem can be kept at bay without the use of potent drugs such as steroids if careful control of fleas is carried out.

Related or similar conditions

- ▶ **Allergy**
- ▶ **Fleas**

Milk sensitivity

Milk is not a necessary food for adult cats, despite the familiar image of a cat lapping from a bowl of it! As cats mature, they lose the ability to digest milk effectively, even though they may still enjoy the taste. In most cats, an occasional drink of milk causes no problems, but some individuals do not cope with it well and have diarrhoea. In these cases, just exclude milk from the diet or else water it down with plain water or provide skimmed milk. See also **Diarrhoea**. Supermarkets and pet stores also sell cat milk which is lactose-free.

Miscarriage

See **Abortion**.

Moulting

Most pet cats seem to moult on an almost continual basis. To some extent the loss of hair on chairs, carpets, etc. can be reduced by regular grooming. Nothing can be done to prevent this natural loss of dead hair, and there is no abnormality unless actual bald patches or excessive itching are associated with it. See also **Baldness**.

Mouth and tooth problems

Mouth problems are common in cats and it is likely that many pet cats suffer in silence from chronic grumbling pain caused by diseased teeth or inflamed gums. The extent to which this sort of discomfort can bring cats down is often only apparent after the mouth has been treated – many older cats take on a completely new lease of life after removal of painful teeth. Even if nearly all of the teeth have to be removed, eating will be easier and many cats with very few teeth still seem to enjoy biscuits.

Many cats also get a condition called tooth resorption, affecting any or all of the teeth, but usually starting on the premolars. In this problem, the tooth crown develops open defects which become filled with granulation tissue due to loss of hard enamel near the gum margin. This exposes the sensitive structures underneath and leads to inflammation and pain. It is a particularly unpleasant condition and extraction of affected teeth is required. X-rays of the cat's mouth often reveal the involvement of multiple teeth. All affected teeth should be removed.

The yearly booster vaccination is a good time to give the mouth a 'once over' examination to look for developing problems and hopefully catch them before they become too severe.

Aside from tooth and gum problems, other mouth conditions include **Ulcers**, caustic **Burns** (from lapping chemicals), **Foreign bodies** (especially threads, fish hooks, etc.) and **Tumours**. These are all less common than straightforward build up of tartar (mineral deposits from food) and tooth resorption or other dental disease.

Signs of mouth pain include reduced or no appetite (but possibly with a desire to try to eat), poor grooming of the coat, drooling, pawing at the mouth, general irritability and bad breath (halitosis). Mouth diseases are occasionally associated with other health problems – a common association is bad breath/ gum disease and chronic renal failure (discussed on page 132). **Gingivitis/stomatitis** is another troublesome condition of inflammation in the mouth; treatment can be difficult.

☎ Urgency

Mouth problems become urgent when food intake stops, because **Dehydration** then becomes a risk. As most routine mouth problems are seen in older cats, dehydration can worsen any other health problems that may also be present at a low or undiagnosed level, e.g. **Kidney disease**. It is obviously best to be able to treat a sore mouth before it gets to the stage where the unfortunate cat finds eating too painful.

If you notice signs of mouth pain (typical ones are trying to eat and then shying away quickly, pawing at the mouth or chewing on one side of the mouth) seek an early routine appointment.

✚ First aid & nursing

Offer soft or liquidised food to the cat with a sore mouth. Warming this up helps release aromas which may encourage the cat to try eating, and warm food is also less painful for sensitive teeth. Homemade blenderised food is ideal and highly flavoured foods (e.g. sardines in tomato sauce) can be used together with, e.g. smoked ham, chicken and some added water. If there is dribbling/drooling, bathing the mouth and lips with a tepid solution of salty water can help.

Once the painful teeth have been treated, regular (2–3 times weekly) use of a pet toothpaste can help slow down future build up of tartar again. It is worth trying with this but admittedly, not every cat will cooperate. For those that can be persuaded to, the bonus is fewer visits to the cat dentist!

Veterinary treatment

- Dental surgery can be time consuming and, therefore, expensive, but is often a very necessary treatment with great benefits for the cat's overall health and welfare. In older patients, blood tests may be advised before any prolonged anaesthetic, and intravenous drips are quite often used in elderly patients. Afterwards, antibiotics and painkillers are usually given while the mouth heals.
- Cosmetic dentistry is not performed in pets – the emphasis is always to relieve pain and discomfort.
- Mouth tumours are fortunately quite rare (they are usually malignant) but chemical burns to the mouth and tongue occasionally occur, either because the cat licks caustic substances directly or – more frequently – because it cleans these from a contaminated coat. If severe,

these burn injuries may need to be treated by resting the mouth completely and feeding the cat through a temporary tube inserted into the oesophagus or stomach. Although this sounds drastic, most cats tolerate tube feeding extremely well and are spared the pain of trying to eat through a painful mouth.

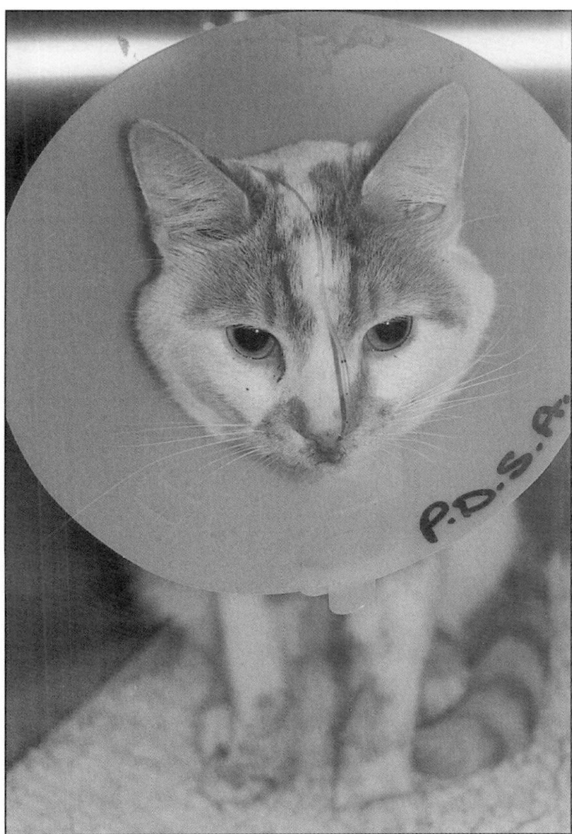

Boris fell two storeys off a balcony. He had been sleeping on the railing but a sudden noise woke him with a fright and he lost balance. He fractured his jaw and hard palate and eating was very uncomfortable so a small feeding tube was placed via his nostril, allowing the injured areas to be rested while they healed, but still ensuring Boris didn't go hungry. He was almost fully recovered after two weeks.

Tip: A few hints for successful tooth brushing

- *Days 1–3*: Just get the cat used to sitting still while you gently lift the lip margins. An assistant helps to steady the cat. Spend no more than 5 minutes a day. Reward well and give attention afterwards. It should be a calm and pleasurable experience for the cat!
- *Days 3–5*: Smear a tiny amount of cat toothpaste along the gum margins on each side of the mouth. Allow the cat to lick and swallow. Don't brush at this point.
- *Days 5–7*: Introduce the toothbrush very gradually and gently, slowly building up pressure used. Finger tip brushes are often easiest for cats and most veterinary practices sell suitable kits.
- *Day 8 onwards*: Try to brush at least 2–3 times weekly but daily is even better. Try to cover all areas of the mouth (not necessarily at the one treatment session).

Related or similar conditions

- **Appetite (abnormal)**
- **Gingivitis/stomatitis**
- **Kidney disease**
- **Salivation**

N

Nail problems and scratching behaviour

Most cat owners live with the consequences of cats' natural tendencies to want to scratch things – usually the most expensive chair in the house or the most visible area of carpet or wallpaper! Cat scratching posts can help, since cats tend to return to the same area for scratching and if they can be encouraged to use a post they are then less likely to damage furniture. This gives us a clue as to why cats want to scratch in the first place – it is partly a marking behaviour which provides a visual indication of a cat's presence as well as leaving scent on the surface scratched (there are scent and sweat glands on the bottom surface of the cat's paws and scratching places this scent on the object). Permanently indoor cats are likely to scratch around the house more than those going outside, who are probably expressing their behaviour against various trees, etc. in the vicinity.

Scratching also serves to shed loose top shells from the nails, leaving the pristine new ones underneath – obviously this is an important feature in animals which are designed to be efficient hunters. The scratching action also mimics the movements that are required during hunting and climbing. Overall then, this sometimes inconvenient behaviour is an important part of a cat's natural behaviour and one we have to understand properly, especially if it is necessary to try to limit scratching in certain areas.

Aside from this, medical problems with the nails are infrequent. Some claws have a tendency to curl and grow inwards (especially the small dew claws on the front feet) – these should be checked regularly and trimmed if needed since they can grow deeply into the surrounding skin if left, causing excruciating pain. Nail bed infections sometimes occur in cats, and these too are painful and require lengthy treatment.

☎ Urgency

Nail problems are not usually urgent and simple first aid is appropriate for most routine injuries. Excessive scratching around the house may be part of a more general behaviour problem associated with anxiety.

+ First aid & nursing

'Pulled' nails occur when the nail is partly or fully detached from the underlying claw, usually with minor bleeding also being present. If the nail is literally hanging by a thread, it can be pulled off or trimmed with nail cutters, providing the cat's temperament allows this (if not, leave this job for the vet or veterinary nurse). The area underlying will be pink and tender for a few days, until the tissues harden up, and it will be some weeks before the nail itself regrows. Bathing with warm salty water can help. No treatment beyond this is usually needed.

Trimming the nails is quite possible at home providing you have suitable equipment, patience and a willing assistant to hold the cat. If it all becomes a struggle, abandon attempts and let the vet do it, however with care, most cats will tolerate nail trimming. When starting off, only do a couple of nails at each sitting to avoid confrontations!

Nail trimming: 10 tips

1. Have the cat restrained in a sitting position (for the front nails) at a convenient working height. Make sure the surface that the cat is on is not slippery. Be calm and relaxed about it.
2. Take the paw and hold gently but firmly. The assistant helps by extending the leg through pushing from behind the elbow – this means you don't have to pull on the paw to get it forward, which some cats resent. Remember old cats may have pain from arthritis.
3. Use sharp nail cutters. Human ones are suitable or ask which type to buy at your veterinary practice. Avoid those that are too big and clumsy as an accurate cut will be difficult due to the small size of cat nails.
4. Extend the claw from its sheath by pressing the surrounding skin back to expose the whole nail.
5. In white nails, look for the 'quick' – this is the pink area that shines through the nail. It contains blood vessels and nerves and you want to avoid this. In black nails, you have to make an 'educated guess' as to the amount that can be removed (see the diagram) since the 'quick' is not visible. Err on the side of caution or else get your vet or veterinary nurse to show you a suitable length of cut.
6. Cut at about 1–2 mm below the end of the 'quick' or where you think it might be.

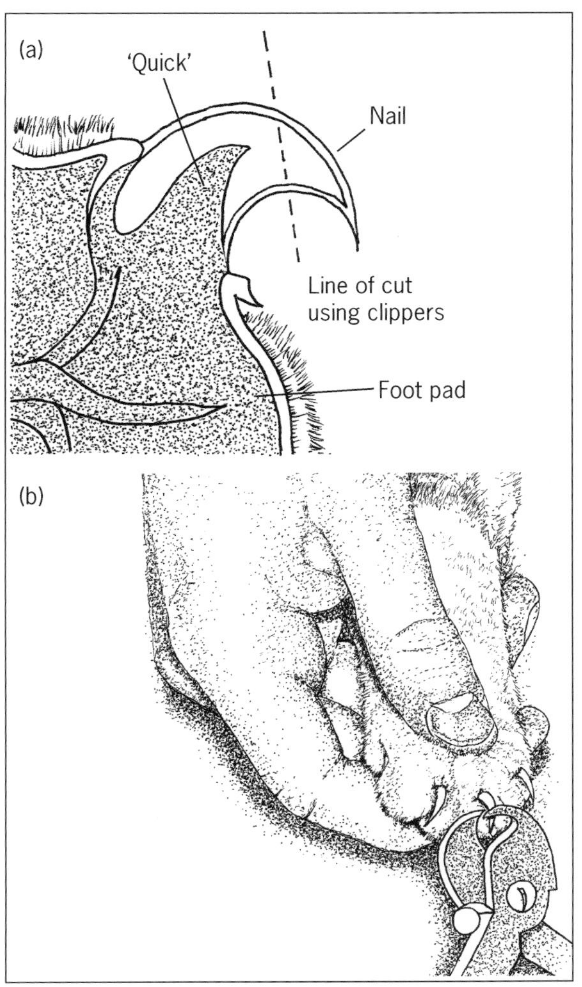

Trimming nails: an assistant is helpful.

7. Repeat on all nails and check the dew claws (small nails on the inside of the front paws). A few cats also have dew claws on the back paws. These often hang very loosely and nearly always over-grow; back dew claws are better removed at the time of routine neutering since they frequently get caught up on furniture, fences etc.
8. Reward the cat!
9. If you accidentally hit the 'quick', your cat will react and there may be slight bleeding. This always stops quickly. If necessary a small piece of cotton wool or light bandage can be put over the bleeding area for an hour or two. No further action is needed, however your cat may remember this when you try to trim the nails again.
10. Back nails are less often overgrown, but can be trimmed with the cat lying down on either side, or restrained in an assistant's lap, with the back feet supported.

First aid for nail or foot infections involves warm water salty baths every few hours until the foot is examined by a vet. Avoid putting on dressings since it is usually better to allow air to circulate. The cat may want to lick the foot – this is natural but if excessive (e.g. non-stop licking) a 'buster' collar can be put on.

Veterinary treatment

- Removal of the nails or declawing is not carried out unless for medical reasons (e.g. deep infection, severely traumatised toes/nails etc.).
- Nail bed infections often require lengthy courses of antibiotics to clear these up, otherwise they tend to recur. Several weeks is not unusual.
- Excessive scratching of furniture caused by anxiety behaviours can sometimes be helped using pheromone (synthetic cat hormone) sprays from the veterinary surgeon. These must be used in conjunction with proper behaviour advice for best chances of success (see Tip and also the sections listed below).

Tip

Never punish a cat for scratching behaviour. Instead, place a scratching post close to the favoured areas. Make sure it allows the cat to stretch right up to full height when standing on the back legs. Once the cat has adopted the post for scratching, it can be gradually moved to a convenient location if you wish. If making your own, avoid covering the post with carpet or fabric – wind round thick rope or use a wooden post (carpet might encourage the cat to scratch other areas of carpet or fabric in the house).

Related or similar conditions

- **Anxiety/fear**
- **Behaviour problems**
- **Lameness**

Neoplasia

Neoplasia, meaning 'new growth of cells' is the medical term for **Cancer** and is dealt with under that section.

Nephritis

Nephritis literally means inflammation of the kidney. It is a slightly older term used by some vets. See under **Kidney disease**.

Neutering

Neutering is the surgical operation to prevent breeding and associated sexual behaviours. In males, this is referred to as **Castration** (removal of both testicles) and in females as spaying or ovariohysterectomy (removal of the ovaries and uterus). When these organs are removed, the hormones that they produce no longer circulate in the body and sexual and reproductive behaviour ceases.

The majority of pet cats are neutered, usually at around 6 months of age, and the operations require a full general anaesthetic. Castration is a very quick procedure but spaying is a more major operation as the abdominal cavity has to be entered. No stitches are used in cat castrations unless one or both of the testicles is in an unusual position; for spay operations in females, both internal and skin stitches are used, though quite often the skin stitches may be 'buried' so that they are not visible on the surface. Female cats are spayed through an incision in the (usually) left flank area, or on the underside of the abdomen. Hair clipped from the surgical site has normally regrown by two months after the operation.

Is neutering unnatural?

In one sense, neutering is unnatural as it involves removal of body organs which were designed to stay with the cat for its life. The operation is performed largely for the convenience of the pet owner, rather than specifically for the welfare of the individual cat. Neutering does have broader welfare implications in that it stops continual breeding and production of kittens which exceed the number of good homes available, and neutering of feral cat populations helps control numbers of stray cats which exceed the available food supply. In general, neutering of feral cats is though to be a more humane method of controlling numbers than mass extermination or allowing the excess to die off from hunger. Humane control programmes combine neutering with vaccination and feeding of stray city cats, aiming for a stable or naturally reducing population.

For pet cats, neutering is the option favoured by most owners who are not professional cat breeders and it is recommended by nearly all veterinary surgeons.

There is nothing inherently wrong with having an unneutered (entire) cat, but you should remember than unneutered males may be responsible for the production of many kittens by mating with different female cats; not all of these may find good (or any) homes. Entire tom cats also tend to fight frequently, making them prone to bite **Abscesses** and **Feline immunodeficiency virus** (FIV). Most owners also find the pungent smell of their urine unpleasant.

Unneutered queens will almost certainly become pregnant unless they are kept indoors all the time. Oestrus behaviour (referred to as 'calling' – usually alarming wailing or crying sounds that can sound just like a human baby crying and lead many owners to think their cat is in severe pain) will still usually be shown regularly, even in indoor cats, and some may argue that it is possibly inhumane to deny a female cat the opportunity to express mating behaviour when such strong instinctual drives cannot be fulfilled. Other signs of oestrus behaviour are back arching, rolling or writhing around (some owners confuse this with fits) and movements of the tail to one side.

Neutering of female cats is sometimes required for specific medical reasons – the main one being uterine infection (**Pyometra**).

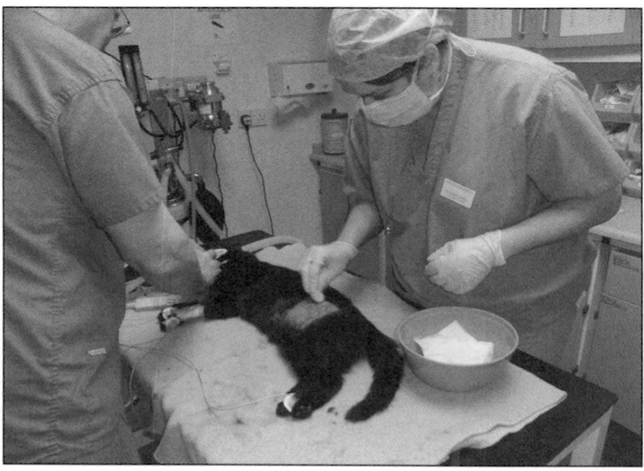

Female cat being prepared for spaying at a veterinary clinic. In the UK, the operation is normally performed through an incision in the flank. In other countries, an incision on the midline of the abdomen (belly) will be used.

☎ Urgency

Unneutered female cats in oestrus (season) are the cause of many emergency telephone calls to veterinary surgeons, mainly because of the blood curdling crying sounds they can make. Owners assume their pet must be in agony. This combined with writhing around, odd facial expressions and general restlessness and irritability present an alarming sight to the uninitiated. The history of a young, unneutered female cat usually allows the necessary reassurance to be given.

In males, urine **Spraying** usually triggers the neutering appointment to be made as tom cats have particularly pungent urine once they reach puberty.

Neutering is an elective operation which is arranged in advance. The preferred age for males is 6 months, and 5–6 months for females. Earlier neutering is also possible and is preferred by many cat welfare and rescue organisations.

✚ First aid & nursing

No first aid is required before routine neutering, but remember that the cat should have an empty stomach before a general anaesthetic. This means no food for at least 8 hours beforehand (water is fine until the morning of the operation). Keep cats indoors the night before the appointment, as they have an uncanny ability to disappear on the morning of their operation!

After any surgery, the cat should be kept indoors for 24–48 hours and it is preferable to keep female cats in for a few more days. The home environment should be warm and quiet. A small tempting meal can be offered on the same evening after a general anaesthetic and surgery, but do not be surprised if it takes a day or two for the appetite to return fully to normal. Most cats should be bright and alert on discharge from the veterinary practice. While they may sleep a little more at home, they should always be rousable and responsive to their surroundings. If you are worried there may be a problem (e.g. depression, apparent pain, breathing problems, straining) contact the vet for advice.

In female cats the wound should be inspected daily. If there is any seepage, redness or parting of the skin edges, seek veterinary advice. In male cats, stitches are not used for routine castrations and it is not easy to see where the small operation has taken place, but there should certainly be no bleeding or major swelling around the area below the anus where the incision was made into the scrotum.

Veterinary treatment

- Neutering involves a general anaesthetic (albeit a very short one in male cats) and surgery. Painkillers will usually have been given before or after the operation to minimise postoperative discomfort. This is usually very slight in males, but may be slightly more noticeable in female cats owing to the more serious nature of the operation. Nevertheless, most cats make a rapid and smooth recovery.

Related or similar conditions

- ▶ **Oestrus and mating**
- ▶ **Pyometra**
- ▶ **Surgery**

Nose problems

Nose problems take the form of:

- Nasal discharge, which can be clear, cloudy or bloody (or a mix of these).
- Congestion of the nasal passages showing as noisy or spluttery breathing.
- Growths on the nose and, in white cats, sunburn on the nose.
- The nose can also be injured in accidents, fights, etc. – it often gets scratched in fighting male cats, for example.

Clear nasal discharges are usually associated with **Allergy** or mild viral infections; cloudy discharges are associated with more severe infections, usually involving bacteria as well as viruses; bloody discharges are associated with trauma, **Foreign bodies** in the nose, severe **Inflammation** and **Tumours.**
Sun-loving cats are prone to burns on the nose and ear tips and also to a form of skin cancer (squamous cell carcinoma) involving these areas. This is more of a problem in white cats or in those with white patches.

☎ Urgency

Most nose problems are caused by rhinitis/sinusitis associated with the viral infection of **Cat flu**. As such, urgency is not high but the problem should be checked out during an early routine appointment.

Simple wounds can be bathed in salt water to keep them clean. When blood is present, this can indicate a more serious problem. If the cat was involved or suspected of being involved in an accident, the blood could be coming from the nose (not a life-threatening problem) or from the chest/lungs (potentially a life-threatening problem if there is internal bleeding). Blood is also present when there are foreign bodies, e.g. grass seeds, or tumours in the nose. Severe bouts of sneezing in cat flu may result in some blood if a small blood vessel ruptures. Because there are some serious conditions included here, it is always safest to seek emergency advice when blood is seen coming from the nose.

+ First aid & nursing

Sticky discharges can be bathed away using warm water. This will aid breathing and make the cat feel better. If cat flu is suspected, follow the detailed nursing advice given on page 52.

When blood is present, keep the cat warm and quiet (in a basket) until you receive professional advice.

Sunburn can be prevented by restricting access to window ledges etc. when the sun is strong and by applying sun screens. These are really only effective on the ear tips, as cats will almost invariably lick them off from the nose!

Veterinary treatment

- Examination usually allows a provisional diagnosis to be made. X-rays of the nose/nasal passages may be required to rule out foreign bodies and tumours.
- Treatment for **Cat flu** is described under that heading.
- For **Tumours** of the nostril, surgery can effect a cure, though this cannot be guaranteed. The conformation of the face will be altered since usually a large portion of the nose must be removed.

Related or similar conditions

- ▶ **Breathing problems**
- ▶ **Cat flu**
- ▶ **Rhinitis/sinusitis**

Notoedres

Notoedres cati is a mange mite which occasionally causes skin and ear problems in cats. See under **Mange mite**.

Nystagmus

Nystagmus is rapid involuntary eye movement, either from side to side, up and down or in a circle. This happens naturally when the head is moved, but can also be a symptom of disease of the eye or nervous system if it occurs at other times. Veterinary examination is required to try to find the reason.

O

Obesity

Obesity (being overweight) is common in cats. Estimates vary but it is possible that between 10–40% of cats seen by vets are overweight. It can be a serious health problem, making certain diseases worse and increasing the likelihood of acquiring others. It is a problem that is often misunderstood by owners and correcting obesity requires commitment from all members of the family.

Obesity most often arises because the cat is consuming more calories that it is using up. The excess calories are stored in the body as fat. Weight gain can arise from other, medical, causes as well, but these are very much in the minority of cases; probably only around 5% of cats are overweight because of a medical disorder. Although neutering is often cited as a cause of weight gain, this is not invariably the case; most neutered cats are not overweight, and some cats that have not been neutered are. However the hormonal changes brought about by neutering do make certain individuals more prone to weight gain if excessive food is supplied. There is also some evidence that indoor cats are prone to obesity due to lack of exercise.

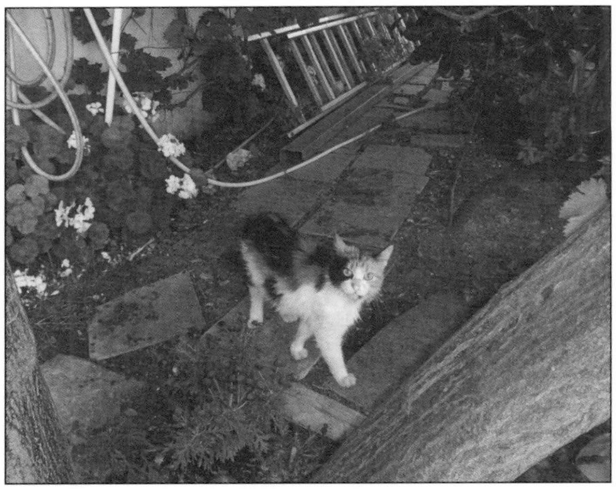

Obesity is less common in cats that take exercise regularly.

Overweight kittens nearly always turn into overweight cats. The fat cells that are produced at this age cannot be removed, so these individuals will always tend to get overweight. The correct feeding of kittens is therefore of great importance. As cats grow older, reduction in the amount of exercise and also a reduction in the 'basal metabolic rate' means that obesity becomes more likely in ageing pet cats. The 'average' pet cat weighs between 3–5 kg, though this does depend on body stature – a small cat could be very overweight at 4.5 kg.

A few diseases cause obesity. Hypothyroidism (underactive thyroid gland) is a well known cause in dogs and people, but cats do not get this condition unless both of their thyroid glands have been removed surgically as treatment for the opposite problem – an *overactive* **Thyroid gland,** which is common in older cats. Even then, it is a rare occurrence to find this complication after thyroid removal in cats; very rare cases of congenital hypothyroidism may also be encountered. Other hormonal diseases may result in weight gain, but they are diagnosed infrequently.

A commoner medical cause is weight gain caused by drugs which are being used to treat other problems. Several commonly used drugs have this effect after prolonged use. Steroid drugs are widely used for allergic conditions of various sorts, including feline **Asthma**, and hormone preparations known as progestagens are also used, although less frequently than 10–20 years ago. Both of these drugs increase the appetite and can lead to considerable weight gain. Long term use therefore always aims to use only the absolute minimum dose required to control symptoms, and usually on an alternate or every-third day basis with steroids.

Diseases caused or worsened by obesity

Obesity reduces quality of life and can worsen or even lead to certain diseases. These associated diseases are mentioned below (see under separate entries).

- *Breathing problems and Bronchitis*
  Any respiratory problem seems to be made worse when the patient is overweight. Cats have to work harder to breathe and the effects of stress and overheating are exaggerated.
- *Heart disease*
  Being overweight places extra strain on the heart. If the heart is already struggling due to disease, this extra strain can make matters worse.
- *Arthritis*
  Joint degeneration is worsened by the extra 'wear and tear' imposed on their joints by overweight cats. The joints were not designed to cope with the excess weight and, as arthritis progresses, serious deteriorations can occur if weight is not shed. In some cats, attaining a healthy weight may mean that most of the symptoms of arthritis disappear, making drug treatment (with its potential for side-effects if long term use is needed) unnecessary.
- *Diabetes*
  Overweight cats have been shown to be more at risk of diabetes than their healthy counterparts.
- *Liver disease*
  Infiltration of the liver with fat is a serious and potentially fatal condition in overweight cats that suddenly stop eating because of other problems, e.g. another disease present.
- *Feline idiophathic cystitis*
  This problem has been shown to be more frequent in overweight cats.
- *Pancreatitis*
  Another unpleasant condition that is predisposed to by obesity in cats.
- *Skin problems*
  Obese cats often do not groom themselves well. They may be physically unable to reach the back or perineal areas, with resulting problems such as urine scald, skin infections, etc. The general coat quality is also often poor, with excess scurf and a dry coat.

- *Constipation*
  Overweight cats are more prone to constipation than their healthy counterparts.

It can be seen from the above how many body systems are affected adversely by obesity, making its prevention and treatment an important part of cat care.

☎ Urgency

Obesity is a non-urgent medical condition, however reduced or zero eating (anorexia) in obese cats is potentially serious due to the possibility of the condition hepatic lipidosis (see under **Liver disease**) developing. Any overweight cat with no appetite should receive a veterinary examination promptly in case this serious condition develops.

✚ First aid & nursing

The most important aspect here is to ensure that everyone who might possibly feed the obese cat (including neighbours) are aware of the nature of the condition and the necessity, for the cat's own health and welfare, to achieve controlled weight reduction. Involving these people in the whole process, by means of keeping and recording weights and targets, etc. can help to ensure success, otherwise the good work of everyone else might be undone by one person who does not understand what is trying to be achieved.

It is worthwhile keeping regular checks on weight at home. This is simple to do on bathroom scales – weigh the cat in his basket and then weigh the basket alone. Keep a note of the basket weight and make sure the same blanket is always inside it so that the subtraction remains the same. Keep a record chart of weight on a weekly basis and remember that a gradual steady weight loss is healthier than large sudden reductions, which can be dangerous.

Weight reduction is best performed under the supervision of a vet or veterinary nurse, who can give individual recommendations on the diet, including, if necessary, the supply of prescription reducing diets for severe cases. A routine health check is performed at the same time to make sure there are no obvious diseases going on which may be influencing the cat's weight.

Veterinary treatment

- Any underlying diseases will need diagnosed and treated, and treatment may also be needed for problems which obesity is directly contributing to, e.g. arthritis.
- As for the obesity itself, a careful programme of weight reduction is needed. Starvation could be fatal due to fatty infiltration developing in the liver, so if an obese cat is put on to a new diet food and he refuses to eat for more than 24–48 hours, veterinary advice should be sought rather than just leaving the cat without any sources of food.
- Usually an initial target weight will be set. This may not be the ideal weight for the cat, but will be chosen as the initial goal to work towards. Usually the target weight will be about 10% less than the current weight: so a 7kg cat may be given a target weight of around 6.3 kg, to be achieved over a 3–4 month period. Once this weight is achieved, a further target will be set and worked towards. Once the ideal weight for body size is attained, a programme to maintain the weight at this level will be devised.

A few tips for weight-watching cats

Tip	Reason
Feed several small meals	More energy is burnt off during the digestion process than if one large meal is given; this can help with weight loss to some extent.
Encourage exercise	Can help burn off calories – BUT this is less important than regulating the diet, and some obese cats cannot exercise more without making other problems worse, e.g. **arthritis**. Encouraging more outdoor exercise or indoor playing is useful in moderation.
Weigh frequently	Keeps up motivation! Remember that slow, steady progress is what is being aimed for.
Keep in touch with the veterinary practice	Diet clinics are often run – these can be helpful and assist to keep motivation up. Any health problems can be acted on quickly.
Make sure all humans are 'on board' with the aims and objectives	One person feeding the cat inappropriately can ruin a carefully planned diet programme.

- Advice on the cat's diet will be given at all stages. Sticking to the cat's usual food but just feeding less of it is one approach but this is not always ideal, and indeed nutrient deficiencies can result from this approach due to the nature of the nutrient and energy balance in regular commercial cat foods. For these reasons, veterinary reducing diets are often recommended – these diets are specifically designed to meet the overall nutrient needs of dieting cats, whilst providing fewer calories, thereby allowing weight loss without any risk of deficiency symptoms developing.

Related or similar conditions

- **Arthritis**
- **Asthma**
- **Constipation**
- **Cystitis**
- **Diabetes**
- **Heart disease**
- **Liver disease**
- **Pancreatitis**

Oedema

Oedema (also spelt edema) is the medical term for abnormal fluid accumulation in the body. A variety of problems can lead to this, including low blood proteins, liver disease, heart disease, abdominal tumours and allergy. Oedema can be localised and slight, e.g. a patch of skin oedema after a burn, or oedema on the eyelid after a sting – these forms show as skin puffiness or swelling. Oedema can also be much more severe and general, e.g. large amounts of fluid accumulating in the abdomen as a result of heart or liver failure, showing as a swollen or pear-shaped abdomen that may feel like a water-filled balloon when gently touched. Oedema on a limb or tail would result in that part becoming swollen and tubular in appearance. All such problems should receive prompt veterinary attention. See also **Allergy**, **Bites**, **Burns**, **Feline infectious peritonitis**, **Heart disease**, **Liver disease**, **Stings** – for examples of some conditions where oedema may commonly be seen in various severities.

Oestrus and mating

Oestrus (also spelt estrus) is the term used to describe the sexual cycle of the entire female cat (queen), during which she is receptive to mating by entire tom cats and can become pregnant. Cats enter oestrus repeatedly (approximately every 3 weeks) during their breeding season, which is triggered by increasing day length in temperate climates. Behaviour alters during the oestrus phase, and female cats show several unusual behaviours which signify sexual readiness:

- **'Calling'** – an alarming noise which female cats make to attract toms. This sound uncannily resembles the cry of a human baby. Inexperienced owners often assume their cat is in severe pain or distress.
- **Rubbing, rolling and affectionate behaviour** – the female cat in oestrus may be suddenly much more affectionate than usual, in an overtly demonstrative way. This behaviour can become quite agitated and some owners think their cat is having a kind of fit or funny turn.
- **Back arching, tail deviation and treading** – this behaviour is designed to make mating easier. It can often be stimulated in the receptive cat by stroking gently along the back area. The cat adopts the posture automatically.
- **Altered appetite** – when in season, the female cat may have a reduced appetite due to hormonal influences.

The loud noises, scent dispersal (by rubbing, etc.) and other behaviours ensure that maximum chances are available to attract a mate. Usually, a cat in season will have neighbourhood entire tom cats attracted to the house and, quite likely, spraying urine in the vicinity.

The mating process itself proceeds by the tom cat mounting the female (made easier by her position) and taking hold of the scruff area of the queen in his mouth. This is a natural part of the process, not a sign of aggression, and the queen reacts in much the same way as kittens do when picked up through the scruff by their mother. The tom cat's penis has backwardly directed barbs on it, and when withdrawn after ejaculation these barbs stimulate the lining of the queen's genital tract. This process is necessary to induce ovulation (release of an egg) in the queen, to allow fertilisation to take place. It usually provokes an aggressive response towards the tom and the queen may wail loudly at this point, before writhing around on the ground for a few minutes.

☎ Urgency

Oestrus and mating behaviours are natural phenomena and no veterinary involvement is needed, however many emergency telephone calls arise because of the plaintive sounding noises that queens in oestrus make, and because of the unusual rolling behaviours which owners can find alarming. Usually, taken with the age of the cat and the knowledge that she has not yet been spayed, the necessary reassurances can be given.

✚ First aid & nursing

None is needed, save for the occasional small wounds that may appear in the scruff area of the queen after mating. These may now and again form **Abscesses** which need to be treated in the usual way.

Veterinary treatment

- This is not needed unless mating produces some injury, or unless the frequency or duration of oestrus cycling is abnormal.
- The best time to spay entire queens is between oestrus periods.

Related or similar conditions

▶ **Neutering**
▶ **Pregnancy**

'Off colour'

Being 'off colour' is one of the commonest symptoms owners tell veterinary surgeons about their cats. It is a very vague symptom which can mean any or all of the following things:

- Having a poor appetite
- Not interacting as much with humans or other pets
- Not going out as usual
- Not grooming as usual
- Seeming 'unhappy'
- Being lethargic
- Being irritable
- Being reluctant to move around the house – wants to stay in the same place all the time

None of these things point to any one disease – a cat with symptoms like this could be suffering from almost any medical condition and a veterinary surgeon will rely on other additional symptoms to guide him or her towards a possible diagnosis, e.g. vomiting, drinking to excess, irregular breathing, etc.

Many cats that seem off colour have a high temperature, and this usually indicates infection caused by either a virus or a bacterium.

☎ Urgency

Because so many problems are possible, both slight and serious, it is difficult to give strict guidance about urgency. However you should consider the situation urgent if:

- Symptoms have been present for more than two days
- There has been no food or water intake for 1–2 days
- The cat's condition appears to be worsening
- Breathing is irregular

- No urine or faeces has been passed for 24–48 hours
- The cat seems in severe pain when moved or lifted
- Gums are pale (rather than salmon pink in colour)

✚ First aid & nursing

General nursing care is appropriate. This means keeping the cat indoors, in a comfortable temperature and with sufficient bedding. Litter tray, food and water should be nearby and the **Appetite** should be tempted. A close watch and records should be kept for urine and faeces passed, respiratory rate (see **Breathing problems**), any **Vomiting** or **Diarrhoea**, and food and water consumed. If you know how and are able, the **Temperature** can be taken – most owners are advised not to attempt this unless experienced however.

Veterinary treatment

- The emphasis will be on making a diagnosis. In many cases, this will be possible after a clinical examination but reference to further tests (e.g. blood tests, urine tests, X-ray) may be needed. As mentioned above, many 'off colour' cats have a high temperature.

Related or similar conditions

▶ **Almost any of the medical conditions in this book could be involved.**

Oil on coat

This is a common but serious problem, which can be an emergency. See **Coat contamination.**

Old age problems

Cats are long-lived animals and many domestic companions live well into their teens, with a few old age pensioners still going strong at 20. A cat is usually considered middle aged at around 6–8 years and old aged above 12 years. As they get older, certain changes appear gradually as a result of the ageing process. Elderly cats may spend less time outside and more time in the house or in one particular part of the house. Cats sleep a lot anyway, but older cats will sleep more than younger ones. Niggling health problems may make older cats a little more irritable to other pets or children – the commonest one is **Arthritis** of the limbs or spine and, while not always requiring drug treatment, care has to be taken to ensure that the older cat is not handled roughly by younger more boisterous pets or children.

'Senior' cats take longer to respond to things and to register what is going on, so

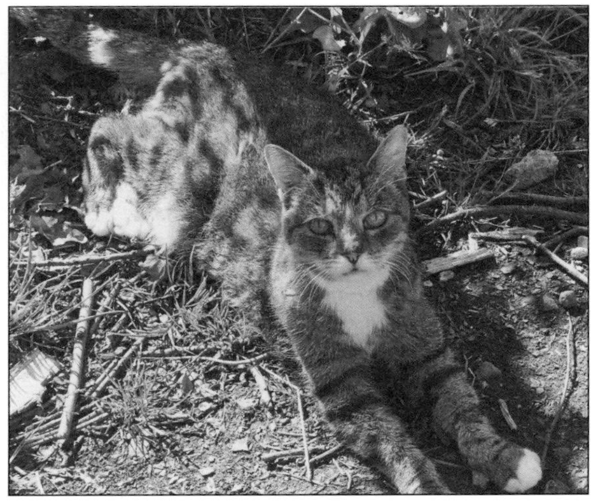

As they get older, cats tend to become less active and lose muscle mass.

allowances should be made for this, and they are less able to adapt to change quickly if, e.g. new additions are made to the household or there is a change in environment due to flitting. To some extent, however, this also depends on the personality of the individual cat. One quite common problem, and something which can cause owners concern, is so-called 'night calling' – when the cat makes bloodcurdling yowls in the middle of the night after everyone has gone to bed and the house is quiet. This happens quite a lot in older cats and although the cat sounds in distress, more often than not when the anxious owner rushes through the house to find it, the cat behaves quite as normal! Night-calling may just reflect a little disorientation, senility or need for reassurance in the older pet and treatment is not usually given.

Physically, cats that are very old lose muscle mass and their coat loses some of its condition and gloss. The face may take on a slightly 'pinched' appearance around the nose and cheeks, again due to loss of muscle, and the eyes will be less bright. Older cats probably become slightly **Deaf** too. Claws may become overgrown due to the cat taking less exercise and the claws may be retracted less effectively, making them more prone to get caught up in bedding etc.

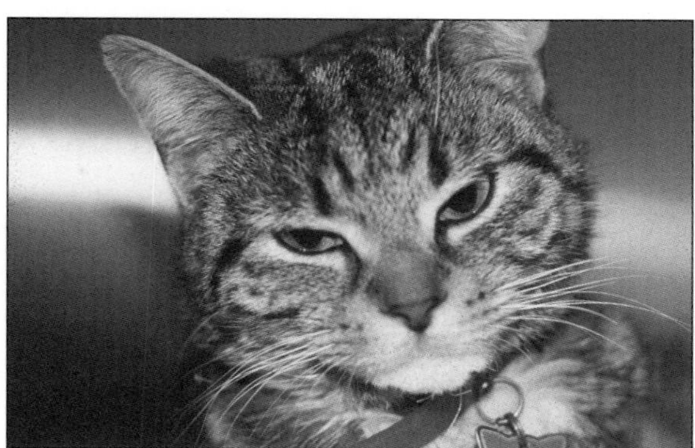

A cat is considered 'senior' at around 10–12 years.

☎ Urgency

Obviously, ageing is a natural and gradual process and you will probably be advised of its effects during yearly health examinations and booster vaccinations for your cat. In older cats, general health problems should never be allowed to go on too long before advice is received because older patients have fewer reserves to cope with the effects of disease.

✚ First aid & nursing

Some quite simple things can make life easier for the older cat. They often prefer warmth more, so arranging a warm bed somewhere will usually be appreciated, e.g. near a radiator. Alternatively you could use a heated cat bed. Extra padding (e.g. foam layers) makes things more comfortable for stiff, arthritic cats. If the cat is having problems getting up on to a favourite chair, providing a step or stool may help. Make sure the nails are kept trimmed and short since long nails are uncomfortable to walk on and may grow into the paw pads.

Make sure cat flaps are not too high or set up so that the older cat has to struggle to push through them. Providing a litter tray indoors means that the cat doesn't always have to go outside in cold weather to relieve himself. Speak to veterinary staff about a suitable diet for the older cat, which takes account of any on-going health problems. When grooming an older cat, soft brushes are often better than combs, which can cause pain if they bump across bony prominences or arthritic joints.

Look out for symptoms of diseases which are particularly common in older cats:

- **Mouth pain or bad breath** – indicating diseased teeth or gums
- **Drinking and passing urine to excess** – indicating **Kidney disease**, overactive **Thyroid gland** or **Diabetes** (and also certain less common diseases)
- **Weight loss** – some weight loss is inevitable with age, but significant loss is common with overactive **Thyroid gland, Kidney disease** and some tumours
- **Changes in appetite** – overactive **Thyroid gland** causes increased appetite (together with weight loss); **Kidney disease** or **Mouth and tooth problems** may cause a reluctant appetite and many other diseases cause poor appetite
- **Pain and stiffness** – signs of **Arthritis.**

Veterinary treatment

- The problems of old cats is an important area of companion animal veterinary medicine and many practices can provide fact sheets and information on old cat diseases and disorders, as well as periodic health checks to look for common problems. It is always best to treat these problems early to gain the best chance of a speedy recovery.

Related or similar conditions

- ▶ **Arthritis**
- ▶ **Diabetes**
- ▶ **Euthanasia**
- ▶ **Kidney disease**
- ▶ **Mouth and tooth problems**
- ▶ **Thyroid gland (overactive)**

Osteomyelitis

Osteomyelitis is a serious infection of bone which may follow injury or surgery. Bone infections are very difficult to cure as antibiotics do not penetrate the dense structure of bone well and pockets of infection can linger even after extensive treatment lasting months. Fortunately, osteomyelitis is fairly rare in cats. The commonest situations would be infection after deep **Bite** wounds or traumatic loss of tissue (e.g. after a road accident), or following orthopaedic surgery for broken bones when a post-operative infection takes hold. Treatment can involve further surgery as well as prolonged courses of antibiotics. In very severe cases, amputation sometimes has to be considered.

☎ Urgency

Any deep wound or open injury suspected of being a **Fracture** should be treated urgently to limit the chances of infection. Remember however that most wounds in cats are much shallower and do not threaten underlying bone.

Osteomyelitis itself is a chronic disease and is usually diagnosed after X-rays and a bone biopsy. In the initial phases of bone infection, the cat may appear unwell with pain and a high **Temperature**. Once the disease becomes established, the cat usually reacts much as normal, apart from not using the affected limb, which may have areas of discharge or swelling. It is this low grade, grumbling nature of the disease that makes it so difficult to completely clear up.

✚ First aid & nursing

Open wounds should be covered with a

clean dressing until a veterinary surgeon can assess them. If it is impossible to keep or hold such a dressing in place, simply transfer the cat to a clean cat carrier and take to a veterinary practice. Look at the sections that give advice on **Bleeding**, **Accident** and **Wounds**.

For the cat under treatment for osteomyelitis, a good plane of nutrition and physiotherapy can be helpful. Ask the veterinary staff for appropriate guidance. All antibiotics must be given as directed, for the entire course, and medication should not be interrupted or stopped without consulting with your vet.

Veterinary treatment

- Osteomyelitis is often a lengthy and expensive disease to treat. Multiple X-rays to check progress, repeat biopsies and sometimes several separate surgical operations are required for complex cases, and treatment can stretch over several months.
- Severe infection with non-healing fractures can sometimes occur and occasionally, the most practical treatment option may end up being amputation. Usually such cases are under the care of specialists, or else amputation is considered earlier for economic reasons. Remember that cats almost invariably cope well with three legs, and can have an excellent quality of life.

Related or similar conditions

- ▶ **Accident**
- ▶ **Bleeding**
- ▶ **Fractures/dislocations**
- ▶ **Lameness**
- ▶ **Wounds**

Overgrooming

Cats can spend around 30–40% of their wakeful time grooming their coat in order to keep this in tip-top condition. If a cat stops grooming for any reason (e.g. **Mouth and tooth problems**, **Arthritis** or general illness) the coat soon begins to look unkempt and a dishevelled cat is nearly always an ill one. Grooming removes loose and dead hair, keeps the skin free of adhered particles and parasites from the environment, reduces scurf build up and also helps with heat loss in hot weather, when the evaporation of saliva produces a cooling effect.

Some cats groom excessively and do this so much that hairless patches appear on the coat and **Fur ball** becomes a potential medical problem due to the increased quantities of hair that are swallowed. When cats are overgrooming and have no symptoms of skin parasites or other obvious causes of **Itching** or skin disease, then the grooming is a displacement activity which is occurring in response to **Anxiety**.

☎ Urgency

The problem is a non-urgent one as it develops over weeks or months.

✚ First aid & nursing

First, make sure excessive time is indeed being spent in grooming. Remember that a large amount of the waking day is normally spent in attending to personal hygiene in cats – they truly are fastidiously clean animals.

Most owners whose cats indulge in overgrooming do pick up and recognise that this occurs in response to stressful situations, and can identify the 'anxiety' type of grooming as opposed to more normal behaviour. It is important to try to acclimatise the cat to the stressful or frightening situations (or avoid them completely if possible) in order to prevent this displacement activity. The precise method used depends on exactly what the frightening stimulus is, but usually a programme of controlled and increasing exposure can be worked out with a veterinary surgeon or behaviour therapist. Gradually, over a period of weeks, the cat is conditioned to accept the stimulus and not to respond in an anxious way. We must remember that cats' sensory abilities are superior to our own, and that they can be picking up subtle cues that we are unaware of. By focusing on these, abnormal behaviours can be modified or reduced. Skilled help is needed in most cases.

Some cats are generally anxious and are frightened by a variety of things. Here, it is important to try to devise practical measures to reduce the anxiety 'load' of the cat. It will probably be impossible to avoid everything that a generally fearful cat is wary of, but by tackling several of the big concerns, substantial improvement in anxiety related behaviours can often be made.

Veterinary treatment

- Common skin diseases need to be ruled out before this problem can be diagnosed. Once behavioural reasons have been confirmed, input from a behaviour therapist or vet with experience in this area will usually be very beneficial. Remember that improvement takes time (and commitment from all members of the family). Do not expect too great an improvement until a couple of months have elapsed.

Related or similar conditions

- **Anxiety/fear**
- **Behaviour problems – general**
- **Fleas**
- **Grooming (poor)**

P

Pain

Pain is a common cause of aggression in cats, and you should always suspect this if a normally placid animal shows uncharacteristic behaviour towards you or another animal. Pain is usually caused by injury or inflammation, but locating the source of pain is not at all easy in agitated cats that resent any interference whatsoever. In these cases, it is safest to leave close examination to the veterinary surgeon, who has the option of sedating the cat to allow careful checking of all body parts. Look at the general advice on dealing with nervous, fearful or aggressive cats (**Aggression** on p. xviii).

One of the commonest causes of pain in cats that can roam outside is a bite **Abscess** or cellulitis (painful muscle or tissue infection/inflammation), but pain from diseased teeth and arthritis is also very frequently seen, especially in middle aged or older cats. Urban cats are also more prone to falls, road accidents and, unfortunately, malicious injuries such as kicks and air gun pellets.

☎ Urgency

Any cat showing signs of severe and unrelenting pain needs emergency treatment. Common examples of such situations would be pain from a **Fracture** after a road accident or fall, post-operative pain that seems to be worsening and not easing off (as expected), pain from any eye injury or inflammation, and pain that seems to be coming from the abdominal area.

Some minor injuries are characterised by a brief period of very intense pain/aggression which then wears off over 30 minutes or so, during which time the cat may want to hide away somewhere. Cats who have their paws stood on or their tails caught in the door often behave in this way. Given a short period of time, if the injury was not too severe, they return more or less to normal – or perhaps retain a slight limp or tail droop. This sort of injury is not life-threatening and can safely be left until morning if it occurs at night and the cat seems well otherwise. Quite often, by morning the cat is completely back to normal.

Remember that very vocal cats can appear in pain but sometimes are not. The commonest example of this is the ear-piercing yowls made by entire female cats in season (see **Oestrus**) and the 'night calling' that is shown by many cats in **Old age**. Both of these are easily confused with a response to pain by the inexperienced owner.

✚ First aid & nursing

Always ensure you are in no danger from being bitten or scratched and, if in doubt, leave the cat quietly alone for a period to see if he becomes more amenable to handling or close observation.

If possible, see if you can tell where the pain seems to be coming from:

- Is there an obvious lameness or lifting of a paw?
- Is the tail carried as normal?
- Is the cat able to and does she want to move around?
- Can you see any swellings on the body or evidence of bleeding?
- Do the eyes and ears appear normal?
- Is there blood or saliva coming from the mouth?
- Is the breathing quiet and relaxed?
- Does the cat seem to be straining or 'clamping' her abdomen?

All of these will provide helpful clues to your vet.

If there is lots of distress, coax or place the cat in a cat carrier or box (wear thick gloves and a long sleeved coat if necessary) until you can arrange for transportation to a clinic.

Veterinary treatment

- Diagnosing the source of the pain allows treatment to be started to control the underlying disease or injury. While that is working, painkillers can also be given to make the patient more comfortable. Good nursing and psychological reassurance is an important part of the nursing process in the hospital and at home.

Related or similar conditions

▶ **Accident**
▶ **Bites**
▶ **Fractures/dislocations**
▶ **Surgery**

Pancreatitis

The pancreas is an important organ which lies near the stomach in the abdomen. It secretes enzymes and hormones and is essential for normal digestion and metabolism. Inflammation of the pancreas (pancreatitis) occurs in cats and is a painful and unpleasant condition. Typical symptoms are of a subdued cat, with poor appetite, vomiting and sometimes diarrhoea. Dehydration and a high temperature are frequently seen. The cat may show signs of pain in the abdomen and may 'guard' the area or hiss/bite whenever anyone tries to lift him or her up. Very severe bouts of pancreatitis can be life-threatening due to additional complications of the severe inflammation occurring within the abdomen and the nearness of all the other important organs. Pancreatitis can also be a chronic condition and can be associated with other inflammatory disease, for example in the bowels.

☎ Urgency

Pancreatitis may occasionally result in an emergency appointment but more often, the cat has been ill for a day or two with symptoms that are not improving or even getting worse, and owners bring their pet in for a routine visit complaining of no appetite, vomiting and lethargy. Owners of cats that have suffered the problem before often recognise the symptoms, however the symptoms themselves are not particularly specific for pancreatitis and other problems, including less serious ones, can also show in this way.

✚ First aid & nursing

See also **Vomiting**. If the cat is able to tolerate fluids by mouth, without vomiting these back up, small volumes of water or glucose solution should be given every 1–2 hours. Around 10 mls is adequate, and will help to protect against Dehydration. Most cats will not eat, or will only take a mouthful or two, and they will be keen to lie quietly somewhere. If there is severe vomiting, do not attempt to feed or syringe fluids into the cat; phone for advice straight away. Make sure a litter tray is nearby and that the cat will not get disturbed by children or other animals.

When cats are discharged home for convalescence, careful reintroduction of a bland diet is required, with observation for any further vomiting. Diets rich in carbohydrate (pasta, rice) are better since the recovering pancreas has to 'work' less hard in dealing with these foodstuffs. Sometimes a low fat diet is recommended to try to limit any future attacks.

Veterinary treatment

- This consists of no fluid or food by mouth for several days, so affected cats require hospitalisation and intravenous fluid therapy (a drip), to correct dehydration and restore normal balance of body fluids and electrolytes while the inflamed pancreas is settling down.
- A battery of tests are usually used to help diagnose pancreatitis and separate it from other possible diagnoses – these often include blood tests, X-ray and ultrasound.
- Other drugs used in pancreatitis include antibiotics, painkillers, and in severe cases sometimes even plasma or blood transfusions.
- Once vomiting has stopped and the cat is tolerating fluids by mouth, they can usually be discharged home with dietary advice.

Related or similar conditions

- ▶ **Appetite (abnormal)**
- ▶ **Dehydration**
- ▶ **Vomiting**

Panleucopaenia

This term means a reduction in the numbers of protective white blood cells circulating in the bloodstream. This arises as a consequence of infection with **Feline infectious enteritis**. The virus results in depletion of the numbers of white cells, laying the infected cat open to worsening or complicating infections. The disease feline enteritis is sometimes referred to as feline panleucopaenia because of this effect it has on the cat's white blood cells.

Panting

Panting (an increased breathing rate through an open mouth) is a natural means of heat loss in healthy cats in very warm or hot environmental conditions. It is also a reaction that is frequently seen in stressed cats during travel or in unfamiliar surroundings, e.g. at a veterinary clinic. In this sense, in otherwise healthy cats, it is not an abnormality as such but a response to stimuli coming from the surroundings.

Panting, however, should not be ignored, especially in sick or old cats. This is mainly because cats in general pant far less readily than dogs and when it occurs it can occasionally mean that the cat is near the limit of its respiratory and circulatory capacities. Efforts should be made to cool the cat down or reduce the stress that is being experienced as soon as possible. Cats that are suffering from various diseases will often pant as they try to cope with the effects of added stress, and a fairly small amount of stress may provoke the panting response. This is quite common in cats with overactive **Thyroid gland** or **Heart disease** – they manage well when relaxed and quiet, but additional stimulation can push them towards the edge of their ability to cope. Obviously, in these individuals, sustained stress showing as panting could be dangerous.

☎ Urgency

If your cat starts panting at home, the first thing to suspect is that the environmental temperature is simply too warm. However, cats are naturally hot climate animals and tolerate high temperatures well, so if *you* are not finding the conditions in the house warm, it is very unlikely that your cat is panting for this reason unless it has been hugging the fire excessively or lying near a hot radiator.

Stress may be causing the panting. Have there been loud noises or other stressful occurrences? If so, giving the effects of these time to wear off may be all that is needed. A cat that has been chased outside may rush in through the cat flap in a great flurry of activity and pant as much from fear as from shortness of breath. It should be settling down after 20 minutes or so.

If you feel that neither of the above two reasons are applicable, then you should seek emergency advice regarding your cat. The reason is the same as that mentioned above: cats pant infrequently; when it occurs it must be taken seriously as there may be severe respiratory or circulatory problems occurring.

+ First aid & nursing

The first rule is *avoid all further stress*! Additional fear or excitement can very occasionally be enough to tip the balance and push a sick and already stressed cat into respiratory or heart failure. If you know what is stressing the cat, take steps to remove it or place the cat in another place. A quiet, dark, cool environment is ideal – if the cat is in a cage carrier, place this in a quiet place, cover with a towel or blanket and observe unobtrusively. In cases of severe heat stress, a wet towel or blanket can be used to cover the cage and a cool air fan can be directed towards it if available. Bathing the face, ears and paws in cold water or with damp cotton wool can help reduce heat build up.

Veterinary treatment

- Examination and tests should reveal the cause of the panting, and emergency treatment to stabilise the cat may be needed for heart or respiratory problems. Hospitalisation for oxygen therapy and emergency drugs may be needed.
- Once the cat has been brought on to a level plane, further treatment can be planned as needed.
- Stress or heat associated panting should quickly stop (within 10–20 minutes) when the cat is moved out of the environment that is producing the symptoms.

Tip

If you are worried your cat is severely stressed in a vet's busy waiting room, tell the nursing or reception staff you are concerned and they will be able to help by letting the cat wait in a quieter area or even outside.

Reassurance from someone the cat knows can also go a long way to alleviating stress and fear.

Related or similar conditions

- **Asthma**
- **Breathing problems**
- **Fever/high temperature**
- **Heart disease**

Paralysis

Paralysis means temporary or permanent loss of function of a part of the body due to damage to its nerve supply. For example, a paralysed limb cannot be moved at will and may have no sensation (feeling) in it. In cats, limbs and the tail are the most commonly paralysed parts of the body and this is usually the result of accidents, e.g. road accidents, falls.

The bladder can also become paralysed. This is a frequent complication after pelvic fractures or lower back injuries in cats and if not treated, or if the initial nerve damage has been very severe, incontinence can result. Urine accumulates and distends the bladder enormously, but the cat has no sensation of needing to urinate owing to the paralysis. Eventually the severe over-distension destroys the bladder's natural ability to contain and control urine flow. If treated early enough (by expressing the bladder manually or under sedation to prevent over-distension) this type of paralysis can clear up once the nerves recover. In another (more severe) form of bladder paralysis, the bladder remains completely flaccid and undistended at all times and urine simply leaks out continuously. It all depends on how serious the initial nerve injury to the bladder was as to which type of paralysis occurs.

Paralysis can be caused by diseases too – a tumour or severe inflammation which involves a nerve or the spinal cord may result in paralysis of the part of the body that the nerve supplies; also, certain forms of surgery may result in accidental nerve damage, leading to temporary or permanent paralysis.

☎ Urgency

If you notice paralysis in your cat, e.g. a dropping tail with no sensation when you pinch the tip, or a cat which cannot use any of its limbs, seek advice immediately. Whilst tail paralysis is not life-threatening, there may be other injuries to consider (especially breathing or bleeding problems in traumatised cats). Early treatment may be able to save a leg in limb paralysis but this very much depends on the underlying cause of the problem.

Some cats with apparently paralysed limbs which are not being moved may be found to have fractures, but the cats are not showing the expected degree of pain that one normally expects after a limb fracture due to the effects of physical or psychological shock.

✚ First aid & nursing

Little in the way of practical first aid can be carried out, however you should ensure that the cat does not accidentally damage the paralysed part. There may be no sensation in it at all, hence it could easily become traumatised because the protective effect of pain is lost. Keep the cat in a secure place while you arrange veterinary attention. Treat any other injuries following advice given elsewhere in this book.

Parasites

Parasites are small organisms which usually live off, and feed from, much larger animals, known as their hosts. They may spend all of their life-cycle on the host (lice and skin mites do this), or they may visit the host for shorter spells at a time in order to feed (fleas and ticks do this). 'Visiting' parasites complete their life-cycles in other places (in your carpets and soft furnishings in the case of fleas!). While adult intestinal worms remain in the intestines, their eggs or larvae are passed out in the faeces to infect other cats, sometimes via complicated life-cycles involving intermediate hosts (e.g. mice), which are then eaten by other cats.

Most people cringe or scratch at the mere idea of parasites but really efficient parasites cause very few problems for their hosts, e.g. many stray or feral cats will carry some fleas as well as internal parasitic worms, which appear to have no visible effect on the cat's health. If the fleas or worm numbers were to increase a lot, however (and this could happen in overcrowded conditions or if the cat became ill for other reasons), then medical symptoms may appear. In most situations a 'balance' is reached and host and parasite live together without any problems.

For these reasons, treatment of parasites may not always be a good thing in stray or feral cats, because the host-parasite balance is upset and will only reestablish later anyway – it may be better to leave things as they are in the first place. But in pet cats parasitic diseases are nearly always treated, except in very ill animals who could not tolerate the drugs used, because a few parasitic diseases can cause problems in people (see also **Zoonoses**).

Most of the skin parasites cause irritation if present in significant numbers and the commonest parasite by far in the cat is a skin one: the common cat flea, *Ctenocephalides felis*. This parasite also affects dogs, even though dogs have their own species of flea. In fact, the cat flea is such a successful parasite that it is found much more frequently on dogs than the dogs' own species of flea!

Other common parasites which may affect cats are:

- **Skin mites** – living within the top layers of the skin or in the ears; there are several varieties of skin mite, causing various degrees of itchiness
- **Lice** – living on the hair coat, a particular problem in neglected or debilitated cats
- **Ticks** – attached to the skin surface (often resembling small warts or growths)
- **Worms** – living in the intestines, and termed roundworms or tapeworms
- **Ringworm** – a fungus which causes skin irritation and is commoner in long haired cats
- **Giardia** – a protozoan (microscopic animal) parasite which can cause diarrhoea and weight loss.

Each of these parasites is discussed fully under the appropriate section. The important thing to remember is that all parasites are best diagnosed by a veterinary surgeon, who can then prescribe appropriate treatment. Although many antiparasitic products may be bought 'over the counter', and may be cheaper than a veterinary surgeon's fee and prescription, reliable treatment depends on an accurate professional diagnosis. Shop-bought products may not be as successful – if this is the case, owners are sometimes then prompted to repeat treatment, or use a higher dose, risking toxicity (poisoning). This happens frequently when ineffective flea control products are used on cats – not only do the cats still have fleas, but serious symptoms from absorption of excessive amounts of the insecticidal chemicals used can occur.

Related or similar conditions

- **Roundworms**
- **Skin problems**
- **Tapeworms**

Peritonitis

Peritonitis is a severe disease of inflammation in the lining membrane of the abdomen. It can arise for various reasons and is always serious. Damage to internal organs such as the stomach, bladder or bowel can lead onto peritonitis, and the condition is also a major complication arising after any abdominal surgery. Trauma or injury which leads to damage or rupture of abdominal organs carries the risk of peritonitis; it can be rapidly life-threatening with affected animals spiralling down in condition and succumbing to shock, dehydration and sepsis.

Peritonitis may not be easy to recognise as the symptoms, though severe, can be vague in nature. The affected cat may simply be extremely subdued, possibly vomiting, with abdominal pain and rapid breathing. Usually the prior history of the cat may lead to its suspicion, e.g. recent abdominal surgery, trauma or severe infection.

Feline infectious peritonitis is a specific disease of cats, which presents in a different way to the non-infectious causes mentioned above.

☎ Urgency

This is an urgent condition since peritonitis can pursue a relentless course, even with treatment. If you suspect the problem (e.g. you take your cat home after abdominal surgery and he seems to be deteriorating instead of improving) contact your veterinary surgeon for advice.

✚ First aid & nursing

As long as there is no vomiting, fluids (water and glucose solution) can be given by mouth at the rate of 5–10 mls every hour. The cat should be kept warm and quiet whilst advice is sought. Note if vomiting occurs, what the breathing rate is while at rest (see under **Breathing problems**), and whether there seems to be any internal pain when you gently touch the belly area. Keep a check on the demeanour of the cat; if he appears to be becoming unresponsive or in progressive pain, the situation is worsening.

Veterinary treatment

- Peritonitis may be suspected if the cat has a recent history of abdominal injury, wounds or surgery, and clinical symptoms match those often associated with the problem.
- Blood tests, X-rays/scans, and tests on small samples of fluid withdrawn from

the abdomen may be used to confirm the condition.

- Many cases require surgery to repair damaged organs, stop leakages and remove areas of contamination. Intensive aftercare is usually required and repeat anaesthetics and operations may be required to ensure that the condition is being brought under control.
- Peritonitis always carries a 'guarded' prognosis owing to the severe nature of the condition.

Related or similar conditions

- ▶ **Feline infectious peritonitis (FIP)**
- ▶ **Foreign body**
- ▶ **Pyometra**
- ▶ **Vomiting**

Plants (eating)

Cats are carnivorous animals, but all carnivores require (and enjoy) eating vegetable material to gain essential nutrients, roughage and vitamins. Many wild carnivores, once they have killed a prey animal, eat the digestive organs first and take in partly digested vegetable matter in that way. Carnivores, cats included, will also 'graze' on wild plants outside (or houseplants if kept indoors). Chewing on rough and indigestible stems may encourage the cat to vomit and thus aid in the bringing up of **Fur balls** or indigestible material from hunted animals that is present in the stomach. There is also some evidence to suggest that selective eating of various plants and herbs can be a natural response to certain diseases or deficiencies owing to 'cravings' developing in the sick animal. Instinct seems to direct the animal towards the appropriate herbal remedy. (Note that dietary deficiencies are rare in pet cats fed a good diet).

Eating plant material and grass is therefore a natural and healthy occupation for all cats, even although some do seem to indulge in it more than others!

Tip: Some plants are toxic

In most cases, your cats will damage your plants, and not vice versa. However many plants can cause toxic symptoms in cats if consumed. If you have cats, it is safer to avoid certain plants or else keep them in rooms to which the cat does not have access. Toxic species include:

- Lilies (particularly toxic)
- Azalea
- Poinsettia
- Delphinium
- Hydrangea
- Begonia
- Oleander; and various others.

If you provide your cat with 'kitty grass' it is likely that he or she will prefer this to houseplants anyway. The plants will be spared and any (small) risk of toxicity avoided.

Depraved appetite (the medical term is pica) can show as a willingness to eat or chew odd things. See **Wool eating**, a recognised behaviour in cats, for example. Other things may be chewed or eaten. Sometimes, this can be part of an underlying behaviour problem. Especially if additional medical symptoms are present, diseases of organs such as the **Liver** may need to be considered because these can lead to unusual appetite cravings.

Pneumonia

Pneumonia is a serious disease of inflammation of the lungs and air passages which leads to breathing difficulty, cough, high temperature, lethargy and, in severe cases, death. It is much less common than other respiratory diseases, especially **Cat flu** and feline **Asthma** (feline bronchitis). Pneumonia can arise as a complication of other diseases, especially in very debilitated cats, or it can be caused directly by viruses or bacteria.

Instead of being full of air as usual, the lungs in pneumonia become fluid-filled and the lung tissue gets thickened, leading to increased breathing rate, increased effort in breathing and moist noises during breathing. In severe cases, rasping or gurgling noises will be heard (termed moist rales).

Cats with pneumonia will be very subdued, off their food and reluctant to move. The breathing patterns will be clearly abnormal.

☎ Urgency

This is an urgent condition, as is any severe breathing problem in cats. Seek advice without delay.

+ First aid & nursing

The most important thing is to avoid stressing the cat. Even small amounts of stress can push a struggling cat over the edge of compensation into respiratory failure. The difficulty in breathing is itself probably making the cat somewhat anxious and the constricting sensation of having to fight for breath is very unpleasant.

Handle the patient slowly and gently and stop if distress seems to be caused. Keep the cat in a well ventilated area; air fans can help and if the cat seems hot, bathe the face, ears and paws with cold water.

Count and keep a note of the respiratory rate when the cat is at rest, and note whether there is any increased effort in breathing (see under **Breathing problems**).

Veterinary treatment

- Tests used to confirm pneumonia include X-rays and blood tests.
- Treatment depends on the severity and can include antibiotics, intravenous fluids (a drip) and hospitalisation for rest and oxygen therapy. Severe pneumonia can be life threatening.

Related or similar conditions

- ▶ **Asthma**
- ▶ **Breathing problems**
- ▶ **Cat flu**
- ▶ **Cough**
- ▶ **Heart disease**

Poisoning and toxicities

Cats are generally fastidious eaters and are not so likely to consume poisons or toxins as dogs. The main means whereby cats are poisoned are:

- Eating rodents which have themselves been poisoned
- Cleaning contaminated coat or fur by licking (common)
- Accidental overdosing by owners using flea control products (common)
- Administration by owners of human pain killing drugs, e.g. paracetamol – which is extremely toxic to cats; they

also have a much lower toxic dose of aspirin compared to other animals
- Malicious poisoning

Symptoms vary a lot but may include such things as incoordination, staggering, abnormal twitches, fits, vomiting, salivation and diarrhoea.

☎ Urgency
If you suspect poisoning or overdose has occurred, seek urgent veterinary attention.

✚ First aid & nursing
It is usually too difficult to attempt to make the cat vomit (using, e.g. a strong salt solution). In addition, if the substance swallowed was a caustic one, vomiting will cause further damage to the oesophagus by the regurgitated chemical. Rapid transport to a veterinary premises will generally be safer. If at all possible take details of the toxic product consumed or been in contact with, e.g. a product label, a drug bottle, or supply any other information that might help the vet find out the nature of the product so that appropriate treatment can be given.

Any coat contamination means that licking of the fur must be prevented, even if it means the cat is held wrapped in a towel or blanket all the time.

Veterinary treatment
With any poisoning the approach is to:

- Limit absorption of further poison
- Support the cat's essential organ functions and control dangerous symptoms
- Find out the degree of damage already done to vital organs, and whether this may be reversible or compatible with life.

This treatment usually requires hospitalisation and various tests and investigations.

Tip
Never give any human drugs to cats in an attempt to relieve pain or cure symptoms. Cats' metabolism of drugs is very different from that of human beings, and drugs which are safe in people can be fatal in cats.

Related or similar conditions
- ▶ **Brain damage**
- ▶ **Coat contamination**
- ▶ **Fits**
- ▶ **Kidney disease**
- ▶ **Liver disease**
- ▶ **Vomiting**

Pregnancy

Pregnancy in the cat lasts an average of 63 days. Except for professional breeders, few cat owners will know the exact day of mating, so there is usually an element of guesswork involved in a cat that is found to be pregnant! The majority of pet female cats are neutered at an early age (around 5–6 months) and so pregnancy does not of course occur. There is no merit in deliberately allowing a cat to have one litter of kittens before routine neutering (spaying) of females.

False pregnancy (pseudopregnancy) can occur after a mating which does not result in fertilisation, or sometimes it can result even when there is no mating. A cat which has a false pregnancy will not return into heat (oestrus) as expected in 3 weeks – the next heat period will be after about 40 days. Unlike dogs, cats with false pregnancies do not usually produce milk in their mammary glands.

Pregnant cats show a steady weight gain throughout the course of their pregnancy, this being especially marked during the last third of the pregnancy, when development of the breasts (mammary glands) also occurs in preparation to feed the kittens. Activity levels decline and the cat may need to eat more frequent meals. Generally, food should be available ad lib to pregnant cats and they will regulate their own intake. No supplements are required. Just before birth the abdomen is usually huge in cats (movement of the kittens may be detectable through it), the nipples will be prominent and red and milk may be expressible.

☎ Urgency

Pregnancy is a natural condition and no treatment is required unless problems develop. But see the section on **Birth** for information. Most cats have no difficulties, and make good mothers. Minimum human interference is generally the best approach.

✚ First aid & nursing

The pregnant cat should be treated largely as normal. Be prepared for weight gain and lowered activity levels, especially towards the end of pregnancy. Have food and water available at all times, since nutritional needs do increase. Seek advice from your veterinary surgeon regarding worming during pregnancy, and make sure all vaccinations are up to date prior to any planned pregnancy.

Towards the end of pregnancy, provide opportunities for the pregnant cat to choose a nest area in which to have the kittens. Ensure there is adequate space and peace for the cat to rest without agitation from other animals or children.

Veterinary treatment

- No veterinary treatment is required beyond advice on worming and confirmation of pregnancy if this is desired. Veterinary care during birth problems is discussed under **Birth**.
- The time to spay a female cat following pregnancy is soon after the kittens have been weaned. Seek veterinary advice.

Related or similar conditions

- ▶ **Abortion**
- ▶ **Birth**
- ▶ **Pyometra**

Prolapse

A prolapse is a displacement of tissue or an organ out of its normal position, usually caused by disease, injury or abnormality of some type. Organs that may be prolapsed in the cat include:

- The eye, after severe trauma. The eyeball displaces forward out of the socket and protrudes.
- The uterus, in cases of problems at birth (parturition). The uterus protrudes out of the vagina and is visible as a large mass of pink tissue.
- The rectum, occasionally in cases of disease or injury. The pink or red rectal tissue protrudes out of the anus (commoner in kittens with digestive problems).

The danger with all prolapses is that the protruding tissue is damaged, sometimes irreversibly, due to restriction of its blood supply. This rapidly leads on to further problems. Additionally, severe prolapses can cause medical shock and tissue or general infection.

☎ Urgency

All prolapses are urgent and should be classed as emergencies.

✚ First aid & nursing

The prolapsed tissue must be protected from drying out and further trauma. This is best achieved by covering the area with swabs moistened in warm saline or water. Use non-adherent material, e.g. cotton or cloth, rather than cotton wool, which can adhere to the tissue and cause problems later. Keep adding further moisture to the covering so that the area stays wet. Water-based lubricating jellies such as K-Y Jelly (but not Vaseline) are very helpful also – place a thick layer on the tissue.

In the case of the eye, if the prolapse is very recent, it is sometimes possible to immediately replace the eye by parting the eyelids and exerting gentle backwards pressure on the eye through a moistened or lubricated pad. Two confident handlers are required: one to steady the cat and the other to deal with the eye. In most cases, due to anxiety in the cat and lack of nursing experience of the owners, this is neither possible or safe, and the best course of action is to seek professional help as soon as possible. However if you are an experienced cat handler and the cat is cooperative, this action may well save the eye.

Veterinary treatment

- The main emphasis is to save the cat's life, by attending to the most severe injuries first, and to try to save the prolapsed and damaged tissue, or else remove it so that further problems do not develop.
- For the eye, this often unfortunately means removal of the eye, however cats cope extremely well with one eye. If the uterus has prolapsed, an emergency Caesarian section and hysterectomy is the usual course of action. Rectal prolapses can be corrected if the damage is not too severe, followed by temporary sutures (stitches) to hold the replaced tissue in its normal position.

Related or similar conditions

- ▶ **Accident**
- ▶ **Eye problems**
- ▶ **Pregnancy; birth**
- ▶ **Shock**

Pyometra

Pyometra is a condition of infection in the uterus (also sometimes called metritis or pyometritis). It is a problem that is found in older, un-neutered female cats, and is potentially serious due to the possibility for complications such as toxaemia (blood poisoning), peritonitis and kidney failure. In pyometra, the uterus becomes filled with fluid (pus) and can increase to an enormous size, and even rupture.

Cats that have been neutered (spayed) cannot develop this condition unless a portion of uterus has been left behind, in which case a so-called 'stump pyometra' may result. This is not very common in cats.

Symptoms of pyometra in cats can be vague and include some or all of:

- Lethargy and poor appetite
- Abdominal swelling
- Vomiting
- Drinking to excess
- Vaginal discharge (yellowish, blood-stained or white colour)

The problem usually needs to be considered in older un-spayed females that are showing associated signs of illness, but other conditions can mimic it, e.g. **Diabetes** and **Kidney disease**.

☎ Urgency

In most cats, symptoms of pyometra come on gradually over a period of a few days, and include some of the features mentioned above. These usually prompt a routine visit for a check up, when the condition may be suspected. If early signs are not very obvious or picked up, sudden deteriorations can occur (possibly caused by rupture of the enlarged, pus-filled uterus and development of peritonitis) – these are rapidly life-threatening and emergency attention is needed. Symptoms would be those of **Peritonitis**.

✚ First aid & nursing

If you suspect this condition, complete rest is needed and the cat should be kept indoors and handled carefully, especially when touching the abdomen. Dehydration is a threat, and if the cat is not vomiting, water and glucose should be given by mouth (5–10 mls every hour). If the cat is vomiting, a drip is probably required.

Most cats with this condition have a poor appetite, but if not vomiting may eat a little when hand fed with appetising foods. Seriously ill cats should always receive urgent attention since this condition can be life-threatening.

Veterinary treatment

- A diagnosis is usually made after clinical examination, possibly supported by X-rays, scans and blood tests. It is often useful to know how other organs (especially the kidneys) are coping when a cat is suffering from pyometra.
- The priority is to take the patient to surgery as soon as she is fit, but this can mean a spell on a drip beforehand to help correct dehydration and electrolyte imbalances, and so reduce the risks of major surgery in an already ill patient. Usually a few hours of drip fluids is deemed sufficient; most vets are keen to operate as soon as they can since this carries the best chance of success.
- After surgery, good nursing care and antibiotics will be required. Despite the severity of this problem, and the major abdominal surgery required, many cats go on to make an excellent recovery. Very old patients may have additional problems (especially **Kidney disease**) which could affect their chances of a full recovery.

Related or similar conditions

- ▶ **Dehydration**
- ▶ **Kidney disease**
- ▶ **Neutering**
- ▶ **Peritonitis**
- ▶ **Vomiting**

R

Rabies

Rabies is a fatal viral illness that affects man and animals, and occurs all over the world except in certain rabies-free areas such as the United Kingdom, Australia, Spain, Portugal, Norway, Sweden, Japan, Taiwan and Iceland.

The disease is spread in the saliva from a bite by an infected animal. It causes brain inflammation (encephalitis), which is unpleasant and fatal.

Although most people associate rabies with the image of a 'mad dog' foaming at the mouth, the disease actually has a wide variety of symptoms, making it difficult to diagnose. Such is the seriousness of the condition, that even suspected rabies is enough to bring into action public health control measures designed to stop any potential spread of the disease.

Rabies can produce symptoms of:

- Changes in behaviour – a normally friendly animal becomes aggressive, or vice versa
- Subdued behaviour
- Salivation and problems swallowing
- Weakness, altered gait or paralysis

These symptoms tend to progress quickly once they start to be shown, but the incubation period (time from bite by infected animal until first symptoms are shown) can vary enormously from days to months, depending on where the bite was received. Bites on the extremities, e.g. feet/toes, have the longest delay because the virus must move slowly along the nerve fibres to the brain before symptoms start to be seen. Once symptoms appear, death usually occurs within about a week (unless the animal is humanely destroyed beforehand). There is no specific test for rabies in the living animal. Confirmation of diagnosis requires a post-mortem examination.

Note: If you are ever bitten by an animal which could have rabies, the bite area should be vigorously scrubbed with soap or detergent for 10 minutes, preferably using a nail brush or similar. This is likely to destroy the virus which, despite the severity of the disease, is very fragile. Immediate medical advice should also be obtained.

☎ Urgency

Rabies is not common in pet cats in developed countries, and in areas of the world free from the disease, it can effectively be disregarded – other problems can cause any of the symptoms mentioned above, and are much more likely. However, with recent relaxation in regulations allowing transportation of pets between countries, vigilance for this serious disease must be kept up. Also, people visiting countries where rabies is endemic may encounter an animal suffering from it, so some basic knowledge about the disease is useful. In less well developed countries, rabies still exerts a large death toll on animal and human life.

✚ First aid & nursing

None is appropriate for rabies as the disease is invariably fatal. Any attempted treatment would normally be illegal.

Non-travelling cats residing in rabies-free countries do not require vaccination. Cats do seem slightly more sensitive to adverse effects of rabies vaccination, but modern vaccines have reduced this to a minimum.

Veterinary treatment

- If rabies is suspected, veterinary surgeons come under government orders to report the possibility. Public health regulations then come into force and the animal is quarantined and, possibly, euthanased if the disease could be present.
- The veterinary surgeon's usual role is in vaccination against the disease and coordinating the blood testing, micro-chipping and administrative requirements for international travel of pets.

Tip: Rabies vaccination

Rabies is protected against by vaccination, the vaccine having first been developed in the 1880s. Rabies vaccination is mandatory for animals travelling between countries, and is often carried out routinely in pet animals kept in countries where the disease is present.

A first vaccine is given at 12 weeks (or in adult cats at a suitable time before intended travel), repeated a year later and then boosted every 1–3 years. Note that detailed regulations are in force in the United Kingdom and many other countries regarding the blood testing, micro-chipping and vaccination protocol to be followed before any international travel by cats. If travel is planned, time must be allowed to complete all the necessary formalities otherwise the cat will not be allowed to leave the country (or enter the country travelled to). For more advice, speak to your veterinary surgeon or contact government animal health departments.

Related or similar conditions

► **Brain damage**

Rheumatism

See under Arthritis and **Bone/joint** problems.

Rhinitis/sinusitis

Rhinitis means inflammation of the nasal passages, and is a common condition in cats where it is often associated with **Cat flu**. Sinusitis – inflammation of the bony spaces in the skull – may accompany rhinitis and is also quite common in cats with flu. Other causes of rhinitis/sinusitis also occur, as detailed below, albeit less frequently than the viral illnesses of cat flu. See also **Nose problems**.

Most forms of rhinitis result in a nasal discharge. This can vary from being clear, thin and watery, through thicker consistency and a cloudy or yellow colour, to being blood-stained, depending on the underlying cause.

A mild allergy or early stages of viral infection might be expected to produce a clear thin discharge. Later stages of virus infection, or chronic cat flu, can produce thick tenacious discharges which cake and matt up around the nostrils.

Foreign bodies lodged in the nose will cause a discharge and usually also intense sneezing and irritation of sudden onset. Blood tinges may be seen. Perhaps the most frequently observed foreign body in the cat nose is a piece of grass or plant that has migrated into the nose area via the throat after being chewed but not properly swallowed.

Infections in the nose can result in discharge, and those caused by yeasts (usually an organism called *Cryptococcus*) may take many months to clear up. Bacterial infections are a common complication of cat flu.

Tumours can arise in the nose area but are thankfully quite rare in cats, as they are usually very malignant.

Benign growths (naso-pharyngeal polyps) arising in the pharynx may lead to a nasal discharge and noisy or 'rattly' breathing. These are seen most often in young cats and may require surgery for complete removal, otherwise they tend to recur.

☎ Urgency

Most forms of rhinitis are not urgent problems and can be checked out at a routine appointment. However sustained attacks of severe sneezing and gagging may indicate a foreign body, and prompt advice should be taken to alleviate the discomfort caused.

✚ First aid & nursing

The nose and nostril areas should be kept clean by frequent bathing with warm water or saline. Nursing advice as for **Cat flu** and **Nose problems** should be followed as necessary.

Veterinary treatment

- Diagnosis is made after examination and necessary tests which can include X-rays, endoscopy, blood tests and advance scans such as CT scans and MRI scans.
- Treatment may be surgical, e.g. for polyps, or using drugs, e.g. for yeast infections and chronic bacterial infection associated with cat flu.

Related or similar conditions

▶ **Breathing problems**
▶ **Cat flu**
▶ **Foreign body**
▶ **Nose problems**

Ringworm

Ringworm is an important cause of skin disease in cats. Despite the name, the parasite is a fungus and not a worm. The medical term is dermatophytosis.

One species of fungus is responsible for most cases of ringworm in cats (*Microsporum*). In fact, many cats carry this parasite without showing any symptoms at all, but these carriers can be responsible for infecting other cats, dogs and people with which they come into contact.

Symptoms are most frequently noticed in younger animals, and patchy hairloss is seen (not always in a circular or 'ring' pattern, despite the name). Often, there are not many other symptoms of skin disease such as redness, itchiness, scales and crusts, etc. The commonest areas affected are the head and paws. Other parasites such as fleas may be present too, and if this has occurred itching may be much more intense.

Diagnosis is not always easy; it usually requires samples to be submitted for culture and specialist identification, which may take some time. If another cat is present in the house (or a dog), they may need to be tested too in case they are acting as carriers.

☎ Urgency

Ringworm is a non-urgent condition. However do not delay following up treatment as the disease is transmissible to humans, and complete elimination of it can take many weeks.

✚ First aid & nursing

It is important to alert the veterinary surgeon to any in-contact animals or people which also have skin disease, as cross-infection with ringworm may have occurred.

Treatment of ringworm can be lengthy, but must be carried out very diligently if the problem is to be eradicated, so all instructions should be followed. Note that all grooming tools, bedding, cages, boxes and toys must be decontaminated on advice from the veterinary surgeon as these items can perpetuate the problem due to spores surviving on them. When possible, such things should be disposed of by burning.

Veterinary treatment

- Ringworm is a problematical disease because it is so difficult to eradicate, and because some cats may act as symptomless carriers. Long-haired cats may need to be entirely clipped out to allow treatment and should ideally be quarantined until they have been proved clear of the disease – this usually requires two negative ringworm tests taken 6–8 weeks apart.
- Drugs used to treat ringworm are strong and potentially toxic. They must be handled with great care, using gloves, and given exactly as directed. Duration of treatment may be up to two months.
- Sometimes skin washes/shampoos are also used. Fractious cats may require sedation for this.
- In-contact animals may also need treated and any humans with skin problems should visit their doctor with a letter from the veterinary surgeon regarding the diagnosis.

Related or similar conditions

- ▶ **Allergy**
- ▶ **Baldness**
- ▶ **Fleas**
- ▶ **Itching**
- ▶ **Lice**
- ▶ **Mange mites**
- ▶ **Skin problems – general**

Rodent ulcer

See under **Granuloma**.

Roundworms

Roundworms (or nematodes) are parasites which live in the small intestine of cats. The scientific name of the cat roundworm is *Toxocara cati*, but another species (*Toxascaris leonina*) may also be present.

Cats become infected when they take in roundworm eggs, within which is contained an infective larva. Once inside the cat, the larva migrates through various of the cat's tissues. Some of the larvae enter muscle tissue and become dormant there; others enter the bowel where they mature into egg-releasing adult worms. Infection can also occur in suckling kittens, and this is an important route. When female cats begin lactation, the larvae that are dormant in their muscle tissue re-activate and migrate to the mammary gland (breast). They are released into the milk supply and thus, by an ingenious mechanism, infect the kittens. As all cats have some larvae dormant in their muscles, *all* suckling kittens are assumed to be infected in this way.

Infection can also occur when cats consume prey animals, in which larvae have become dormant, where they are 'waiting' until the prey animal is eaten by a hunting cat.

Despite their elaborate life cycle, roundworms are an infrequent cause of disease in adult cats, but heavy worm burdens in kittens can produce digestive upsets, a pot belly, failure to grow well and general signs of poor condition such as a bad coat.

Urgency

Worm infestation, though undoubtedly upsetting if you see worms present in cat faeces or sometimes vomit, is not an urgent problem. Arrange a routine veterinary appointment for a worming prescription.

✚ First aid & nursing

Kittens should be wormed regularly from 2 weeks of age and until weaning using a product obtained from a veterinary surgeon. A worming schedule should also have been discussed during pregnancy for the female cat.

Regular weighing of kittens helps keep track of their weight gain, which should be steady. Coat quality, activity levels and general demeanour should also be monitored, as all of these may be affected by a particularly heavy worm burden.

Veterinary treatment

- It is always best to obtain wormers from your veterinary practice, when appropriate advice can also be obtained from the vet or nurse.
- Adult cats are usually wormed 2–3 times yearly unless they are regular hunters, when 4 times yearly may be advised. Tapeworms may also need to be considered.

Related or similar conditions

▶ **Tapeworms**
▶ **Weight loss**

S

Salivation (drooling)

Salivation or drooling/dribbling is of course quite normal in anticipation of food, and some cats will do this, though it is much more a feature of dog behaviour – cats generally react to food with more dignity!

A much commoner non-medical reason is the cat which salivates when it is cuddled or stroked. This is often combined with a rhythmic kneading action of the fore paws and loud purrs of contentment. This affectionate behaviour is a vestige of kittenhood – the cat feels the type of warmth and security it experienced as a kitten suckling from its mother, and some cats will go so far as to suck on clothing or owner's skin. The kneading with paws stimulated milk flow from the mother cat's mammary glands and is also a part of this behaviour. It is essentially a harmless, if inconvenient, response and most owners do not mind it greatly. Stopping the stroking session before dribbling gets too intense is one solution, as is trying to encourage slightly more independence in the cat – by not always responding to requests for affection.

Medical causes of salivation are also possible and anything which irritates the lining of the mouth could cause it, e.g. caustic **Burns** (by lapping chemicals or cleaning them off contaminated fur), dental disease and mouth ulcers (see **Mouth and tooth problems**). **Fractures** of the jaw or hard palate have to be considered in cats that may have been involved in an accident, and sometimes cats with other medical problems such as **Kidney** or **Liver disease**, or **Poisoning**, will salivate due to nausea. Problems in swallowing can also lead to accumulation of saliva in mouth and hence dribbling.

☎ Urgency

Most owners can recognise the affectionate type of salivation mentioned above. Other causes may be urgent, especially if there is a possibility that an irritant chemical has been swallowed. It is safer to have salivating cats checked over immediately, or at least obtain veterinary advice by telephone – the problem may turn out to be a relatively minor one, but the possibility of more severe disease has to be taken into account.

+ First aid & nursing

If your cat will tolerate it, it may be possible to examine inside the mouth. Have an assistant steady the cat and control the forelegs in the sitting position. Press on the lower jaw at the incisors and tilt the cat's head back – the mouth will open, but keep fingers well clear of the inside. You may be able to see injuries, red areas of inflammation or lodged objects.

Cats that are salivating profusely can become dehydrated. Their fluid intake should be encouraged with water or glucose solution until they are seen by a vet. Give 5–10 mls by mouth every hour if possible.

Veterinary treatment

- Clinical examination will reveal the cause in most cases of salivation. It is important to try to find out if there has been any exposure to potential toxins, e.g. overdosage of flea control products, chemicals on the coat that may have been licked off.
- Blood tests may be used to assess organ function and test for viruses such as **Feline immunodeficiency virus** (FIV).

Related or similar conditions

- ▶ **Appetite (abnormal)**
- ▶ **Burns**
- ▶ **Feline immunodeficiency virus (FIV)**
- ▶ **Foreign body**
- ▶ **Mouth and tooth problems**

Scabs

Scabs are hard, dry deposits that form over and protect wounds while they are healing naturally. They can also arise due to irritation from skin disease, especially when there has been much scratching. See **Skin problems**. Scabies is a skin disease caused by parasitic mites – see under **Mange mites**.

Scratching

Every cat scratches itself now and again as a normal part of the grooming process. Minor skin irritation and itches can occur and pieces of plant material may get lodged in the coat and irritate the skin. This can be a severe problem in long haired cats, who should be checked over regularly for items trapped in the fur. When scratching is excessive, it damages the skin and hair coat and is usually a sign of skin disease. See under **Itching** and **Skin problems**. Scratching at the ears may be a sign of ear mites and this is dealt with under **Ear problems.**

Scratching of furniture, walls, etc. can also be a feature of cat behaviour. See under **Nail problems and scratching behaviour**, where the scratching of inanimate objects is covered in some detail.

Scratching of other animals or people is a behavioural response of fear or aggression. Many cats are treated for scratch wounds incurred in fights. They are usually minor and superficial injuries, though can be painful. Occasionally **Abscesses** may form, or severe damage to sensitive structures such as the eye may result. See **Aggression, Anxiety/fear**.

Note that cat scratches in people should not be ignored. Seek medical advice whenever a deep scratch has occurred.

Season

This is one word used to describe the sexually receptive period of the un-neutered female cat, which is characterised by mating behaviours and responses. See under **Oestrus**.

Senility

See under **Old age problems**.

Shock

Shock is a specific medical term used to describe a series of changes that occur in the body following injury, inflammation, infection or the consequences of other diseases. If progressive and uncorrected, medical shock can be life-threatening as the body enters a spiralling circuit of complications which affect organ function.

A cat 'in shock' is not therefore just one that has had a severe fright (although the mental effects of trauma should never be underestimated), but is a patient that is suffering severe disruptions in essential body functions and balances arising from some major event which has initiated the sequence. The basic hallmarks of shock are failure of the circulation leading to low blood pressure, mental depression, coldness of the skin and mucous membranes (gums) and a high heart rate. If sustained, general organ and brain damage and death occurs.

Many different types of shock are recognised, e.g. allergic, cardiac (heart), toxic and traumatic. A cat involved in a road accident may enter a state of shock owing to loss of blood, either to the outside (from a major bleeding wound) or else internally. A cat experiencing an acute allergic reaction can enter the state of anaphylactic shock, initiated by a serious malfunctioning of the immune system and a cascade of inflammation affecting many organs and tissues. A cat in acute heart failure can enter shock due to a precipitous fall in blood pressure owing to poor output from the heart.

Shock can be reversible and responsive to appropriate treatment or irreversible, in which case death supervenes.

☎ Urgency

From the above, it can be seen that shock is a very urgent condition. Rapid treatment is essential to try to limit the effects and prevent a vicious circle of deterioration.

Important signs of shock are:

- Inactivity
- Reduced mental awareness
- Cold ears, paws, tail and gums
- Pale or bluish gums

Advice should always be sought immediately and in any cat known to be involved in an accident but which appears normal, a careful watch should be kept for any deterioration which may indicate delayed shock reactions.

✚ First aid & nursing

The cat in shock should be warmed up by wrapping in warm, soft materials (e.g. towels, jerseys, etc.) – insulating bubble wrap is ideal to incorporate underneath as body heat is well conserved by this substance. Warm water bottles can be placed around the cat. Take care that the chest is not constricted by wrapping the cat too tightly or placing water-filled bottles over the rib cage. Take care also that the bottles are warm and not hot, otherwise skin burns may result if the cat is unable to move away from the heat.

If the cat is conscious, providing stimulation by talking to her and stroking the head can help maintain awareness. First aid should be carried out for wounds or breathing problems as described under **Accident** and **Collapse**.

Veterinary treatment

- Medical treatment for shock centres around intravenous fluid therapy (a drip), emergency drugs, oxygen and restoring body temperature. Severely bleeding wounds are attended to but other problems such as fractures are considered secondary until the cat's condition is stabilised.
- Usually, a response to treatment can be assessed after an hour or so, but it may not be possible to give definite reassurances until 24 hours have elapsed. At this time, other injuries may need to be assessed and dealt with.

Related or similar conditions

- ▶ **Accident**
- ▶ **Bleeding**
- ▶ **Breathing problems**
- ▶ **Collapse**

Sinusitis

See under **Rhinitis/sinusitis**.

Skin problems

Overall, skin problems are encountered less frequently in cats than in dogs, where allergic skin disease is very common indeed. However there are a number of important skin disorders in cats. These are discussed in detail separately in the following sections:

- **Allergy**
- **Baldness**
- **Burns**
- **Coat contamination**
- **Dermatitis**
- **Fleas**
- **Granulomas**
- **Grooming (poor)**
- **Harvest mites**
- **Itching**
- **Lice**
- **Lumps**
- **Mange mites**
- **Miliary eczema/dermatitis**
- **Moulting**
- **Overgrooming**
- **Ringworm**

By far the commonest problem is fleas, and a range of skin complaints can be associated with these parasites. For example, most cases of **Miliary eczema** (gritty nodules in the coat) are caused by fleas, with a much smaller percentage being traced to food or other allergy.

The commonest sign of a skin problem is scratching which, if severe, leads to hair loss and skin damage. Some cats are not seen to scratch very much but still show loss of hair. In these patients, the hair may be getting removed by **Overgrooming** or, in a small number of cases, may be falling out due to other reasons such as hormone imbalance.

☎ Urgency

Apart from burns and coat contamination (which should be considered emergencies), skin problems are not urgent and a routine appointment is usually advised.

+ First aid & nursing

See the appropriate sections. An Elizabethan collar can be used in many situations to prevent self-trauma and licking of damaged skin or contaminated coat.

Veterinary treatment

- A professional diagnosis is necessary for all skin problems. Diagnostic procedures may be quite involved and courses of treatment lengthy, but careful attention to detail and completion of all treatments is necessary to give the best chances of success.

Related or similar conditions

▶ **See the list of individual skin problems above.**

Snake bite

Most snakes avoid larger mammals but cats, with their superior abilities in stealthy hunting, may interact with snakes and provoke a strike. Usually the head or front feet areas would be bitten. In temperate climates there are fewer species of dangerous snake. Adders are found in the United Kingdom but in warmer climates a range of other venomous species may be present.

Following a bite, there can be considerable swelling of the affected tissues, which is often very rapid in onset. Absorption of toxins into the body can then result in other symptoms appearing. These symptoms depend on the quantity of toxin absorbed and the species of snake that has bitten, but vomiting, disorientation, fits, dilated pupils and shock/collapse are all possible.

☎ Urgency

Urgent advice should be sought in case the quantity of venom received was large. This will hopefully allow treatment to be started before major symptoms begin.

+ First aid & nursing

Take care that the snake is not still in the vicinity as it may strike out again.

Collapsed cats should be resuscitated (see Accident) and transported quickly to a veterinary clinic. If you know the species of snake, or which ones are common in the area, this information may be useful as in areas where bites are common, antitoxin may be kept.

Veterinary treatment

- Antitoxin may be administered if this is available, otherwise general supportive treatment for shock and collapse will be given and other symptoms dealt with as they appear.

Related or similar conditions

▶ **Allergy**
▶ **Collapse**
▶ **Shock**
▶ **Poisoning**

Sneezing

Sneezing is a common symptom of **Cat flu** but can also occur in **Allergy**, in dusty environments and in cats exposed to fumes and cigarette smoke. Sitting too close to gas fires may also provoke sneezing bouts and the use of air fresheners, carpet cleaners and fabric conditioners may irritate the sensitive nose of some cats, provoking sneezing.

Isolated bouts of sneezing are of little concern, but repeated episodes could indicate a problem that needs treated. In a few cases, the cause may be a **Growth** or **Foreign body** lodged in the nose.

☎ Urgency

The problem is not urgent unless the bouts are relentless and continual, e.g. the cat sneezes constantly in paroxysms for 30 minutes or so. This may indicate a nasal obstruction due to a foreign body. Otherwise a routine appointment should be made if the sneezing seems to be becoming a regular occurrence. The most likely explanation is a viral infection, i.e. cat flu.

✚ First aid & nursing

Remove the cat from dusty, smokey or perfumed environments and see if the problem settles down. Examine the nostril area for any discharges or blood and let the veterinary surgeon know what you find.

Veterinary treatment

- Routine examinations normally point to the cause but if a foreign body is suspected an anaesthetic may be required.

Related or similar conditions

- ▶ **Allergy**
- ▶ **Cat flu**
- ▶ **Foreign body**
- ▶ **Rhinitis/sinusitis**

Socialisation

Socialisation is the process by which cats learn to interact with other cats, people and to a lesser extent other animals (e.g. the family dog or rabbit). It is an important activity since if it goes wrong, the resulting behaviour problems can prove difficult to correct. Badly socialised cats may be unusually nervous, aggressive or unpredictable in their responses.

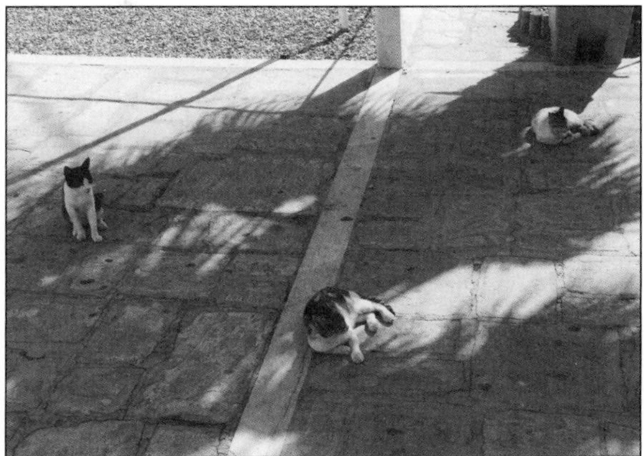

Socialisation determines how the individual cat relates to others.

Not all cats are the same, of course, some are naturally shy and retiring whereas others are outgoing extroverts – one of the joys of cat ownership is understanding and appreciating your own cat's individuality. When do personality 'differences' become problems, i.e. when is a boisterous extrovert cat a nuisance? This depends on many factors, not least the wishes and expectations of the owner and the situation in which the cat is kept. A shy, timid cat may suit an older person living alone very well, but would be miserable in a house full of children and other pets.

When does socialisation start?

It starts when the kitten is very young (around 3 weeks), and some of the basic personality tendencies may be inherited.

Kitten no.	Sex	Behaviour	Possible problem in future?
1	Male	Bold, inquisitive	Very confident or dominant; could be a problem with other pets or, e.g. a frail elderly owner. Might suit a busy household with children very well.
2	Male	Objects to handling	Could be awkward to groom if long-haired.
3	Female	Very shy and retiring	Timid; fear responses or fearful aggression may be shown, especially at first.
4	Female	Approaches given plenty time	Needs to be 'won over'; may not suit a busy family but could be ideal for single owner.

Once kittens begin to move around independently, personality differences can be picked up by the experienced observer. For example in a litter of five 8-week-old kittens, you might find the following distribution of behaviours (see table above).

The invented examples which follow in the table are simplifications, but do help illustrate what to look out for. The important thing is that, while kittens and young cats, good socialisation can help to limit possible future problems and maximise all the positive aspects of the kittens' behaviour.

Pointers to help socialisation

A few general pointers can be given.

- Encourage short periods (10–15 minutes) of handling by adults and children of both sexes from 2–3 weeks of age. Repeat daily. Get the kitten used to be picked up and being gently stroked and spoken to.
- Try to get as many different types of people as possible to interact with the kittens – this is an important responsibility for the person who has bred the kittens, since this crucial early period occurs in the first home.
- Get them used (gradually) to household noises (vacuum cleaners, washing machines, phone, etc.).
- Encourage play between kittens once they start to become independent and, in the new home after weaning, playing with the owner and other people using objects/toys is useful.
- Meeting new cats and dogs is an important part of socialisation. See the advice under **Behaviour problems** and **Jealousy** regarding introducing a new cat to the household. If you keep rabbits, it is important to begin socialisation with them as soon as possible so that the very young kitten recognises the rabbit as a companion and not a prey animal.
- Introduce the cat basket or carrier and associate it with rewards (food or play) afterwards. Start off by leaving the

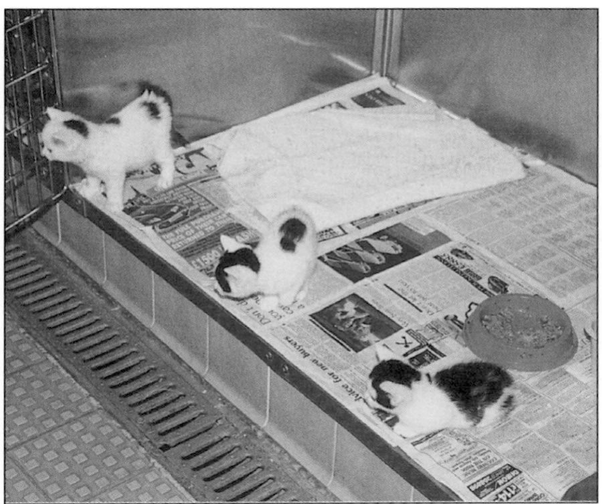

Exploration and play behaviour in young kittens. *Below:* The more dominant kittens tend to take the lead!

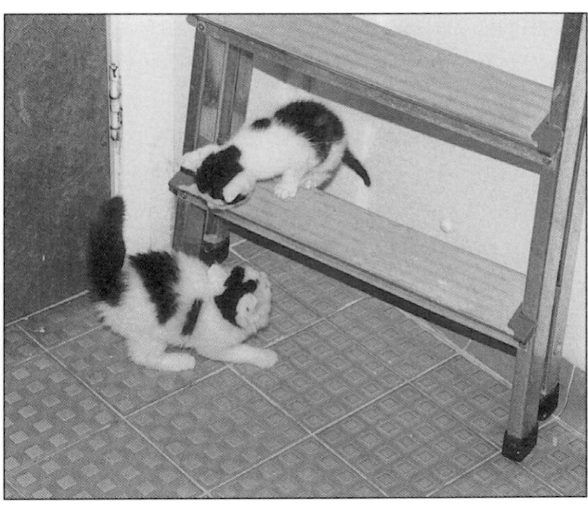

Play and investigation of the surroundings is a vital part of socialisation. It should be encouraged, and is also fun to watch!

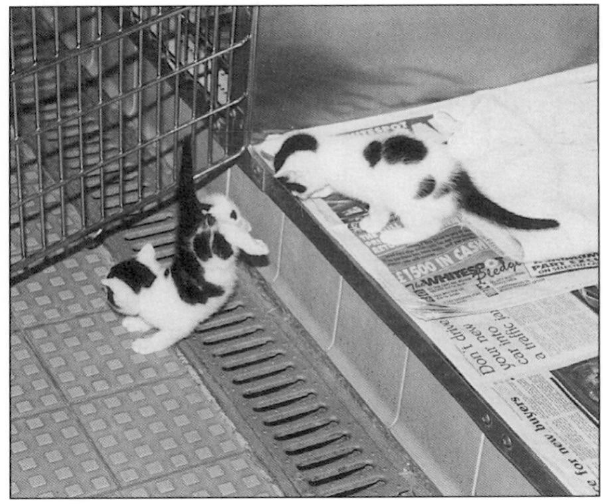

Socialisation with people should be started as soon as possible.

kitten enclosed in the basket for 5 minutes. Repeat every few days, building up the time to 10, 20 or 30 minutes. In the basket, use a sheet or cat bed that the kitten has been familiar with elsewhere in the house (see under **Travel fears and sickness** for a step-by-step guide to introducing the cat carrier). This is useful because, otherwise, the cat may only associate the carrier with unpleasant events (e.g. going to the vets or cattery).

- Start very short car journeys once the kitten is thoroughly used to the basket or carrier. Literally spend only a few minutes at a time to begin with – the first few times, you may only have the engine running without actually driving anywhere. Gradually extend the length of the journey. It is a great bonus to have a cat which travels well without signs of severe anxiety and stress – the time to introduce this is in the young kitten.

- Continue the above for the first few months of the cat's life, by which time the majority of the cat's behavioural tendencies will have developed. Remember that kittens should not interact with unvaccinated cats, nor spend time in places where unvaccinated cats may have been, until their innoculations have been completed (usually at 12 weeks).

Related or similar conditions

Problems that may be associated with socialisation are dealt with under **Aggression**, **Anxiety/fear**, **Bereavement**, **Jealousy**, **Loneliness**, **Overgrooming** and **Spraying** (**urine**) – see the relevant sections.

Spaying

This is the operation to prevent reproductive behaviour and breeding/pregnancy in female cats. It is normally carried out at 5–6 months. See under **Neutering** for full details.

Spinal injury

Spinal injuries nearly always arise after severe trauma, e.g. a road accident or fall, but the spinal cord can also be injured by serious infection or invasion by a **Tumour**.

Spinal injuries show as weakness or paralysis – the cat will be unable to move properly and may completely drag a limb or limbs. The tail may hang loosely and there could be incontinence. Because sensation can be lost, damage to the paralysed part is a risk as the cat will be completely unaware of further injury.

☎ Urgency

Spinal injuries, or suspected ones, are always urgent and emergency attention should be received. Quite often, in cats which drag their hind quarters, the damage turns out to be a fractured pelvis – a very common injury in traumatised cats – but spinal damage may also be present to a greater or lesser degree.

✚ First aid & nursing

Prevention of further damage is important and this is best achieved by confinement of the cat in a well padded cat cage or carrier. Take care when lifting as the cat may be in pain or distress – thick gloves and a long sleeved coat are advisable. Use a makeshift stretcher.

Veterinary treatment

- Treatment for shock is usually required, followed by assessment of the severity of the spinal damage. Total permanent paralysis of one leg or the tail can be treated by amputation, and most cats do extremely well. When more than one leg or the bladder is irreversibly damaged, the outlook is very poor and euthanasia is the kindest option.
- Referral to neurological specialists is possible for complicated cases.

Related or similar conditions

- ▶ **Accident**
- ▶ **Fractures/dislocations**
- ▶ **Paralysis**
- ▶ **Shock**

Sprain/strain

Sprains or strains affect muscles, tendons and ligaments – the soft tissues which connect bones together and span joints. *Strain* refers to the muscle and ligament damage that occurs, and *sprain* refers to the damage that may result around a joint by stretching or disruption of the joint capsule and associated structures.

These injuries usually arise from overexertion or incoordinated movement. They are not all that common in cats, because cats move with astonishing grace and coordination most of the time. However older or overweight cats do incur joint sprains and cats involved in trauma may have severe strains or sprains without any associated fractures or dislocations, if they have been fortunate.

☎ Urgency

These are uncomfortable injuries but, when occurring alone, are not emergencies. The problem is that owners are often unaware whether it is just a sprain or strain, or whether something more serious has occurred. Any cat in significant pain should therefore be seen by a vet.

✚ First aid & nursing

Rest and warmth are important so keep the cat indoors. For many minor injuries, this is all that is needed, and normal function returns after 12–48 hours of rest.

Note that **Abscesses** and **Bites** can show in a very similar way due to muscle inflammation (cellulitis), so a thorough check through the coat for any puncture wounds is sensible.

Sprained joints may benefit from alternated hot and cold treatment using warm packs and, e.g. frozen peas. Apply for 5–10 minutes at a time four times daily, but only if the cat tolerates this well.

Veterinary treatment

- X-rays may be taken to rule out fractures and dislocations.
- Severe sprains and strains are treated with painkillers and rest. Sometimes bandaging is used to support the limb, but most cats rest sensibly when they have these injuries.

Tip

Do not be tempted to administer human painkillers to cats – poisoning is likely as cats cope with these drugs in a quite different way from humans and very small doses can be toxic.

Related or similar conditions

- **Abscess**
- **Bites**
- **Fractures/dislocations**
- **Lameness/limp**

Spraying (urine)

Deposition of urine on prominent surfaces is an important means of communication for all members of the cat family. Passage of urine in this way is not carried out in order to relieve a full bladder, but as a specific means of communication in the same way as male dogs 'cock' their leg against lamp posts etc. to deposit scent markings (bitches also communicate using urine).

Cats will spray urine droplets irrespective

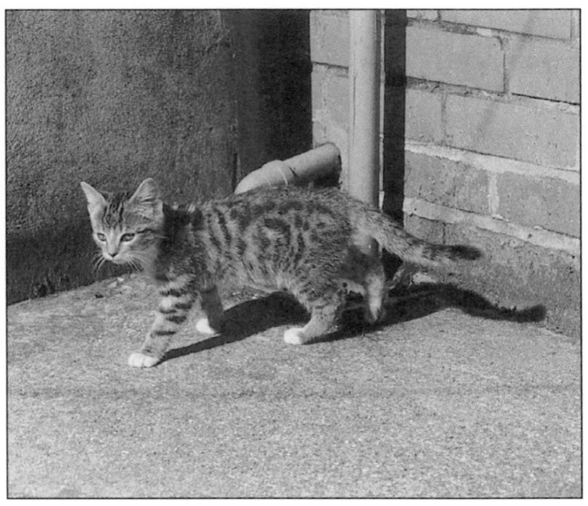

Young male cats will usually begin to spray urine as territory markings at around 6 months of age.

of how full their bladder happens to be at the time and adopt a very characteristic posture while doing so. The urine is deposited in short jets from a standing position with the tail elevated (compared to the squatting position adopted when passing urine to relieve a full bladder).

It is an activity which is practised by both sexes of cat, and by neutered animals. Spraying occurs against vertical surfaces, e.g. trees, fence posts, garden tubs and – unfortunately for some cat owners – areas around the house. There is no doubt that urine spraying in the home is a major source of distress for many cat owners, and it can sometimes be a difficult problem to solve. No one wants to live in a house where there is an all pervasive odour of cat urine.

In entire male cats, the problem is often stopped by **Castration**, and this should be carried out at about 6 months of age in young tom cats. Older entire tom cats may also cease this behaviour after castration, though it may take some weeks to come about. So castration is always the first step in male cats which are spraying.

A sign of insecurity

Spraying in neutered males and females is considered a behavioural problem associated with **Anxiety**. These cats have

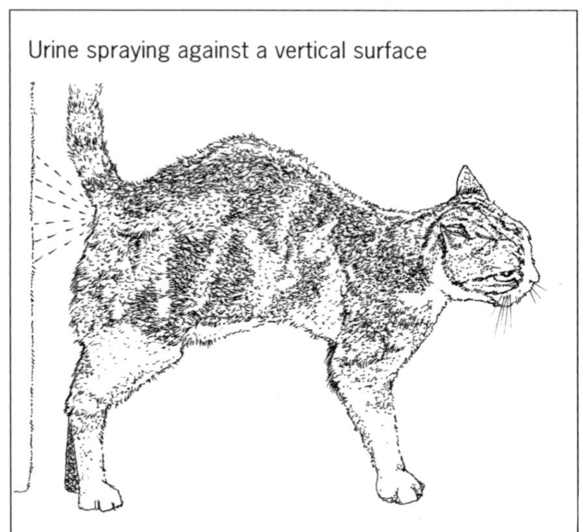

Urine spraying against a vertical surface

Urine spraying againt a vertical surface

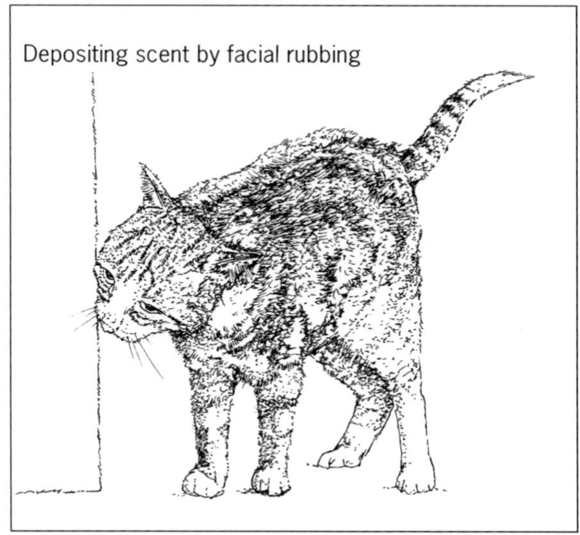

Depositing scent by facial rubbing

Depositing scent by facial rubbing

psychological problems, of which urine spraying is a manifestation.

They are likely to spray repeatedly in the house as well as pass urine in the litter box, and this is often confusing and frustrating for owners who do not understand the underlying reasons for the behaviour. For example, some owners even believe the cat is being deliberately naughty and 'getting back' at them for a perceived grudge or resentment on the cat's part. Nothing like this is the cause and it is important to emphasise the difference between voiding urine to empty the bladder (in the litter box) and spray-marking of urine to deposit scent (on household surfaces) as a means of gaining reassurance for the underlying anxieties.

Also, male cats with urethral obstruction (feline lower urinary tract disease [FLUTD] – see **Cystitis**) may also urinate – or attempt to – frequently, including outwith the litter tray, when suffering from this emergency condition.

In both these cases, cats would be expected to squat rather than adopt the typical spraying stance (see illustration) but it is not always possible to catch the cat in the act of passing the urine and so find out what posture was taken. It is therefore important to seek veterinary advice when in any doubt about urination behaviours as the area is truly a complex one.

☎ Urgency

Urine spraying behaviour is a non-urgent condition, but any activity suspicious of urinary obstruction is an emergency. The obstructed cat will be perpetually restless, calling out and attempting to pass urine with little result. They are often in and out of the litter box, but only ever succeed in releasing a few drops. The abdomen will be tense and hard, and the cat's overall condition will be deteriorating to collapse after 12–24 hours. Obstruction is essentially a male cat problem owing to the long and narrow urethra. Female cats may be agitated with cystitis, but rarely develop obstructions.

✚ First aid & nursing

Behavioural advice for spraying

Once it is understood that the trigger is anxiety, then efforts can be made to locate the cause of the anxiety and take measures to reduce it. The cause can vary between cats and in difficult cases input from a pet behaviour specialist is strongly recommended. Fairly common possibilities are:

- A new cat, pet or person in the house
- A new cat in the neighbourhood
- Flitting
- House alterations resulting in new scents in the house
- Cats which have always had a tendency towards this behaviour and occasionally lapse into it for reasons not picked up by the owner.

See under **Jealousy** and **Behaviour problems** regarding ways of introducing a new cat to the household in a non-threatening way. Similar gradual exposure techniques can be used for dogs and indeed people, although in these cases confining the incomer to a cage for a while may not always be appropriate! Instead, limit exposure and introductions to short periods when you are present, and then place the cat in an area where he feels secure. Build up tolerance very gradually over several weeks.

When spraying is occurring generally within the home, initial steps are to simplify the cat's environment and remove access to sprayed areas. Restricting the cat to one or two familiar rooms which are not sprayed in, or to an indoor kennel area when left alone, are useful. Suitable kennels can be bought from pet stores and suppliers and are large enough to include litter tray, bed area and room for some toys. Use familiar bedding and bowls in the kennel. (Some veterinary practices have such kennels available for loan). Around a week should be spent in the restricted environment, although it is usually fine to allow the cat out and into one or two rooms while you are there, unless spraying occurs at these times too.

Next, begin a programme of gradual extension into other areas of the house, including those previously sprayed in (these must be cleaned first as outlined below). When introducing the cat to these areas, the cat's main human contact should always be present to establish security and the cat should not be left alone. Gradually build up exposure and tolerance. Feeding the cat in these areas can be helpful.

It is vital that any sprayed areas are cleaned properly, otherwise the cat will be prompted to return and 'top up' the fading scent. The chemical nature of the pheromones present in urine means that only certain cleaning methods are reliable. You should:

- Clean the area thoroughly and repeatedly with a warm solution of biological washing powder.
- Rinse thoroughly after the last wash and allow to dry.
- Next apply an alcohol, e.g. surgical spirit to the whole area, by spraying on. Proprietary products based on enzymes are also available.
- Again allow to dry.
- Only then allow the cat access.

Other cleaning agents, e.g. those containing chlorine, stimulate the cat to return to the area, as do strong scented agents. If you have expensive fabrics, test the cleaning procedure on a small area first to check that no discolouration results. Severely contaminated fabrics may however need to be replaced completely.

In order to prevent re-spraying, as well as applying the behavioural measures outlined above, it can be helpful to leave small bowls of food in the appropriate places. Most cats are very unlikely to spray in areas where food is present, and the food itself acts as a reassuring stimulus. Synthetic pheromone sprays are also available from veterinary practices and proper use of these, when combined with behaviour techniques, can be very successful in stopping this behaviour.

If you are having problems, veterinary or behavioural advice should be sought as this can be a complex problem and many owners may get frustrated and disheartened when trying to cope on their own.

Tip

Any form of punishment is quite ineffective for this problem and is likely to make the situation worse by adding to insecurity.

Veterinary treatment

- This involves ruling out causes of urinary system disease that may lead to abnormal urination patterns that could mimic spraying, and also liaising with any behavioural specialists brought on to the case. (Many practices have staff interested in behaviour problems present 'in house').
- Sedative drugs are not the answer to this type of problem and are rarely used, but pheromone sprays often show good results if other aspects of behaviour modification as outlined above are also tackled.

Related or similar conditions

- ▶ **Anxiety/fear**
- ▶ **Behaviour problems – general**
- ▶ **Bereavement**
- ▶ **Cystitis**
- ▶ **Incontinence**
- ▶ **Loneliness**
- ▶ **Neutering**
- ▶ **Urination problems**

Sting

Stings are quite common in pet cats owing to their inquisitive nature and tendency to play with insects. Bees or wasps trapped in the house are very likely to become objects of attention for the pet cat, and in the garden many cats will amuse themselves by chasing and attempting to catch them.

Stings often occur around the head/face or front paws. The area becomes swollen, painful and, if near the eye, distorted in appearance. Cats may paw or rub at the affected area after a sting and behave unpredictably.

☎ Urgency

Most stings are uncomfortable but non-urgent. First aid treatment is appropriate. The exceptions are the infrequent cases when a sting occurs actually in the mouth or throat, because severe swelling here can obstruct the airway – an emergency situation. Stings close to the eye should also be considered urgent.

✚ First aid & nursing

The affected area can be bathed in iced water to reduce swelling and ease discomfort. Cold packs can be applied. Swelling usually subsides in a matter of hours.

If you know a bee has stung, bathing the area in a dilute solution of bicarbonate of soda is helpful (the alkaline solution neutralises the acidity of a bee sting); wasps stings can be bathed in a dilute acid such as vinegar or lemon juice (they are alkaline). In most instances, cold water works just as well.

For breathing obstruction and collapse, apply the 'ABC' routine as described under **Accident** for resuscitation and seek immediate help.

For eye stings, a cold water swab can be held against the eye whilst taking the cat to a clinic.

Veterinary treatment

- If specific treatment is needed, anti-inflammatory drugs may be administered for a few days.

Related or similar conditions

- ▶ **Allergy**

Straining

Straining can be an important symptom and it is important to try to discover what is causing it. There are a number of possibilities:

- **Straining to pass urine** – when only small amounts of urine are passed frequently (in or out of the litter tray); when there may be blood in the urine; or when, despite straining frequently, no urine at all is passed.
- **Straining to pass faeces** – confusingly, this can occur with both **Constipation**, when faeces are not passed, or only small amounts of hard and dry faeces are passed; and also **Diarrhoea**, when loose or liquid faeces are passed. The amounts of diarrhoea may be large or small and the straining comes from irritation in the rectum and a sense of 'urgency' that this produces. Many owners at first think their cat with diarrhoea is actually constipated because of the straining that frequently occurs.
- **Straining for other reasons** – for example, during birth in pregnant cats, or because of abdominal pain or, occasionally, full **Anal glands**.

Often, close observation allows you to make a decision as to what is going on but sometimes only the vet can decide.

Some of the problems above are very urgent. Straining associated with the urinary system is generally more urgent than that associated with the bowels, as if no urine is being passed there is always the risk of an obstruction, especially in male cats. If neglected, this can be life-threatening.

Each of the problems above is discussed fully in appropriate sections. See:

- **Anal glands**
- **Birth**
- **Constipation**
- **Cystitis**
- **Diarrhoea**
- **Enteritis**
- **Urination problems**

'Stroke'

'Stroke' is a condition seen in people, but one which is not really recognised in cats, although the term may occasionally be used loosely by some vets to mean a brain or balancing disorder, with symptoms of incoordination, wobbliness and sometimes head tilting. This general pattern of symptoms seen can also be caused by **Ear disease**, and by a variety of other disorders such as **Poisoning**, **Liver** and **Kidney disease**, **Diabetes**, etc. So, as far as possible, common diseases must be ruled out in trying to diagnose a cat with symptoms like this. If brain disease is considered likely, treatment may be tried to reduce the severity of symptoms.

Cats do suffer from a specific disease called feline idiopathic vestibular syndrome, which is quite common. Symptoms are loss of **Balance** (this can be severe, leading to rolling over), a head tilt and abnormal flickering eye movements. This is a distressing disease for owners to witness, but usually carries a good outlook. The cats start to improve within a few days and have usually largely recovered by 2–3 weeks after initial signs. Treatment may be given, although it is not known if this materially affects the duration of the problem as cats usually recover spontaneously no matter what type of treatment is given.

See also **Brain damage** and **Ear problems**.

Stud tail

This is a skin condition of the tail top area that is sometimes encountered in unneutered tom cats. Symptoms are of inflammation, hair loss and crusty deposits in this area. Veterinary diagnosis and treatment is required.

Sunburn

Most cats love sun and will sun bathe frequently on window ledges, in conservatories and out of doors. This is a natural and in many ways healthy activity, but there are some dangers. The cat's hair coat protects most of the skin from the damaging effects of ultraviolet light except on unprotected areas, especially the nose and ear tips. Too much exposure on these areas produces a unpleasant skin inflammation with redness, pain, swelling and itchiness. As well as this, chronic inflammation and ulceration of this type can lead on to malignant skin cancer (squamous cell carcinoma) in cats. White cats are especially prone and the ear tips are the most commonly affected sites. Affected areas would be red, ulcerated, angry looking and painful.

☎ Urgency

The condition develops due to long term exposure to ultra violet light waves and so is non-urgent. However you should seek attention at an early stage if you notice skin changes (redness, skin scales) on the ear tips or nose. The **Cancer** does not develop immediately but only after a period of pre-cancerous inflammatory and ulcerative stages, so there is scope for preventative treatment.

✚ First aid & nursing

If possible, try to limit exposure to sun, e.g. block off spaces on window sills or restrict access to conservatories. Sun barrier cream is very useful (high protection factor sun block). When applying this, put it on before feeding or playing with the cat to try to discourage immediate rubbing off – its use is obviously more suited to the ear tips than the nose, and the ear tips are a much commoner site for this problem anyway.

Veterinary treatment

- This condition does need monitoring, owing to the possible progression to squamous cell carcinoma of the ear tips. If this is suspected or anticipated, amputation of the ear tips below the hair line may be carried out. Although this does distort the ear and alter appearance, it can prevent the development of this serious cancer.

Related or similar conditions

- ▶ **Burns**
- ▶ **Skin problems**

Surgery

Surgery involves cutting, removing or repairing animal tissues as a means of treating injury or diseases, or as preventative medicine. **Neutering** comes into the category of 'preventive medicine', where surgery is used to prevent breeding and associated reproductive behaviours in healthy animals, and is the commonest operation which vets perform on pet cats.

Surgery is a vital part of animal medicine and treatment, and many lives are saved every day by surgical procedures. Surgery is carried out in controlled conditions under local or (more usually) general anaesthetic, which ensures the cat feels no pain and enables the surgeon to examine and treat the situation in a systematic way.

Modern anaesthetic techniques, combined with skilled monitoring and observation, means that the risks of surgery are minimised, such that many procedures are now considered 'routine'. Nevertheless, for ethical reasons, you will always be asked to sign an anaesthetic and surgical consent form before any treatment is started. Untoward happenings, though rare, do occur and owners must be made aware of this. (This applies to any anaesthetic you receive in a human hosptial also, and similar treatment consent forms are required.) The only exception is if, in delaying treatment because signed consent was not available, the animal's life would be put at further risk – in these circumstances, veterinary surgeons can proceed with appropriate treatment as quickly as necessary, since it is envisaged that this would be the preference of any caring owner.

Of course, many animals receiving surgery may be ill for various reasons, and depending on the nature of the illness, surgical risk may be affected. Gradings such as 'high risk', 'medium risk' and 'low risk' may be used by some vets, but they can only ever be approximate. Decisions about when (or if) to embark on surgery therefore requires good communication and understanding about what is hoped to be achieved by the procedure. Delaying surgery unnecessarily can compromise the chances of the cat making a full recovery.

In some forms of surgery, the objective is clear, e.g. to place a metal pin in a broken leg and thus help it to heal. In other situations, however, the veterinary surgeon may only have a hazy idea about what is wrong, and is hoping that surgery (by allowing direct examination of internal organs) will clarify the situation and at the same time allow treatment, e.g. exploratory surgery of the abdomen to remove a suspected intestinal obstruction or collect a biopsy for further diagnosis.

Occasionally, unpleasant surprises occur during surgery, such as discovering unsuspected and untreatable cancer in the abdomen when another sort of problem was expected. In these difficult situations, decisions about what to do can be very hard, since it may be judged kinder to perform euthanasia while the patient is still asleep rather than allow him to waken up after major surgery which has not been able to help the cat. Whenever possible, all eventualities will be investigated before surgery is embarked upon but, disease being what it is, and medicine an imperfect science, it is not always possible to predict accurately what is going on before the cat receives their surgical operation.

☎ Urgency

The urgency of surgery varies enormously. For example, urgent operations to control bleeding or treat internal organ rupture or damage may be needed in order to save a cat's life. Similar lifesaving procedures may be needed if the airway is blocked or if there is major chest damage. Without such emergency surgery, death could quickly result. The risks of such rapid surgical intervention are high, because patients will already be in a critical state, but the risks of *not* going ahead may be even higher.

Most surgical operations, however, fall in to a less urgent category. Whenever possible, it is preferable to make sure that the cat is prepared properly for a surgical procedure and can therefore cope with the effects of this in the best way. Thus an cat which has broken a leg in a road accident may be treated for shock first, and only when considered stable (e.g. 48 hours later) may the necessary orthopaedic surgery be carried out. Major surgery on the ear may be planned well in advance to follow a course of antibiotics in order to try to limit infection before the operation, since this will reduce the chances of a worse infection developing after surgery.

Each case is different and complex in its own way, and veterinary advice and decision-making should be followed.

✚ First aid & nursing

Proper preparation of the patient is very important before surgery, and all advice should be followed. The standard protocol followed by most veterinary surgeons is:

- No food for 8–12 hours before the admission to the veterinary hospital, e.g. remove all food bowls at 8 pm the night before and keep the cat indoors.
- Allow water until the morning of the operation.
- Ensure there is a litter tray available overnight.
- Report any changes in your cat's condition to the veterinary staff on the morning of the operation, and take along all tablet bottles currently being used.

An empty stomach is important before elective anaesthetics since it reduces the risk of vomiting while under anaesthetic, and consequent problems caused by that.

After surgery, you will be given specific instructions which will depend on the nature of the operation that was carried out. But all cats require to rest in a quiet area at a comfortable room temperature, where they can be easily observed and where they will be free from interference by other pets or children. Water and food can usually be given and a litter tray provided within easy reach. Tempting food (e.g. chicken/fish) is usually appreciated after an anaesthetic and surgery, and do not be surprised if it takes a few days before appetite and bowel habits are back to normal.

Any adverse or worrying signs should be reported to your vet as soon as possible.

Veterinary treatment

- The act of surgery is one part of the veterinary treatment. It is likely that diagnostic tests and procedures will have been used beforehand (e.g. X-rays), and that post-operative treatment will also be needed (e.g. antibiotics, painkillers, bandages).

- Surgery often involves some degree of hospitalisation (except for routine neutering) and major surgery can necessitate a lengthy hospital stay. Visiting the cat can help keep up demeanour and encourage a positive attitude during this important phase of recovery.

Tip: Causes for concern

Most cats recover smoothly from anaesthetics and surgery and young cats are often very much their normal selves even a few hours after routine neutering. Older cats, and those experiencing more major surgery, can take much longer to recover fully. If any of the following occur, phone for advice.

- Seems to be becoming *less* active and mentally aware instead of more, as the anaesthetic wears off fully over 4–6 hours.
- Severe vomiting or diarrhoea.
- Bleeding or seepage from a wound that is in excess of what the veterinary staff led you to expect.
- Apparent severe pain (do not administer any human painkillers).
- No urine passed 24 hours after admission (it may take longer for faeces to be passed).

Related or similar conditions

- **Bleeding**
- **Bruising**
- **Fractures/dislocations**
- **Neutering**

Swallowing

Problems with swallowing can result from tooth/gum pain, mouth or tongue ulcers (see **Mouth and tooth problems**), caustic **Burns** from chemicals or the cleaning of these by the cat off contaminated areas of fur (see **Coat contamination**), throat inflammation and enlargement of the throat glands (often accompanies infections or certain forms of **Cancer**).

Objects stuck in the mouth/throat, though fairly unusual in cats, can also lead to swallowing problems – one possibility is needle and thread that is being played with and then swallowed. This can lead to serious internal problems if the thread becomes stuck around the base of the tongue but the needle is swallowed on down the digestive tract. Surgery is needed.

Many generally ill cats may dribble and appear to have problems swallowing. Conditions such as **Kidney disease** and **Feline immunodeficiency virus** (FIV) may have to be considered as throat inflammation can accompany such diseases.

Signs of swallowing problems are mainly salivation, repeated attempts at swallowing and sometimes regurgitation of undigested food. Cats may gag or retch repeatedly and paw at the mouth. The throat area may be tender and gentle touching of it provoke a spasm of retching and gagging.

☎ Urgency

A sudden onset of swallowing difficulty should always be investigated promptly because the symptoms are unpleasant and can lead on to further complicating problems if not treated.

+ First aid & nursing

This is limited owing to the difficulty in examining the mouth and throat of the conscious cat. If you see thread hanging from the mouth, this should *not* be pulled as to do so can cause worse internal damage – seek urgent veterinary advice and keep the cat calm meantime.

If there is a risk of coat contamination and licking of this, further licking and intake of poison must be avoided, even if it means holding the cat constantly to prevent this. An Elizabethan collar, if available, should be fitted.

In other instances reassurance and keeping the cat as quiet and relaxed as possible are important. Excess saliva can be wiped away from the mouth and nose.

Veterinary treatment

- Full examination of the mouth and throat often requires a general anaesthetic, and sometimes further tests are needed to diagnose rarer causes of swallowing problems which can have underlying medical or neurological reasons.
- Most of the causing conditions are discussed in detail in the appropriate section of this book.

Related or similar conditions

▶ **Burns**
▶ **Cat flu**
▶ **Choking**
▶ **Coat contamination**
▶ **Foreign body**
▶ **Mouth and tooth problems**

T

Tapeworms

Tapeworms are a rare cause of medical symptoms in cats, although several different species exist. Adult tapeworms of the species *Taenia* live within the small intestine and absorb nutrients from the cat's digestive processes, but usually cause no symptoms at all in the cat. Tapeworm eggs are passed out to the environment in the cat's faeces. The eggs are inadvertently eaten by 'intermediate' hosts (e.g. rodents). The intermediate hosts are then eaten by another cat, which becomes infected with the tapeworm that is present in the rodent's tissues. Due to the complex life-cycle involving intermediate hosts, these tapeworms are always commoner in hunting cats.

A tapeworm called *Dipylidium* has a life-cycle which uses the cat flea (or louse) as its intermediate host. Fleas or lice consume the tapeworm eggs which are passed by the cat. The tapeworm then develops inside the fleas or lice, which are subsequently swallowed by cats during grooming, thereby infecting themselves.

As with *Taenia*, very little adverse effects are caused to the cat by the adult tapeworms living within the small intestine. Sometimes irritation may be caused at the anal area as mobile segments from the tapeworms migrate about on the fur (this is the usual sign that tapeworm is present), but this is not very common.

However because of the close alliance between tapeworm and fleas/lice, it is important that control measures against both types of parasite are carried out, under veterinary advice, if tapeworm segments are noticed on a cat or its bedding.

☎ Urgency

This is not an urgent problem and can be dealt with at any routine appointment.

✚ First aid & nursing

No first aid is required, but the cat's bedding can be washed thoroughly and on obtaining a suitable product from a veterinary surgeon, the house can be treated against fleas, which are an intermediate host for the common *Dipylidium* tapeworm, as explained above.

In general, it is best to avoid shop bought worming products as their effectiveness may be variable and the dosing instructions can be complicated.

Veterinary treatment

- Safe and effective worming medicines are available. Note that **Fleas** may also need to be treated as fleas and tapeworms have a linked life-cycle. Regular hunters may need to be wormed 4 times yearly for tapeworms.

Related or similar conditions

- ▶ **Anal glands**
- ▶ **Fleas**
- ▶ **Lice**
- ▶ **Roundworms**

Tartar

Tartar is the medical name for the yellowish mineral deposit that builds up on teeth. When severe, it can cause gum inflammation; associated problems include tooth loosening and irritation/pain. Tartar is removed from otherwise healthy teeth by the dental treatment of 'descaling' and polishing. Tooth brushing can then help prevent its build up again. See also under **Mouth and tooth problems**.

Temperature

See under **Fever/high temperature** or **Hypothermia** (low body temperature). The normal body temperature of a cat, measured using a clinical rectal thermometer, is 38.6°C.

Thirst

Excessive thirst is an important symptom in cats and is always taken seriously. It can however be difficult to pick up, especially in cats which go outside and may therefore be drinking at these times from puddles or other natural sources. Eventually, even in outdoor cats, water intake may become so excessive that owners notice extra drinking when in the house.

Common signs of excessive drinking

- Cat found often in the sink or bath drinking drips from tap
- Water bowl needs filled more often
- Excessive urination – litter tray wetter than normal
- Cat drinking from dog's bowl, plant waterers, etc.

Excessive thirst often goes hand in hand with excessive urination: the symptom of polydipsia/polyuria in medical jargon. Never attempt to limit excessive urination by depriving the cat of water – serious **Dehydration** can result as the cat is probably unable to control its water balance effectively, this is why the excess urination is occurring in the first place.

Many conditions can result in increased thirst. The commonest are:

- **Kidney disease**
- **Thyroid gland (overactive)**
- **Diabetes**
- **Liver disease**

These will probably be the first conditions your vet is considering. If they are ruled out, other causes will need to be looked into. Keep a watch for other symptoms – those which are commonly associated with excessive water intake are:

- Weight loss
- Vomiting
- Diarrhoea
- Variable appetite (poor to excessive)
- Changes in activity levels
- Irritability

☎ Urgency

On its own, increased thirst is not an urgent condition, but it does need investigated with a routine appointment since most cats are not seen to drink that often. Usually, the thirst has gradually increased over a period of weeks to months until it has finally become noticeable to the owner.

✚ First aid & nursing

Measuring the water intake carefully is often helpful for the vet. This is most reliable in indoor cats where there are no other pets. A careful measurement, taken over several 24 hour periods, and then averaged, is needed. The easiest method is to fill a large bowl full of water and mark the top level. Throughout the 24 hour period, keep topping this up as necessary, noting down the volume you have used to top up each time. At the end of the 24 hours, add up the total volume you have used and keep a note of it. Repeat 3–4 more times and then average out the water intake by dividing the grand total by the number of days you have measured over.

Clinical polydipsia (excessive drinking) is diagnosed when the cat consumes more than 100 ml water per kg of body weight. For a 3.5 kg cat, therefore, a water intake of more than 350 ml per day would be excessive and a symptom of disease. Below this quantity, it may just be caused by individual preference, diet or perhaps early stages of an undiagnosed illness.

Account does need to be taken of the diet: cats fed on dry food will drink more water than those fed tinned meat, however it is *changes* in the water intake that are significant. If your dried food-fed cat begins to start drinking more than previously, and nothing else has changed, something may be wrong.

Collecting a urine sample and taking this to the appointment will also be appreciated by the vet. To collect a sample, place polystyrene chips in the litter tray (or washed aquarium tank gravel) and decant a urine sample into a cleaned and rinsed bottle. The fresher the sample is, the more accurate will be the results of various tests carried out on it.

Veterinary treatment

- Reaching a diagnosis is the priority and the main means of doing this is by testing urine and blood samples initially. Moving on to further tests may be necessary if results are inconclusive. In most cases, blood tests point to the cause.
- Treatment is detailed under the individual conditions.

Related or similar conditions

▶ **Diabetes**
▶ **Kidney disease**
▶ **Liver disease**
▶ **Thyroid gland (overactive)**

Thyroid gland (overactive)

This condition, also known as hyperthyroidism, is a common diagnosis in older cats. The problem arises due to excess amounts of thyroid hormones circulating in the body. These hormones are produced by the two thyroid glands in the neck, and in hyperthyroidism, the glands become overactive owing to a benign enlargement of one or both glands.

It is unusual for younger cats (e.g. up to 6 or 7 years) to develop hyperthyroidism, and most cats are around 12 or 13 when the disease is first diagnosed. The excess levels of thyroid hormones produces a fairly characteristic pattern of symptoms, but not all cats show the full collection of symptoms. Some individuals may only show one or two signs, and severity also depends on how long the disease has been present before diagnosis.

Characteristic symptoms are:

- A good or even exaggerated appetite
- Good or exaggerated activity levels (a few cats show lowered activity levels)
- Weight loss
- Irritable or aggressive behaviour
- Drinking and urinating to excess
- Occasional vomiting (often after rapid eating)
- Occasional diarrhoea or more frequent defaecation than usual
- Rapid heart rate and tendency to pant when stressed or warm
- Poor looking coat

Many of these symptoms are picked up by observant owners but sometimes recognition of the problem by the owner is delayed because, unlike many other cat diseases, hyperthyroidism does not usually result in a poor appetite.

☎ Urgency

Hyperthyroidism develops over a period of months and so symptoms will gradually worsen, prompting a routine veterinary appointment, usually with concerns about the progressive weight loss despite a reasonable appetite.

Cats with well established hyperthyroidism can suffer from secondary heart problems, and are prone to adverse effects of stress. Sudden deterioration is possible in these patients if they are exposed to excessively warm or stressful circumstances. If collapse of this type were to occur, it is an emergency situation.

+ First aid & nursing

Providing the vet with a clear picture of all the symptoms, together with an indication of their duration, is helpful. Measuring the water intake (see **Thirst**) is a good idea, as is regular weighing of the cat to track weight loss (and weight gain once under treatment). Also note approximate frequency of vomiting/diarrhoea.

Avoid all stressful situations and overheating. If the cat does become stressed and starts panting or breathing heavily, place in a quiet, dark and cool place. The ears and paws can be bathed with cool water and an air fan directed at the cat. Advise the veterinary staff if being in the waiting room proves stressful for the cat.

Veterinary treatment

- Blood tests are needed. As well as revealing the excess levels of thyroid hormones, these tests commonly throw up several other abnormalities. Commonly, some degree of liver dysfunction is detected – this is often considered related to the hyperthyroidism and may not be treated specifically, but when treatment for the thyroid problem is underway it should improve. Many older cats have poor kidney function also, and attention may need to be given to this as well as the overactive thyroid gland.

- The changes in blood pressure caused by the over-active thyroid gland can sometimes mask kidney disease so that the latter only becomes apparent when the thyroid problem is brought under control.
- If associated heart problems are deemed significant, tests such as X-rays, scans and ECGs may be recommended. The heart problems usually improve well once the overactive thyroid gland is brought back under control however.
- Four methods are used to treat overactive thyroid gland in cats:

  1. In very old or sick cats, drugs are given in the form of tablets to control the condition. These drugs must be given for the rest of the cat's life. Drugs are also used for a few weeks before surgery to remove the thyroid gland when that option for treatment is used, since this improves the safety of the necessary anaesthetic.
  2. Surgery is used to remove the overactive gland. Either one or both glands can be removed. If only one is removed, there is a risk that the second gland will become hyperthyroid later, requiring additional treatment (drugs or further surgery). However, the treatment to remove both glands at the one operation is more complex, so a decision has to be made as to which option to go for. More and more, both glands are being removed during the one operation as it is the best long term option and improved knowledge about treating this disease helps limit potential problems. Surgery has the advantage that no drugs need to be given afterwards – a helpful thing if administering tablets in the food or by mouth is not easy! However it is important that the cat is stabilised well before surgery since this is an operation of medium or, in some cases, higher risk, due to the adverse effects of the condition on the heart and circulatory system. Most cats do well however.
  3. The third method is, in many ways, the best one but is not widely available, though this is improving all the time. This technique involves the injection of radioactive iodine into the cat by a straightforward subcutaneous injection (as with the annual booster vaccination). The iodine is taken up by the overactive gland and the gland is destroyed. The treatment is simple and painless, but requires that the cat is hospitalised for 4 weeks until radiation levels have reduced. Not many hospitals are licensed for this treatment, but you may be able to be referred to one that is.
  4. Using an iodine-restricted prescription diet. This newest method of treatment has shown some encouraging results, and may become popular in future.

- Treatment of overactive thyroid gland, though seemingly complex, is well worth the effort as most cats respond well and can live out the rest of their lifespan with a good quality of life.

Related or similar conditions

▶ **Diabetes**
▶ **Heart disease**
▶ **Kidney disease**

- ▶ **Liver disease**
- ▶ **Old age problems**
- ▶ **Thirst**
- ▶ **Blood pressure (high)**

Ticks

Ticks are blood-sucking parasites which attach themselves to the host for an extended period of time, during which they grow in size. Eventually, once feeding is complete, they drop off to complete their life-cycle on the ground.

Owners often mistake ticks for 'skin growths' as they can resemble small lumps on the skin surface. Round the point of attachment of the tick to the skin, there is often an area of skin reddening and mild irritation. This can persist for a while once the tick has dropped off or been removed.

Ticks can be found anywhere on the skin surface or in the ears, and there are many species in different parts of the world. As well as being unsightly, they can cause some irritation and may also spread diseases between animals.

☎ Urgency

Ticks are not an urgent problem. You can remove them yourself (see below) or else arrange a routine veterinary appointment. Ticks are far less common on cats than dogs, since cats groom themselves so fastidiously.

✚ First aid & nursing

Ticks are removed using forceps or fingers (wear gloves) and pulling them slowly but firmly. A slightly turning action can help detach the tick. Many veterinary practices have small tick removing tools which usually work well. Despite rumours to the contrary, it is rare for the 'head' or mouthparts to remain in the cat's skin. Any inflammatory reaction that persists after removal is much more likely to be an immune-mediated reaction to the tick's saliva than the result of retained pieces of tick.

Another option for removal is to apply parasitic products obtained from a veterinary practice which are suitable for the age and size of your cat. Prevention of attachment of ticks is also possible, again using suitable products from your vet. This is useful if you are taking your cat to an area where you know there are many ticks, e.g. the West Highlands of Scotland!

Veterinary treatment

- Suitable products can be used to remove or repel ticks. Always follow dosing instructions carefully and obtain any products from your veterinary surgeon.

Related or similar conditions

- ▶ **Fleas**
- ▶ **Lice**
- ▶ **Lumps**

Tonsillitis

This is not an easy problem to diagnose in the conscious cat, since it is very difficult to examine the tonsils adequately. However severe redness at the back of the throat, along with relevant clinical symptoms, may be taken as an indication of infection and inflammation here. An anaesthetic may be needed to confirm the diagnosis, and rule out other problems (e.g. a **Foreign body**). Tonsillitis is a condition that is not diagnosed with high frequency in pets. Treatment would be with antibiotics. See also under **Swallowing**.

Tooth problems

This is discussed fully under **Mouth and tooth problems**

Toxoplasmosis

Toxoplasmosis is a potentially important human disease associated with cats. *Toxoplasma gondii*, the organism which causes the condition, only rarely produces obvious disease in whatever animal it infects, and many species are susceptible to it. Most cases of illness are seen in very young animals or those with deficient immune systems (e.g. due to **Feline immunodeficiency virus**, FIV). When illness occurs it can take the form of diarrhoea or neurological (nervous system) symptoms such as tremors, weakness, fits and paralysis.

Around 40 per cent of cats will have experienced this infection, mostly without anyone being aware of it (and on sampling, they will be found to have antibodies to this disease). Infection is spread via cysts that are passed in cat faeces, and this has important implications for pregnant women. The cysts are very durable and can last a long time on the ground but are not infectious until 24–48 hours after excretion in the faeces.

If a human were to be infected with *Toxoplasma* it is unlikely any symptoms would be produced unless this was a pregnant woman, in which case there would be a risk of abortion or birth abnormalities. For this reason, the disease, or potential for it, must be taken seriously.

Suitable precautions for pregnant women who are in contact with cats are therefore:

- Avoid dealing with the cat litter tray. This is a sensible precaution to take, even although faeces are not infectious when freshly passed: it takes at least 24 hours for the cysts to become infectious.
- Do not allow faecal matter to accumulate in the cat litter tray.
- Take care in the garden, where contamination with cat faeces is a possibility. Wear gloves while gardening and thoroughly soak and wash all raw vegetables before consuming them.

The disease must be kept in context – it is rare – and is not a reason to avoid keeping or acquiring a cat while pregnant as long as precautions are followed.

☎ Urgency

It is unlikely to present as an urgent condition, except in a cat having fits or seizures. Even then, other conditions would be suspected first unless a disease like feline immunodeficiency virus (FIV) had been diagnosed beforehand.

✚ First aid & nursing

General supportive care is appropriate, depending on the specific symptoms being shown by an affected cat. Encouraging the appetite and reducing stress are important. Good hygiene precautions are needed, although cats that are exhibiting symptoms of toxoplasmosis are no longer considered fully infectious for this disease to spread to other cats or people.

Veterinary treatment

- Diagnosis is difficult and usually requires a biopsy. Blood tests are less reliable as many cats will have experienced this disease without any symptoms and so will be carrying antibodies, which makes the usual blood test results harder to interpret.
- Testing for **Feline immunodeficiency virus** (FIV) an **Feline leukaemia virus** (FeLV) is usually recommended as these infections can lay the cat open to toxoplasmosis in the first place.
- Certain antibiotics are effective against toxoplasma but the outlook for any cat showing overt symptoms of this disease is unfortunately poor.

Related or similar conditions

- ▶ **Brain damage**
- ▶ **Feline immunodeficiency virus (FIV)**
- ▶ **Feline leukaemia virus (FeLV))**
- ▶ **Fits**

Travel fears and sickness

Travel sickness is somewhat different from anxiety about travelling, although there is undoubtedly considerable overlap between the two problems. Acclimatisation to travel is best started in young kittens, since they adapt better and learn quickly, and the acclimatisation process can be as gradual as needed. This can work in older cats too, and is worth tackling if frequent travel becomes necessary (see below for a suitable programme).

Remember that, for a cat, to be placed in an unfamiliar cat carrier, taken into a noisy and unpleasant-smelling car (or bus/train) and subjected to continual movement and agitation before arriving at a threatening and strange destination, must surely be extremely stressful. There are many unfamiliar experiences here of sight, sound, smell and movement – all conspiring to upset an otherwise happy and secure feline. It is amazing that travelling cats are not more terrified than they appear, though in some cases the 'coolness' that is shown may be merely masking considerable inner turmoil.

It is likely that many cats, with their superior sense of smell, also experience severe nausea due to fumes and vapours from transport fuels, and also from the unusual motion over which they have no control. This is especially likely in infrequent travelers.

☎ Urgency

The problem is not an urgent one, though undoubtedly unpleasant for the cat. Attempts should be made to acclimatise the cat to all aspects of travel beforehand by a very gradual process of increased exposure to the experience, starting literally with just a minute or two.

✚ First aid & nursing

Try to limit the length of necessary journeys by careful planning. Ensure the cat carrier is large enough for your cat – some cats prefer it to be covered, others like to see out to some degree. Make sure that familiar blankets are inside the carrier and reassure the cat during movement.

Try to visualise things from your cat's

perspective, e.g. when carrying your cat in its carrier down a street, you may be moving in such a way that the cat, at your knee level, feels it is approaching the large dog that is being walked towards you head-on, and with no means of escape! Unable to retreat, feelings of panic can arise. On public transport, have the open end of the carrier facing towards you and away from walkways or passages.

Veterinary treatment

Sedatives and anti-sickness drugs are available. Their effectiveness is somewhat variable in cats, but they can be worth trying in severe cases. Gradual behavioural acclimatisation is a better long term objective.

Sedatives are not appropriate for air travel as the effects of lowered blood pressure can occasionally cause problems at altitudes. Specific veterinary advice should be sought before air travel is contemplated.

Tip: Acclimatisation to the basket and travel in kittens and cats

Try the following technique.

Session 1: Bring out the cat basket, leave it open in a visible place, but do not put the cat in it. Allow the cat to explore and investigate. Place a familiar blanket inside.

Session 2: Place some food treats in the basket. Allow the cat to go in after them.
Repeat Session 1 and 2 several times, a few days apart.

Session 3: Providing reassurance, place the cat in the basket. Give food treats and attention. Close the door for a few minutes. Reassure the cat through the door.
Repeat Session 3 6–10 times in total, twice a day on different days.

Session 4: With the cat in the basket, carry around the house between rooms.
Repeat Session 4 several times on different days.

Session 5: Venture outside, only for a few minutes at first, but then extending the times and distances.
Repeat Session 5 as many times as necessary on different days until your cat seems relaxed.

Session 6: Introduce the car (or public transport). Again, only for a few minutes (or one bus stop!) before returning home.

In this way your cat's confidence and tolerance will be built upon in a controlled way. If more anxiety is shown at any stage, further repetitions can be built in to reinforce that Session and improve confidence. It is necessary to keep up familiarity with the basket once the cat is 'trained'. This can be achieved by repeating any of the individual sessions every few weeks or so, you do not have to go through the whole process again!

Related or similar conditions

- **Anxiety/fear**
- **Panting**
- **Socialisation**

Tumour

A tumour is an abnormal growth of cells which increases in size and may affect surrounding and even distant organs and tissues in the cat's body. Other words which are used to describe this problem are cancer, lump, mass, growth and neoplasia (the medical term, meaning 'a new growth of cells'). Tumours can arise in any organ or tissue and may be present on the body surface or internally.

Tumours can be benign or malignant. Benign tumours have a low tendency to spread and cause disease elsewhere, whereas malignant ones have a higher tendency to do this. Malignant and spreading cancer can be fatal when it involves vital organs such as the lungs, liver or brain/nervous system. Unfortunately, detecting if or when a malignant tumour has spread is not always very easy as some tumours behave unpredictably, but general guidelines can usually be provided.

Tumours are diagnosed using various techniques including examination by the veterinary surgeon, X-ray and biopsy. Biopsy is the most reliable technique since it allows a pathologist to examine the abnormal tissue and classify it. This helps in trying to provide reliable advice about the outlook (prognosis) of the disease, which is what every cat owner whose pet has been diagnosed with a tumour would like to know.

For more general information, see under **Cancer** and **Lumps**. Tumours are mentioned frequently elsewhere in this book, usually when considering relevant areas of the body, e.g. bone, lung, liver, etc. See the index if you have a specific site in mind.

U

Ulcers

Ulcers are painful areas of inflammation affecting the skin, eye or membranes such as the gums and nose. The affected tissue becomes swollen, red and often moist and angry looking. Various things can trigger an ulcer: trauma, infection or allergy being the commonest. Corrosive chemicals can also be responsible and if swallowed these can ulcerate the throat, oesophagus and stomach, giving very unpleasant symptoms. Ulceration of the ear tips (see **Ear problems**; **Sunburn**) is common in white cats which sun bathe a lot.

In cats, the commonest ulcers are mouth ones (often caused by viral infection) and corneal (eye) ulcers.

☎ Urgency

Ulcers are unpleasant and should be dealt with during an early routine appointment unless there are eye problems, in which case an emergency appointment should be sought.

Any suspected intake of chemicals is also an emergency. This includes chemical contamination of the coat.

✚ First aid & nursing

The affected parts will be red, swollen and extremely tender, so you should certainly avoid applying any antiseptics, creams or powders to the area unless they have been prescribed by a vet.

The eye can be bathed with boiled and cooled water if there is a discharge, and skin areas can be gently rinsed in saline solution if the cat will tolerate this (if not, best leave alone until a vet has checked). Application of an artificial tear product (e.g. Visco-Tears) can greatly help alleviate the pain with eye ulcers and is a very helpful first aid measure. These products are available from pharmacies.

Veterinary treatment

- Some ulcers require surgery for treatment, others respond to antibiotics and anti-inflammatory drugs. Removing the underlying cause of the ulceration is obviously important too, whenever this is known.

Related or similar conditions

- ▶ **Cat flu**
- ▶ **Coat contamination**
- ▶ **Eye problems**
- ▶ **Inflammation**
- ▶ **Salivation**
- ▶ **Wounds**

Urination problems

Problems passing urine are always potentially serious, especially in male cats, who are prone to obstruction of their long and narrow urethra (the tube that leads from the bladder to the outside, via the penis). Urinary obstruction leads inevitably to collapse and death from kidney failure within 12–48 hours. Emergency treatment is therefore required to relieve the obstruction and treat complications.

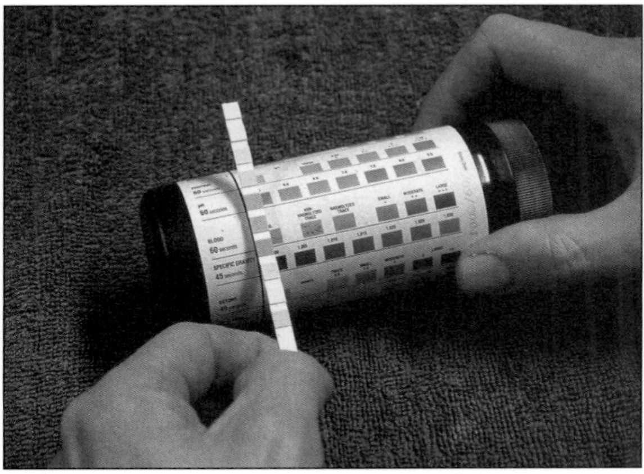

Urine samples are commonly tested for blood, protein, glucose and other substances.

Female cats have a shorter and wider urethra and are hence not so likely to have obstructions, but inflammation of the bladder (cystitis) can cause symptoms of frequent urination, straining to urinate and blood in the urine. General irritability may also be caused.

Some cats form mineral stones within their bladders which produce similar signs to cystitis and, in older cats, tumours have to be considered.

These important conditions are discussed fully under **Cystitis**, where the common problem of feline idiopathic cystitis (FIC) or feline lower urinary tract disease (FLUTD) is detailed.

After traumatic accidents, damage to the bladder nerve supply can occur, and this will lead to problems in urinating. See under **Paralysis**.

Urticaria

Urticaria is the medical term for nettle rash and describes the allergic skin symptoms that can occur when contact with an irritant or stinging plant takes place. Urticaria can also be a general allergic response to foods or drugs that the cat has consumed – a similar sort of skin rash breaks out as if the cat had been stung by nettles.

Affected skin areas are raised into soft circular plaques several centimetres in diameter. The face, ears and eyelids may be swollen.

☎ Urgency

Urticaria and associated allergic reactions are urgent if there is any chance the throat may be affected as this can interfere with breathing. In most cases, breathing is not endangered but a close watch should be kept on the cat. If symptoms appear to be worsening, seek professional advice because urticaria can represent part of a severe generalised allergic reaction, which may require prompt treatment.

+ First aid & nursing

Bathing affected areas with cold water or applying ice packs can help reduce the swelling, which usually takes several hours to completely subside.

Veterinary treatment

- Treatment using adrenalin and powerful anti-inflammatory drugs may be carried out if there are concerns about a severe allergic reaction and possible interference with breathing or the development of allergic shock. Most simple cases caused by contact with plants resolve by themselves.

Related or similar conditions

- **Allergy**
- **Plants (eating)**
- **Skin problems**

V

Vaccination

Vaccination is the process of preventing disease in animals or people by exposing them to the same disease in a 'safe' form. This controlled exposure allows the immune system to learn to recognise the disease so that if encountered in its real, dangerous form in the future, a rapid immune response can be mounted before serious effects of the disease are seen.

Vaccination was one of the milestones of medical history and the process started to be investigated by Jenner in the eighteenth century and Pasteur in the nineteenth. Early vaccines were not however without risk – sometimes the risk of bringing about the disease they were intended to prevent, which totally defeats the purpose. However, with advancing techniques, new methods were found to inactivate viruses so that they became far less harmful but still acted as useful 'practice targets' for the immune system to respond to. Modern day vaccines are generally considered safe and it is easy to forget the enormous impact they have had on devastating diseases, both animal and human.

Domestic cats are usually vaccinated against some or all of the following diseases:

- Upper respiratory viruses (feline calicivirus and feline herpesvirus), known commonly under the blanket term of '**Cat flu**'
- **Feline enteritis**, also known as panleucopaenia
- **Feline leukaemia virus** (FeLV)
- **Chlamydia** infection
- **Rabies**, in travelling cats only in the United Kingdom, but in all pet cats in some other countries

These diseases are all discussed in detail under their individual entries.

Most vaccinations require an initial course of two injections, given several weeks apart, followed by regular boosters to top up immunity and keep protection active. The first three of the above diseases are the ones most commonly vaccinated against currently, but this list has been added to as new vaccines are developed, e.g. vaccines for **Feline immunodeficiency virus (FIV)** and **Feline infectious peritonitis (FIP)** are available in some parts of the world.

Is a booster required every year?

This is a frequently asked question. There is the possibility that some cats retain a good working immunity for longer than one year after receiving a vaccine. In order to check this, blood tests would need to be done to determine immune status. These are available but tend not to be done routinely currently.

Vets currently recommend the annual health check as being the best compromise for all cats. If you desire less frequent vaccination, discuss the matter with your vet so that a good informed decision can be made. In some cases booster frequency may vary between 1–3 years.

Very old cats

On occasion, for example very old cats that have been vaccinated all their lives and now live mainly indoors, vets may agree that immunity is probably fine and, particularly if other health problems are present, may decide to advise missing the booster vaccination or even stop regular vaccination altogether. Again, this is a decision that should be reached jointly by vet and owner after discussing the various options, medical, practical and economic that are thought to apply.

Adverse effects of vaccination

Modern vaccines are very safe in the vast majority of patients, nevertheless, as with all medical products and drugs, a small risk remains in their administration. This small risk is considered preferable to the larger risk imposed by the disease being protected against in most cases; in other words a 'risk-benefit analysis' is usually seen as coming out in favour of the vaccine, since some of the diseases being protected against can be fatal. A comprehensive review* of vaccination in cats and dogs continued to support the administration of vaccines and their annual booster in most cases.

Adverse reactions can be variable in nature, from the temporary slight increase in temperature and sleepiness, sometimes associated with lameness, often noticed in kittens at their very first vaccine (see under First aid below), to rarer symptoms such as allergy/hypersensitivity type reactions and even anaphylaxis (an unusual severe allergic reaction which is treated as an emergency).

Reactions at the site of the vaccination injection, usually in the scruff of the neck, are sometimes seen. These can include:

- Swelling where the vaccination was given. This inflammatory reaction usually subsides over a few days to two weeks, and is considered part of the initial immune response.
- An abscess at the site of vaccination. This is treated with antibiotics and surgical drainage, if needed. Any injection of any product carries a slight risk of infection being introduced into the skin; this is not peculiar to vaccinations and can occur after other routine injections.
- Hair loss at the site of vaccination is occasionally seen.
- Sarcoma (a form of malignant skin cancer) at the site of vaccination is a rare though serious complication of some vaccinations in cats.

Vaccine-associated sarcomas in cats are not frequent but are a concern among vets. Lumps at the site of vaccination which have not disappeared by one month, or

*Veterinary Product Committee working group report on canine and feline vaccination. *The Veterinary Record*. Volume 150, No. 5, February 2, 2002, page 126–134.

which are increasing in size, are usually biopsied and, if of concern, they are removed by surgery for further analysis.

Vaccine failure

Another possible adverse reaction is of a different nature – the vaccine does not protect against the disease it was supposed to. This is rare, though distressing when it occurs. One needs to be sure that the cat is actually suffering from the disease the vaccine is meant to be preventing, and not a similar-looking disease that is mimicking it. Vaccination failure can occur because of problems with the vaccine or because of deficiencies in the cat's immune system.

☎ Urgency

Prompt vaccination of newly acquired kittens is an urgent priority, so that full protection is achieved as soon as possible. Kittens receive passive immunity from their mothers in the important first milk (colostrum) that is produced after birth. This immunity lasts for the first weeks of a kitten's life, but by 8–9 weeks, has reduced considerably. This is the age that the first vaccine is normally given; the second dose is given around 12 weeks, and then boosters administered after that. Kittens are considered fully protected 7–10 days after their *second* vaccine.

If kittens have been hand reared and never suckled, then they will not have received any passive immunity in their mother's milk and special precautions should be taken to prevent infection from other cats during rearing. Veterinary advice should be sought and vaccination started at the date suggested by your veterinary surgeon.

Any adverse reaction which follows vaccination should be reported to your veterinary surgeon. These are rare, but should always be recorded so that improved information on all vaccine products is obtained. (See below for the quite common mild symptoms seen in kittens after initial vaccinations.)

✚ First aid & nursing

Owners often report that some young kittens seem quieter than normal, and possibly off their food, for 24–48 hours after receiving their first vaccination. In many cases, the temperature may be elevated – this reflects the activation of the immune system as the 'mock virus' in the vaccine is attacked and an immune response mounted. Slight lameness may also be present. These mild symptoms of sleeping more and reduced appetite pass over within 1–2 days and probably will not be repeated at the second vaccination several weeks later. If there are any concerns, contact the clinic for advice. In most cases, reassurance is all that is needed. The kitten should be allowed to rest quietly and be provided with water, tempting food and a litter tray in easy reach. Keep indoors until back to normal.

Adult cats rarely show any such side-effects after their annual booster vaccinations.

You should, if possible, avoid periods of stress around the time of vaccination, i.e. do not combine vaccination with long journeys, moving house or acquiring a new pet. This applies to both adults and young cats.

Veterinary treatment

- Initial and booster vaccinations are combined with a health check examination during which all body systems are checked over and advice can be given on preventive medicine and treatment of any developing problems.

Tip: Vaccine batch numbers

On your cat's vaccination record card, you will see a set of vaccine batch numbers recorded after every dose of vaccine that has been given. This is so that any defects or problems with the vaccine can be traced to the manufacturer, who take quality control of vaccines very seriously.

Related or similar conditions

- **Cat flu**
- **Chlamydia infection**
- **Feline enteritis**
- **Feline leukaemia virus (FeLV)**
- **Rabies**

Viruses

Viruses are microscopic life-forms of medical significance as causes of disease. Outwith an animal they are inert scraps of protein, but once in a cell they hijack its metabolism and use it to replicate themselves, often destroying the cell in the process. This destruction of cells affects tissues, organs and even the life of the animal itself in severe viral illnesses.

The common cat diseases caused wholly or in part by viruses are **Cat flu, Feline leukemia virus** (FeLV), **Feline immunodeficiency virus** (FIV), **Feline enteritis** and **Rabies**. Many other cat viruses exist, some of them causing intermittent disease, but those mentioned are the ones commonly vaccinated against. See under **Vaccination** and the individual diseases.

Vomiting

Cats vomit easily – much more readily than human beings – and occasional vomiting, e.g. once every few weeks, is not viewed as unusual in many individuals. 'Natural' vomiting of this type is used to eject hair balls, feathers, swallowed grass, and so on. It is not a sign of illness when it is of low frequency in a cat that is showing no other symptoms.

Medical symptoms often associated with vomiting

- Poor appetite or excessive appetite
- Weight loss
- Drinking and urinating to excess
- Low activity levels
- Bad breath
- Poor coat

Vomiting, however, can also be an important medical symptom, so when does it become serious? It is significant if it is happening on a daily basis and if any other medical symptoms are present. It may also be significant in a cat that never usually vomits, but then is seen to start doing so. Severe vomiting is vomiting that is happening every few hours in a cat that appears otherwise unwell, e.g. subdued and in pain.

It is often useful if vomiting can be distinguished from two other similar symptoms: regurgitation and retching.

- **Vomiting** is often preceded by agitation

or loud miaowing, probably due to feelings of anticipation and nausea. The cat adopts a head down posture and then has strong contractions of the abdomen muscles, and material (food, fluid or froth) is forcefully ejected. The process may be repeated 2–3 more times. If food comes up, it may appear partly digested.

- **Regurgitation** is effortless. There are no major contractions of the abdomen. Food appears in a tube shape and appears completely undigested. The cat may behave as if nothing has happened.
- **Retching** is more like choking, although it can sometimes end in a bout of vomiting. Retching usually results in the production of a small amount of saliva or froth. Again, there are no forceful abdominal contractions.

In practice, it may be difficult for you to tell which of the above is which, and it is not that crucial in most instances, as the vet will be correlating the symptom with other tests and results. If you do see your cat performing this behaviour, though, make an attempt to decide which of the above descriptions seems to fit best.

Many diseases cause vomiting, from simple harmless ones such as mild stomach irritation due to overeating on rich food, to severe, life-threatening conditions such as bowel obstruction or poisonings.

How severe is the problem?

Mild problem, arrange a routine appointment

- Occasional vomiting, e.g. 1–2 times daily
- Cat otherwise bright
- Eating normally
- Allows handling
- Gums pink and moist
- No other symptoms
- Cat staying the same

Severe problem, seek attention urgently

- Frequent vomiting, e.g. every hour
- Cat subdued
- Poor appetite
- Resents handling
- Gums dry and pale or bluish
- Other symptoms present, e.g. panting
- Cat worsening in condition

☎ Urgency

See the lists above. In addition, vomiting in kittens should be viewed more urgently than that in adult cats as they may quickly become dehydrated and, if unvaccinated, could be suffering from a serious infectious disease such as **Feline enteritis**.

Whilst small flecks of blood may occasionally be seen in vomit, the presence of anything more is viewed seriously and urgent advice is needed.

✚ First aid & nursing

The danger is **Dehydration**, so if vomiting is not too severe, water, glucose solution or rehydrating salt solutions (e.g. Dioralyte) should be administered. 5–10 mls every hour is about right for an average sized adult cat. Give with a syringe or dropper. The cat should also be kept quiet and warm. Severe and frequent vomiting should not be treated by fluid administration by mouth, as this is likely to simply provoke further bouts of vomiting. These cats usually require hospitalisation for a drip.

Simple dietary vomiting can be treated with 12 hours of dietary rest (i.e. fluids only) followed by the introduction of a bland diet such as chicken or fish plus rice, gradually weaning back on to the cat's normal food over 3–5 days. Avoid giving milk to drink: offer water, glucose or electrolytes instead.

Keep a note of the number of bouts of vomiting the cat has had and let the vet know this. Also, is there anything else which might help with the diagnosis, e.g. was the cat playing with string or toys it could have swallowed? If so, these could be causing obstructions. Remember that frequent vomiting (every 1–2 hours) demands an urgent appointment.

Veterinary treatment

- Examination supported by blood tests, X-rays and other procedures may be used in the serious case to establish the underlying cause of vomiting. The tests chosen depend on what other symptoms are found during examination of the cat. Treatment can then be planned accordingly.

Related or similar conditions

- **Dehydration**
- **Diarrhoea**
- **Feline enteritis**
- **Foreign body**
- **Poisoning**

W

Warts

Warts are small benign growths on the skin surface which often have a characteristic wrinkled appearance. They are common in dogs, less so in cats. All skin growths should be checked out by a veterinary surgeon in case removal is necessary. Warts near the eye may be removed quickly owing to possible interference with the eyelids.

☎ Urgency

Warts and other small skin lumps are not urgent but should be checked at a suitable routine appointment. If they become traumatised, they may bleed but this usually stops quickly and blood loss is minor.

+ First aid & nursing

Simple first aid for bleeding (e.g. direct pressure for 10 minutes or a light bandage) may be required.

If monitoring a wart or growth for the veterinary surgeon, it can be helpful to take a photograph or note down the measurements, since imagination can play tricks on whether the lump is growing.

Veterinary treatment

- Examination is needed to make sure the lump is indeed a wart. Your surgeon's advice should then be followed about whether removal is necessary. Periodic checks may be made on warts that are not being removed, especially those close to the eye.

Related or similar conditions

- ▶ **Cancer**
- ▶ **Lumps**
- ▶ **Ticks**

Wax (ears)

Ear wax is a natural protective substance which, by a gradual process of production, drying and flaking out the ear, keeps the ear canals healthy. Normal ear wax is a pale colour and is not usually noticeable in the healthy ear although it imparts a shiny and slightly tacky surface coating to the ear lining. Some cats do tend to have waxier ears than others and may tend to accumulate wax, even without any other problems; this can cause discomfort. Use of a mild ear cleaner or a few drops of olive or almond oil (at blood heat) in the ears once every two weeks will help.

In cases of irritation in the ear (e.g. due to ear mites, allergy or infection), wax production increases in response to the damage, and then it can become visible and cause problems due to build up. A characteristic sign of ear mites in cats is masses of dry crumbly and dark wax in the ear openings. Itching and head shaking can result.

For more details, and also for how to apply drops or ear cleaner, see under **Ear problems**.

Weaning

Weaning is the gradual process of separation of suckling kittens from their mother, when they start to become independent animals, able to feed and move around actively by themselves. Kittens may begin to show an interest in liquid food at around 3 weeks. By 6–8 weeks, they are usually eating well and receiving very little nutrition from their mothers. Many kittens are rehomed at this time.

Initially, kittens can be introduced to a cat milk replacer at 3 weeks. They will still be largely feeding from their mother at this time, and the milk replacer may end up being as much an interesting messy bath as a source of food! After a further week or so, liquidised and slightly watered down tinned kitten food can be given. The mother cat will eat this as well, and natural curiosity and mimicking behaviour soon ensures that the kittens are eating reliably.

Food should be available more or less constantly, remembering that kittens need to eat small amounts very frequently owing to their small stomachs. At rehoming at 8 weeks, 4 or 5 small meals are usually sufficient, more if the kitten appears hungry. The number of meals is reduced to 2 or 3 over a period of 4–8 weeks. Dried food can be introduced at this time if desired.

Kittens require regular worming, as advised by the veterinary surgeon, until 4–6 months of age, after which they are wormed 2–4 times yearly.

Related or similar conditions

- **Kittens' problems**
- **Roundworms**
- **Tapeworms**
- **Vaccination**

Weight loss

Weight loss is an important symptom in cat medicine and is always taken seriously. Like drinking to excess, it can have a multitude of causes, and several common cat diseases show both excess drinking (and associated urination) coupled with weight loss.

A gradual weight loss associated with advancing age is seen in old cats, due largely to loss of muscle mass, and is considered an inevitable facet of ageing. This causes many very old cats to 'shrink' with time – they become physically smaller and lighter as the years go by. Nevertheless, whenever you detect weight loss occurring it is worth seeking a veterinary opinion, even in old cats with this very gradual loss of weight, since elderly patients are prone to important diseases which can reduce body weight.

More rapid or even sudden weight loss is always a serious matter, whether due to reduced appetite or weight loss occurring despite normal or even increased appetite. An early diagnosis gives the best chance of successful treatment.

The major diseases causing weight loss in cats are:

- **Abnormal appetite** – i.e. reduced food intake. This could be due to being trapped somewhere without access to food, bullying by another cat, mouth pain or some other physical problem making the eating or swallowing of food difficult.
- **Overactive thyroid gland** – a common cause of weight loss in older cats. These patients often lose weight despite maintaining a good, or even voracious, appetite. Thirst is often increased too, and there may be vomiting.
- **Diabetes** – again, there is loss of weight, coupled with increased appetite and thirst and often other symptoms such as poor coat quality, occasional vomiting and recurring infections.
- **Kidney disease** – weight loss is combined with increased thirst, increased urination and a poor or variable appetite.
- **Liver disease** – usually, weight loss is seen with additional vague symptoms of lethargy, occasional vomiting and diarrhoea and poor appetite. Thirst may also be increased.
- **Cancer** – tumours growing in the body very often cause marked weight loss, especially in the later stages.
- **Chronic illness** – virtually any chronic illness, or chronic pain, can cause weight loss due to general suppression of the appetite, demeanour and normal activities.

Most of these problems are discussed in detail in the appropriate sections of this book and, together, they make up the vast majority of diagnoses of weight loss in domestic cats.

☎ Urgency

Weight loss rarely presents as a sudden thing, unless your cat has been missing and returns home having lost a large amount of weight. In most cases, owners notice the problem over a period of a few weeks or months. Other symptoms may also be present.

✚ First aid & nursing

Little in the way of first aid is appropriate until a diagnosis is reached. Try, if you can, to remember when the weight loss may have first started – this can help the vet even if you can only say 'a few weeks', 'a few months', etc. Also, cast your mind back for any other symptoms that may have been showing themselves, however vaguely e.g. 'Recently, he does seem to be vomiting more than just the usual frequency due to hair balls'; 'Her water intake seems to be gradually increasing'; 'She has gone off her usual favourite foods and nothing seems to appeal to her very much', etc. All of this can help with initial diagnosis.

If weight loss is occurring, weigh your cat weekly and keep a chart. Bathroom scales are fine.

Veterinary treatment

- The full spectrum of diagnostic aids may be necessary to trace the cause of weight loss. In many cases, blood profiles and X-rays find the reason, but further investigations may also be needed.
- Treatment can then be decided upon once the nature of the illness is fully understood.

Related or similar conditions

- **Appetite (abnormal)**
- **Cancer**
- **Diabetes**
- **Kidney disease**
- **Liver disease**
- **Mouth and tooth problems**
- **Pain**
- **Thyroid gland (overactive)**

Wheezing

Wheezing is noisy breathing (respiration) and may be accompanied by increased effort during breathing, noticeable by exaggerated movements of the abdomen or chest, and perhaps more rapid breathing than normal. True wheezing is often caused by allergic conditions, especially the quite common condition of feline **Asthma**, but most owners would be unable to differentiate this from similar breathing noises caused by other conditions such as **Pneumonia**. See also under **Breathing problems** and **Panting** for more details.

'Wool' eating

This is a recognised behaviour pattern in pet cats, especially those of Oriental breed, e.g. Siamese, Burmese, and Oriental crosses. It first starts in young adults and shows as a tendency to suck, chew and eat wool and other fabrics, especially clothing items. Individuals vary in the amount consumed, but it can be surprisingly large quantities, and may on occasion cause medical problems due to bowel obstructions.

☎ Urgency

This behaviour problem is not urgent, unless medical symptoms suggestive of obstruction are seen: this would be severe vomiting, poor appetite, lethargy, etc. Behavioural advice is mentioned below.

✚ First aid & nursing

Deficient diet is not the cause of this abnormal appetite in the vast majority of cases. In fact, the underlying cause is not yet fully understood but the higher incidence in certain breeds (and crosses) suggests it may be partly inherited.

Behavioural stresses may also be partly to blame, and wool eating may be a tendency in anxious or over-dependent cats, for whatever reason. If the source of **Anxiety** is removed (or becomes tolerated), the wool eating can stop. However some cats persist with the habit since it seems to prove extremely addictive and rewarding.

Some behavioural guidelines

- Spend less time giving the cat overt attention. Do not always respond when the cat seeks attention or fuss.
- If possible, allow outdoor access for extra stimulation.
- Reduce access to fabrics that may be eaten, e.g. restrict the cat to the kitchen area mainly.
- Treat fabrics with taste-deterrents, e.g. bitter spray (from veterinary practices).
- Allow access to 'kitty grass' in indoor cats, to promote fibre intake. Also supply dry food to cats normally fed tinned.

Veterinary treatment

- Unusual appetite (pica) can be a symptom of disease, especially **Liver disease**, but the characteristic age and breed of cat, and the behaviour pattern, usually makes the diagnosis obvious.
- Referral to a behaviour specialist may be possible in severe cases.
- For cats presenting with obstructions, diagnosis and treatment proceeds as normal – surgery is usually required to relieve the impaction.

Related or similar conditions

- ▶ **Anxiety/fear**
- ▶ **Appetite (abnormal)**
- ▶ **Behaviour problems – general**
- ▶ **Foreign body**
- ▶ **Socialisation**

Worms

Cats are prone to **Roundworms** and **Tapeworms**. Roundworms resemble strands of spaghetti whereas tapeworms appear as small segments which are sometimes mobile. Full details of their life-cycles and preventative treatments are given under the appropriate sections.

Lungworm is uncommon in cats.

Wounds

Wounds are injuries which disrupt or destroy tissues, usually the skin. Severe wounds may also affect underlying structures such as bones or internal organs and gun shot wounds, in particular, can cause massive damage to adjacent structures.

Wounds vary enormously, from small and superficial to extensive and deep, and can sometimes be very deceptive in appearance. For example, bite puncture wounds are often much more serious than large but superficial skin tears, yet a puncture wound may be so small as to be hardly noticeable on the cat's hairy body. Initial impressions might be that the gaping shallow skin wound is the worse injury, it certainly looks more dramatic. However it is often the small but deep bite injury, combined with the crushing effect on surrounding tissue, that causes the most pain and carries most risk of serious complications.

Wounds are usually associated with some degree of bleeding and if a major blood vessel is damaged, bleeding can be severe and even life-threatening. Fortunately, this is not as common as more minor bleeding – though even this, for the inexperienced owner, can be alarming.

Some wounds (like bite punctures as mentioned above) can be very difficult to locate. The only sign may be a limp or resentment whenever you try to touch part of the cat's body. Or perhaps the cat is simply very irritable, grumpy and off his food. Often, careful examination and parting of the hair can reveal an injury but you should not try this if in doing so you risk injury from the cat.

It is surprisingly easy to cause skin wounds when combing or trimming long haired cats, especially since many of the matts occur close to the skin surface. These wounds are treated as below, for first aid, and if large (more than 1 cm) usually heal quicker if stitched.

☎ Urgency

This depends on the size and type of the wound, its location, the response of the cat and your ability to assess the situation objectively. Some general pointers can be given, but if in doubt phone the vet for advice.

- Small, shallow wounds can be treated with first aid until a routine veterinary appointment is possible.
- Bite punctures in a cat that seems reasonably comfortable can also be given first aid; but arrange an early routine appointment as these are unpleasant injuries with some potential for complications.
- Severe bleeding requires emergency first aid measures and rapid veterinary attention.
- Any interference with breathing or wounds to the chest require emergency veterinary attention.
- Deteriorating condition requires veterinary attention even if the injury initially appears minor. Signs of deterioration could be lethargy and poor responsiveness, reluctance to move, rapid or forceful breathing, vocalising of pain, etc.

Remember that the nature and location of a wound is as important as its size, sometimes even more important. Cats have large quantities of loose and mobile skin and superficial injuries often 'sag' open somewhat. Cats with this type of injury, usually to their owner's extreme surprise, often seem relatively unconcerned – the reason is that the injury is not deep, no major blood loss has occurred and the cat is not in significant discomfort. However, a tiny puncture entry wound can cause excruciating pain that radiates out over a wide area, so that touching anywhere near the wound may provoke a severe pain or aggressive response. In these cases the small wound on the surface is only the 'tip of the iceberg'.

+ First aid & nursing

See the important general advice given under **Accident** and **Bleeding**.

Superficial skin wounds are treated by bathing with tepid saline to keep the area moist and clean. It is unnecessary to apply antiseptic creams or ointments if prompt attention (within 24 hours) is being sought. Simply bathe regularly (every 2 hours or so) and keep the cat indoors. Generally, only attempt to apply a bandage if severe or continued bleeding requires this; most wounds are best left uncovered initially as correct bandaging is a difficult task in the majority of cats and improperly applied bandages can do more harm than good. If the cat will allow, trim the hair around the edges of the wound to allow easier bathing.

It is especially important to keep bathing puncture wounds regularly and warm applications, if tolerated, can help with pain relief by a poulticing action.

Deep wounds exposing bone should be considered emergencies regardless of the response of the cat, i.e. even if the cat appears unconcerned, as bone infection is a serious problem to treat.

Veterinary treatment

- Assessment of wounds allows appropriate treatment. Some wounds are left to heal by themselves (by granulation, in medical jargon) – this is often the best course of action for infected wounds, which may tend to 'break down' again when stitched over. Other wounds are stitched closed early on in the treatment and antibiotics prescribed, if needed. Painkillers may also be used.

- Extensive wounds may require complicated reconstructive surgery, and deep punctures may also require extensive surgery to locate and release deep pockets of pus, together with placement of drains and intensive treatment to control infection and allow healing. This may take many weeks in severe cases.

Related or similar conditions

- ▶ **Abscess**
- ▶ **Accident**
- ▶ **Bite**
- ▶ **Bleeding**
- ▶ **Bruising**
- ▶ **Surgery**

Z

Zoonoses

Zoonoses are animal diseases that can also affect humans. Though there are quite a lot of diseases which potentially may affect both cats and people, in practice these are infrequently diagnosed, and they are certainly not a reason to avoid keeping cats. The advantages of cat ownership far exceed any small risk of disease acquired from them, and most of the diseases that could occur are easily treated.

Several of the diseases mentioned in this book can on rare occasions affect people. In general, if you ever have symptoms associated with illness in your cat, you should seek medical advice and also put your doctor in touch with your vet so that the necessary information can be exchanged if needed. If you suffer from a disease affecting your immune system, you should still be able to enjoy the advantages of cat ownership, however seek advice from your specialist after diagnosis or before acquiring a new cat so that you are aware of any special precautions that should apply in your own case.

The diseases mentioned in this book which can affect people, and their typical symptoms in people, are:

- Mange mites – itchy skin rash.
- Flea bites – red itchy bites (quite common if cat is badly infested, though the cat flea does not normally choose humans as its host).
- Rabies – severe illness and brain disease, usually following bite from rabid animal.
- Giardia – diarrhoea and nausea, usually fairly mild symptoms.
- Toxoplasmosis – mild flu-like symptoms; abortion or birth defects in pregnant women.
- Ringworm – itchy skin symptoms.
- Ticks – ticks present on the skin and skin irritation around them.
- Harvest mites – mild itch or rash in summer/autumn.
- Cheyletiella mites – occasional rash, on arms especially.
- Cat bites – painful inflammation and infection following bite; abscess formation. (Always seek prompt medical advice if bitten by a cat).
- Cat scratch disease – lymph gland enlargement, usually mild, caused by organisms carried by some cats.

There are some other diseases which may also affect people, but they are rarely diagnosed.

Available as a paperback edition

WHY DOES MY CAT . . . ?

Sarah Heath

What motivates your cat and how can you change its problem behaviour? This practical and helpful book, written by a practicing veterinary surgeon who specialises in behaviour therapy, provides the answers and explains how understanding feline psychology can help deal with any perfectly natural behaviour that can cause problems.

The A–Z of cat behaviour can be an eye-opener in understanding how a cat's natural instincts motivate her to respond in a certain way to situations in the home. By redirecting the instincts you will make it possible for your cat to be herself without disrupting the household. With many valuable insights and advice on specific problems *Why Does Your Cat . . . ?* will ensure that your free-spirited cat will remain a source of joy and happiness in your family.

"An essential guide for any cat owner."
The Oldie

Sarah Heath lectures at Liverpool University Veterinary School and is a past President of the European Society for Veterinary Clinical Ethology.

"With many fascinating insights, and a valuable alphabetical section of advice on specific problems, *Why Does My Cat . . . ?* ensures that your free-spirited, much loved cat will remain a source of joy and happiness."
Pet Life

Available in ebook and as a paperback edition

WHY DOES MY DOG . . . ?

John Fisher

ALREADY REPRINTED NINE TIMES

This practical and authoritative book, from a leading dog expert, gives you all the answers and explains how to change problem behaviour without resorting to punishment. Using your dog's psychology, the instincts it has inherited from his wolf ancestors, John Fisher provides a fascinating insight into the roots of a dog's behaviour. Written with both dog and owner in mind.

"All dog-owners should have a copy of 'Why Does My Dog . . . ?'
on their bookshelf to refer to when faced with a doggy problem . . .
Presented in an easy-to-find-and-follow A–Z format. All sorts
of common problems are covered in detail."
Your Dog

John Fisher worked professionally with dogs for over twenty years, as a police dog handler and trainer. He was a founder member of the Association of Pet Behaviour Counsellors and was a regular writer for *What Dog?* and *Pet Dogs*.

"This authoritative book, written by a leading dog behaviour expert
with extensive experience, gives you the answers and explains how
to change your dog's behaviour without resorting to punishment."
Petlife

Available in ebook and as a paperback edition

DOGWISE:
The Natural Way to Train Your Dog

John Fisher

John Fisher explains how to train a dog to understand commands, think for itself and to make the right choice, using force-free methods, with the help of clear instructions and guided by the step-by-step photographs provided in *Dogwise*.

Dog training can be natural and easy if you understand how your dog sees its place in the human pack, you are aware of how dogs learn, you reward him for the right reasons and if you use the dog's natural instincts as a basis for training.

"The inspiration for many of today's behavioural dog trainers."
Your Dog

John Fisher worked professionally with dogs for over twenty years, as a police dog handler and trainer. He was a founder member of the Association of Pet Behaviour Counsellors and was a regular writer for *What Dog?* and *Pet Dogs*.

"If dogs could read then I am sure that they would all make certain that a copy of *Dogwise* found its way into their owner's Christmas stocking."
Dog Training Weekly

Available in ebook and as a paperback edition

WHY DOES MY PARROT . . . ?

Rosemary Low

This practical and helpful book draws on Rosemary Low's unrivalled experience to provide valuable guidance for all parrot owners. Using the basic elements of parrot psychology and behaviour, problem behaviour is explained and solutions are offered.

Using an easy-to-use A–Z format, this book will demystify every problem a parrot owner will come across, such as biting, screaming and feather plucking. No other author on parrots has such breadth of knowledge or experience. Along with her professional authority, Rosemary Low also illustrates her solutions to common problems. Now updated and revised to keep abreast of current developments.

"When you are buying your new bird and its cage and toys,
make sure this book is part of your purchases."
Cage & Aviary Birds

Rosemary Low has been the curator of two of the world's largest parrot collections, she was the editor of *PsittaScene* for 15 years.

"Parrot authority Rosemary Low seeks to prevent many common problems
owners have with companion parrots by explaining the basic elements of
psychology and behaviour the birds follow . . . An easy reference tool."
Bird Talk

Available in ebook and as a paperback edition

WHY DOES MY RABBIT . . . ?

Anne McBride

Rabbits are now the third most popular pet in Britain but few owners understand their behavioural problems. Many of the problems that rabbits demonstrate can be avoided if their living conditions are adapted to follow their natural instincts and Anne McBride explains how to do this. She describes how rabbits live and breed in the wild, and the instincts your pet rabbit has inherited, which make it act as it does. With a range of problems, arranged alphabetically for easy-to-use accessibility, this book covers all types of rabbits, from hutch to house rabbits and fully covers the specific problems that can affect them.

"A comprehensive and practical book for rabbit owners that answers all the questions you've ever had about rabbits . . . will leave no questions unanswered and will help to make the relationship between you and your rabbit better than ever before."
Wild About Animals

Dr Anne McBride lectures at the University of Southampton and is a member of The Association of Pet Behaviour Counsellors.

"A practical, authoritative study . . . and it will appeal not only to pet and houserabbit owners but any fancier who wishes to gain a better understanding of this unique and universally lovable animal."
Fur and Feather

Available as a hardback edition

THE LATEST MEWS:
Learn to Speak Cat 2

Anthony Smith

From the cartoonist behind the popular 'Learn to Speak Cat' cartoon that appeared in the *Metro* newspaper comes another compilation of wacky cartoons that will have you purring with delight.

WITH FULL COLOUR ILLUSTRATIONS THROUGHOUT

Discover how your cat views the world. This is how a cat-centric world would look, from Eskimeows to the cat designed refrigerator. Anthony Smith captures the unique humour of cats, making this book the perfect gift for cat lovers.

"Anthony Smith causes the reader to chuckle on every page.
Even dog-lovers will enjoy this clever little volume."
This England

Anthony Smith started life as a cartoonist for Marvel Comics before working in advertising for many years (he wrote and directed TV campaigns for 'Yorkie: It's Not for Girls' and the 'Dairylea Cows'). His cartoons appear monthly in 'Cosmopolitan'.

"Cartoons by Anthony Smith succeed where all the unknown billions
of actual lolcats fail, in that they are genuinely funny."
The Independent